Essentials
of
Geriatric Neuroanesthesia

Essentials
of
Geriatric Neuroanesthesia

Edited by
Hemanshu Prabhakar, MD, PhD
Department of Neuroanaesthesiology and Critical Care
All India Institute of Medical Sciences (AIIMS)
New Delhi, India

Coeditors
Charu Mahajan and Indu Kapoor
Department of Neuroanaesthesiology and Critical care
All India Institute of Medical Sciences (AIIMS)
New Delhi, India

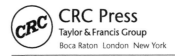

CRC Press is an imprint of the
Taylor & Francis Group, an **informa** business

CRC Press
Taylor & Francis Group
6000 Broken Sound Parkway NW, Suite 300
Boca Raton, FL 33487-2742

First issued in paperback 2021

© 2019 by Taylor & Francis Group, LLC
CRC Press is an imprint of Taylor & Francis Group, an Informa business

No claim to original U.S. Government works

ISBN 13: 978-0-367-77859-0 (pbk)
ISBN 13: 978-1-138-48611-9 (hbk)

Visit the Taylor & Francis Web site at
http://www.taylorandfrancis.com

and the CRC Press Web site at
http://www.crcpress.com

To our grandparents

Karam Chand and Indrawati Prabhakar
Vidhya Sagar and Saraswati Agnihotri

Hemanshu Prabhakar

Amar Nath Gupta and Raj Devi
Jia Lal and Sushila Devi

Charu Mahajan

Dorje and Chimey Angmo
Norbu Gonbo and Tashi Angmo

Indu Kapoor

Contents

Foreword

Is there a need for a textbook on geriatric neuroanesthesia? A similar question was asked four decades ago about the need for a textbook on neuroanesthesia. Now in 2019, there are a substantial number of textbooks on this subject. With complex neurosurgery being undertaken in elderly patients these days, there is a definite need for a comprehensive textbook on geriatric neuroanesthesia.

Life expectancy is increasing all over the world. The global average of life expectancy, which was 48 years in 1950, increased to 70 years in 2012. In India, life expectancy as of 2015 is 68.3 years on the whole—69.9 years for females and 66.9 years for males. In Japan, the figure is 83.7 years for the whole population—86.8 years for females and 80.5 years for males. With increasing life expectancy, more and more elderly patients are likely to present for surgery and anesthesia.

There is a general increase in risk of surgery with increasing age. This has been shown in hip and knee arthroplasty. Despite the increased rate of adverse events, there are gains in terms of pain relief and ability to perform activities of daily living, and overall most elderly groups were satisfied with their surgeries. Thus there are advantages of surgery, though at a higher risk. A similar argument can be held with regard to neurosurgery. Minimizing this risk and offering the advantage of surgery is a big challenge. In a review of octogenarians undergoing neurosurgery, only a small proportion of the emergency admissions were discharged directly to home. Octogenarian patients had higher complication rates and 30-day mortality than those less than 80 years old, demonstrating the additional risk and the need for enhanced perioperative care. Cardiovascular, pulmonary, and metabolic risks increase with age. Added to this, the polypharmacy, drug interactions, and altered response to drugs due to organ dysfunction complicate the management of the elderly patient. Cognitive function might be altered in some elderly patients, and the response of the patient's cognitive function to anesthetics is a matter of great debate.

To address the above issues, Prabhakar et al. have undertaken a massive effort of compiling a textbook of geriatric neuroanesthesia. They have divided the topics to suit the practical requirements of the clinicians. In the initial chapters the age-related changes in neuroanatomy, neurophysiology, and neuropharmacology as relevant to neuroanesthetic practice are discussed, followed by discussion of the individual lesions and various general aspects of management of the elderly, such as fluid and electrolyte balance, pain management, and palliative care. Overall, this book is a practical compendium which will be very helpful to practitioners of geriatric neuroanesthesia.

G.S. Umamaheswara Rao
Senior Professor
Department of Neuroanaesthesia and
Neurocritical Care
National Institute of Mental Health and
Neuro Sciences (NIMHANS)
Bangalore, India

Acknowledgment

We wish to acknowledge the support of the administration of the All India Institute of Medical Sciences (AIIMS), New Delhi, in allowing us to conduct this academic task.

Special thanks are due to the production team at Taylor & Francis Group, CRC Press: Shivangi Pramanik (Commissioning Editor – Medicine), Mouli Sharma (Editorial Assistant), Ritesh Bhutani (Senior Sales Manager – Medical), Rajni Dhingra (Manager – Professional & Textbooks Marketing), and Sunaina Bhullar (Assistant Marketing Manager).

Contributors

Sona Shah Arora MD
Department of Anesthesiology
Grady Memorial Hospital
Emory University School of Medicine
Atlanta, Georgia

Marc Alain Babi MD
Neurocritical Care Fellowship
University of Florida
Gainesville, Florida

Smriti Badhwar BDS MSc
Department of Physiology
All India Institute of Medical Sciences
New Delhi, India

Suparna Bharadwaj MD
Department of Neuroanaesthesia and
    Neurocritical Care
National Institute of Mental Health and Neuro
    Sciences
Bangalore, India

Federico Bilotta MD PhD
Department of Anesthesiology, Critical Care and
    Pain Medicine
Sapienza University of Rome
Rome, Italy

Summit Bloria MD
Department of Anaesthesia and Intensive Care
Postgraduate Institute of Medical Education and
    Research
Chandigarh, India

Brittany Bolduc DO
Department of Neurology
Boston University School of Medicine
Boston, Massachusetts

Anastasia Borozdina MD
Department of Anaesthesiology and
    Intensive Care
Pirogov Russian National Research Medical
    University
Moscow, Russia

Carlo Brembilla MD
Department of Neurosurgery
Ospedale Papa Giovanni XXIII
Bergamo, Italy

Dhritiman Chakrabarti MD DM
Department of Neuroanaesthesia and
    Neurocritical Care
National Institute of Mental Health and
    Neuro Sciences
Bangalore, India

Dinu Chandran MD
Department of Physiology
All India Institute of Medical Sciences
New Delhi, India

Katleen Wyatt Chester PharmD BCCCP BCGP
Department of Pharmacy
and
Marcus Stroke and Neuroscience
    Center
Grady Health System
Atlanta, Georgia

Jason Chui MBChB MSc FANZCA FHKCA FHKAM
Department of Anesthesia and Perioperative
    Medicine
Schulich School of Medicine and Dentistry
University of Western Ontario
London, Canada

Claudia F. Clavijo MD
Department of Anesthesiology
School of Medicine
University of Colorado
Denver, Colorado

Kashmiri Doley MD
Department of Anesthesiology and
    Intensive Care
G.B. Pant Institute of Postgraduate Medical
    Education and Research
and
Maulana Azad Medical College and
    Affiliated Hospitals
Delhi University
New Delhi, India

Christine Dy-Valdez MD
Department of Anesthesia and Perioperative
    Medicine
Schulich School of Medicine and Dentistry
University of Western Ontario
London, Canada

Francesco Ferri MD
Department of Anaesthesia and Critical Care
    Medicine
Ospedale Papa Giovanni XXIII
Bergamo, Italy

Paul S. García MD PhD
Neuroanesthesia Division
Department of Anesthesiology
Columbia University College of Physicians
    and Surgeons
Columbia University Medical Center
New York City, New York

Mikhail Gelfenbeyn MD PhD
Department of Neurological Surgery
UW Medical Center
Seattle, Washington

David M. Greer MD MA FCCM FAHA FNCS FAAN FANA
Department of Neurology
Boston University School of Medicine
and
Boston Medical Center
Boston, Massachusetts

Paolo Gritti MD
Department of Anaesthesia and Critical Care
    Medicine
Ospedale Papa Giovanni XXIII
Bergamo, Italy

Nidhi Gupta MD DM
Department of Neuroanaesthesia
Indraprastha Apollo Hospitals
New Delhi, India

Nishkarsh Gupta MD
Department of Onco-Anaesthesia and
    Palliative Medicine
Dr. BR Ambedkar Institute Rotary Cancer Hospital
All India Institute of Medical Sciences
New Delhi, India

Robert G. Hahn MD PhD
Södertälje Hospital
Karolinska Institutet
Södertälje, Sweden

Leslie C. Jameson MD
Department of Anesthesiology
School of Medicine
University of Colorado
Denver, Colorado

Kiran Jangra MD DM
Department of Anaesthesia and Intensive Care
Postgraduate Institute of Medical Education
    and Research
Chandigarh, India

Indu Kapoor MD
Department of Neuroanaesthesiology and
    Critical Care
All India Institute of Medical Sciences
New Delhi, India

Manpreet Kaur MD
Department of Physiology
Vardhman Mahavir Medical College
Safdarjung Hospital
New Delhi, India

Alan J. Kovar MD
Anesthesiology and Perioperative
    Medicine
Knight Cardiovascular Institute
Oregon Health and Science University
Portland, Oregon

Luigi Andrea Lanterna MD
Department of Neurosurgery
Ospedale Papa Giovanni XXIII
Bergamo, Italy

Abhijit Lele MBBS MD MS
Department of Anesthesiology and Pain Medicine
and
Department of Neurosurgery
Harborview Injury Prevention and Research Center
and
Neurocritical Care Service and Neuroscience ICU
Quality Improvement, Neurocritical Care
Harborview Medical Center
Seattle, Washington

Ferdinando Luca Lorini MD
Department of Anaesthesia and Critical Care
Ospedale Papa Giovanni XXIII
Bergamo, Italy

Ankur Luthra MD DM
Department of Anaesthesia and Intensive Care
Postgraduate Institute of Medical Education
    and Research
Chandigarh, India

Charu Mahajan MD DM
Department of Neuroanaesthesiology
    and Critical Care
All India Institute of Medical Sciences
New Delhi, India

Adriana Martin MD
Cleveland Clinic Foundation
Cleveland, Ohio

Megan McCrohan
Oakland University William Beaumont
    School of Medicine
Rochester, Michigan

Seema Mishra MD
Department of Onco-Anaesthesia and
    Palliative Medicine
Dr. BR Ambedkar Institute Rotary Cancer Hospital
and
All India Institute of Medical Sciences
New Delhi, India

Olivia Johnson Morgan PharmD BCCCP BCGP
Department of Pharmacy
Grady Health System
Atlanta, Georgia

Hemanshu Prabhakar MD PhD
Department of Neuroanaesthesiology and
    Critical Care
All India Institute of Medical Sciences
New Delhi, India

M.V.S. Satya Prakash DA DNB
Department of Anaesthesiology and Critical Care
Jawaharlal Institute of Postgraduate Medical
    Education and Research
Puducherry, India

Ega Qeva MD
Department of Anesthesiology, Critical Care and
    Pain Medicine
Sapienza University of Rome
Rome, Italy

Shobana Rajan MD
Allegheny Health Network
Cleveland Clinic
Cleveland, Ohio

Amy D. Rodriguez PhD
Department of Neurology
Emory University School of Medicine
Atlanta, Georgia

Irene Rozet MD DEAA
Department of Anesthesiology and
    Pain Medicine
UW Medical Center
Seattle, Washington

M. Senthilnathan MD DNB PDF **(Critical Care)**
Department of Anaesthesiology and Critical Care
Jawaharlal Institute of Postgraduate Medical
    Education and Research
Puducherry, India

Kruti Shah PharmD BCPS BCGP
Department of Pharmacy
Grady Health System
Atlanta, Georgia

Daljit Singh MCh
Department of Neurosurgery
G.B. Pant Institute of Postgraduate Medical
    Education and Research
and
Maulana Azad Medical College and
    Affiliated Hospitals
Delhi University
New Delhi, India

Vasudha Singhal MD
Department of Neuroanaesthesia and
    Neurocritical Care
Medanta: The Medicity
Gurgaon, India

Christopher G. Sinon BS
Neuroscience Program
Laney Graduate School
Emory University
Atlanta, Georgia

Deepti Srinivas MD PDF (NA) PDF (NCC)
Department of Neuroanaesthesia and
    Neurocritical Care
National Institute of Mental Health and
    Neuro Sciences
Bangalore, India

Monica S. Tandon MD
Department of Anesthesiology and
    Intensive Care
G.B. Pant Institute of Postgraduate Medical
    Education and Research
and
Maulana Azad Medical College and
    Affiliated Hospitals
Delhi University
New Delhi, India

Swagata Tripathy MD DNB IDCC EDIC
Department of Anaesthesia and Intensive Care
All India Institute of Medical Sciences
Bhubaneswar, India

Zilvinas Zakarevicius MD PhD
Department of Anesthesiology and
    Pain Medicine
UW Medical Center
Seattle, Washington

1

Neuroanatomy: Age-related changes

VASUDHA SINGHAL

INTRODUCTION

The advancement of medical technology, combined with better access to treatment and focus on preventive strategies, has led to an extension of the human lifespan. There is therefore a trend toward an increase in the aged population worldwide. Aging is a physiological process characterized by degenerative changes in the structure and function of every organ system in the body. The age-related limitation of the functional reserve of an elderly patient during times of stress, such as that which occurs at the time of surgery, leads to an increase in perioperative morbidity. An in-depth knowledge of the age-related changes in the brain and its function helps the neuroanesthesiologist to better comprehend the implications of anesthesia in elderly neurosurgical patients.

THE AGING BRAIN

Aging affects the brain at all levels, from molecules, vasculature, and morphology to cognition. With increasing age, the brain shrinks in size and the aging vasculature predisposes to cardiovascular diseases and strokes. Progressive white matter lesions and dementia due to cellular death in regions of the cortex lead to cognitive decline. Changes in the levels of neurotransmitters and hormones result in functional deficits in the elderly, such as a short sleep span, decreased motor activity, mood flattening, altered endocrine function, and declining mental status. The anatomical changes seen in different parts of the brain are delineated in "The Brain" section.

The skull

The skull forms the bony skeleton of the head that protects the brain from external injury. With age, bone remodeling affects the shape of the skull and cortical thickness. Significant cortical thinning occurs in the outer and inner tables of the frontal, occipital, and parietal bones in the elderly (1). In a study evaluating the morphological changes in the skull using three-dimensional geometric analysis from computed tomographic images, it was found that there is a relative expansion of the lateral portions of the skull, primarily in the inferior parietal and temporal regions (2). The anterior and middle cranial fossae compress inward with age, with relative bilateral widening along the lateral edges. This particular structural arrangement alters the biomechanical response of the brain to a head impact and makes the frontal and temporal regions of the brain relatively vulnerable to injury in the elderly.

The brain

Most brain structures decline in volume with age, but at highly different rates. The average rate of decline in the volume and weight of the brain is estimated to be ~5% per decade after the age of 40, and the rate increases with age, especially after the age of 70 (3). This volumetric brain reduction is mostly due to shrinkage of neurons, and reduction in the dendritic spines and total number of the neuronal synapses, rather than neuronal loss. Also, the length of the myelinated axons is reduced by as much as 50% (4).

Age effects on gray matter

A large variety of cross-sectional studies using the magnetic resonance (MR) imaging indicate that the gray matter is reduced with age, and this reduction is somewhat greater in the cortical than in the subcortical structures (5–8). The regional cortical volume decreases with age, with the greatest effects seen in the frontal cortex, followed by the temporal areas, posterior association areas, and occipital areas. The primary sensory regions seem to be relatively preserved (9–11). Among the subcortical brain structures, the pattern of changes is highly heterogenous, with the putamen, thalamus, and accumbens being the most affected. The limbic structures—the hippocampus and amygdala—are substantially affected with age as well. The brain stem is probably the best preserved of all brain structures in healthy aging (12).

The cerebrospinal fluid (CSF) compartments, including the ventricular systems, increase in volume with age, partly due to atrophy in other brain areas like the deep white matter.

From the interpretation of various cortical studies using automated techniques, it is hypothesized that the brain areas which are the latest to develop phylo- and ontogenetically are the first to be affected by normal aging ("last in–first out"). The effects of aging are thus strongest in the frontal and prefrontal areas. As a result, executive functions like working memory, behavioral control, decision making, etc., that rely heavily on the frontal neural circuits (e.g., the frontostriatal circuits) are among the cognitive functions to be most affected by advancing age (13,14). These circuits are involved in various neurodegenerative disorders, such as Alzheimer's disease and Parkinson's disease,

as well as in the pathogenesis of neuropsychiatric disorders such as schizophrenia and depression.

It may be remembered, however, that certain memory performances such as procedural, primary, and semantic memory are well preserved with age, as opposed to episodic and working memory. Cognitive retraining for neural recruitment in the aging brain, also called "compensatory scaffolding," by engaging in social, leisure, and cognitive activities as well as regular exercise, may be used to prevent age-related decline in elderly patients (15).

Age effects on white matter

White matter loss starts at a later stage in the aging brain but is more rapid than gray matter loss, and ultimately exceeds it (16). Myelin breakdown is an aspect of healthy aging, and this breakdown contributes to the loss of white matter volume in the elderly. White matter changes play a causal role in cognitive performance in aging, including mental speed, episodic memory function, executive and flexible cognition, and nonverbal problem solving. Thirty percent of subjects older than 60 years of age demonstrate white matter hyperintensities in the periventricular and subcortical regions on MR studies, and these lesions tend to increase with age (17). These white matter lesions, or leukoaraiosis, occur as a result of atrophic perivascular demyelination secondary to vascular insufficiency in the aged. The presence of white matter hyperintensities has been correlated with signs of cognitive decline (18,19). It has also been shown in recent studies to be a predictor of stroke (20). The identifiable risk factors for these lesions include diabetes, hypertension, decreased respiratory function, high cholesterol, and female gender (21).

Postoperative cognitive dysfunction in the elderly

The basal forebrain cholinergic complex, providing major cholinergic projections to the cerebral cortex and hippocampus, undergoes moderate degenerative changes during aging, leading to cholinergic hypofunction (22). This predisposes the elderly population to cognitive impairment, including Alzheimer's disease, and is also a potent factor in the pathogenesis of postoperative cognitive dysfunction (POCD), as most anesthetic drugs interact with the cerebral cholinergic system (23). Elderly patients may suffer from a wide range of changes in their neurocognitive condition and behavior, such as attention, concentration, memory, and psychomotor speed, for weeks or even months after anesthesia and surgery. Hypotension, cerebral microemboli, and inflammatory mechanisms have been implicated in the development of POCD in the elderly (24) and is most commonly seen after cardiopulmonary bypass surgery.

THE SPINE

Aging leads to degenerative changes in the structural components of the spine with biomechanical consequences, leading to rupture of equilibrium and destabilization.

With advancing age, the permeability of the discal endplate diminishes, resulting in diminished nutrient supply of the disc and tissue breakdown, and loss of disc height and turgor. Mechanical incompetence and disc flattening leads to diffuse disc bulging. Degenerative changes lead to the development of vascularity and innervation of the disc, which is as such avascular—this causes the low back pain frequently seen in the elderly. The nociceptive nerve fibers, sensitized by the cytokines and neuropeptides present in the inner annulus and nucleus of the degenerated disc, primarily attribute to the pain (25). Also, age-related structural changes in the annulus and endplate may lead to a transfer of load from the nucleus to the posterior annulus, leading to pain and annular rupture (26).

The segmental instability due to disc degeneration increases the load on the facet joints, leading to their subluxation and cartilage degradation. Spinal canal stenosis may be caused by facet hypertrophy, osteophyte formation, and apophyseal malalignment. Degenerative spondylolisthesis may occur due to destabilization of the joint. The ligaments surrounding the spine become increasingly weak due to chemical and macroscopic changes with age. The degeneration of ligamentum flavum leads to its increased thickness and bulging. All these factors further contribute to spinal stenosis, and if present in the cervical spine, may progress to myelopathy (27).

Osteoporotic changes in the bony elements of the spine may induce major morphological changes—the densely connected plate-like trabeculae in the cancellous vertebral bone are transformed into discontinuous rod-like structures. The number of horizontal trabeculae, which act as a cross-link in the overall structure of bone, also decreases (28). The mechanical strength of the spine decreases, increasing the risk of vertebral fractures. Because the anterior part of the vertebral body is less strong, anterior wedge fractures tend to be more common in the elderly (29). These osteoporotic fractures cause pain and deformity, compromising the quality of life in the aged population.

CONCLUSION

Aging is associated with changes in brain function as well as brain morphology. Cerebral atrophy and increase in subcortical hyperintensities lead to functional and cognitive decline in the elderly. The spine develops degenerative changes and the bone mineral density reduces, leading to a number of painful and often debilitating disorders. Anesthetic induction and maintenance during neurosurgery should take into consideration the fragile anatomy and physiology of the elderly patient.

REFERENCES

1. Lillie EM, Urban JE, Lynch SK, Weaver AA, Stitzel JD. Evaluation of skull cortical thickness changes with age and sex from computed tomography scans. *J Bone Miner Res.* 2016 Feb;31(2):299–307.
2. Urban JE, Weaver AA, Lillie EM, Maldjian JA, Whitlow CT, Stitzel JD. Evaluation of morphological changes in the adult skull with age and sex. *J Anat.* 2016 Dec;229(6):838–46.
3. Svennerholm L, Bostrom K, Jungbjer B. Changes in weight and compositions of major membrane components of human brain during the span of adult human life of Swedes. *Acta Neuropathol.* 1997;94:345–52.
4. Fjell AM, Walhovd KB. Structural brain changes in aging: Courses, causes and cognitive consequences. *Rev Neurosci.* 2010;21:187–221.
5. Walhovd KB, Westlye LT, Amlien I et al. Consistent neuroanatomical age-related volume differences across multiple samples. *Neurobiol Aging.* 2011 May;32(5):916–32.
6. Courchesne E, Chisum HJ, Townsend J, Cowles A, Covington J, Egaas B, Harwood M, Hinds S, Press GA. Normal brain development and aging: Quantitative analysis at in vivo MR imaging in healthy volunteers. *Radiology.* 2000;216(3):672–82.

7. Bahcelioglu M, Gozil R, Take G et al. Effects of age on tissues and regions of the cerebrum and cerebellum. *Neurobiol Aging*. 2001;22(4): 581–94.

8. Walhovd KB, Fjell AM, Reinvang I, Lundervold A, Dale AM, Eilertsen DE, Quinn BT, Salat D, Makris N, Fischl B. Effects of age on volumes of cortex, white matter and subcortical structures. *Neurobiol Aging*. 2005;26(9):1261–70, discussion 1275–8.

9. Raz N, Gunning-Dixon F, Head D, Rodrigue KM, Williamson A, Acker JD. Aging, sexual dimorphism, and hemispheric asymmetry of the cerebral cortex: Replicability of regional differences in volume. *Neurobiol Aging*. 2004;25(3):377–96.

10. Allen JS, Bruss J, Brown CK, Damasio H. Normal neuroanatomical variation due to age: The major lobes and a parcellation of the temporal region. *Neurobiol Aging*. 2005;26(9): 1245–60, discussion 1279–82.

11. Raz N, Rodrigue KM. Differential aging of the brain: Patterns, cognitive correlates and modifiers. *Neurosci Biobehav Rev*. 2006;30(6): 730–48.

12. Fotenos AF, Snyder AZ, Girton LE, Morris JC, Buckner RL. Normative estimates of crosssectional and longitudinal brain volume decline in aging and AD. *Neurology*. 2005;64(6):1032–9.

13. Schretlen D, Pearlson GD, Anthony JC, Aylward EH, Augustine AM, Davis A, Barta P. Elucidating the contributions of processing speed, executive ability, and frontal lobe volume to normal agerelated differences in fluid intelligence. *J Int Neuropsychol Soc*. 2000; 6(1):52–61.

14. Connelly SL, Hasher L, Zacks RT. Age and reading: The impact of distraction. *Psychol Aging*. 1991;6(4):533–41.

15. Park DC, Reuter-Lorenz P. The adaptive brain: Aging and neurocognitive scaffolding. *Annu Rev Psychol*. 2009;60:173–96.

16. Jernigan TL, Gamst AC. Changes in volume with age—Consistency and interpretation of observed effects. *Neurobiol Aging*. 2005; 26(9):1271–4, discussion 1275–8.

17. Meyer JS, Kawamura J, Terayama Y. White matter lesions in the elderly. *J Neurol Sci*. 1992;110:1–7.

18. Almkvist O, Wahlund LO, Andersson-Lundman G et al. White-matter hyperintensity and neuropsychological functions in dementia and healthy aging. *Arch Neurol*. 1992;49:626–32.

19. Ylikoski R, Ylikoski A, Erkinjuntti T et al. White matter changes in healthy elderly persons correlate with attention and speed of mental processing. *Arch Neurol*. 1993;50:818–24.

20. Kuller LH, Longstreth WT Jr, Arnold AM et al. White matter hyperintensity on cranial magnetic resonance imaging: A predictor of stroke. *Stroke*. 2004;35:1821–5.

21. Liao D, Cooper L, Cai J et al. The prevalence and severity of white matter lesions, their relationship with age, ethnicity, gender, and cardiovascular disease risk factors: the ARIC Study. *Neuroepidemiology*. 1997; 16:149–62.

22. Schliebs R, Arendt T. The cholinergic system in aging and neuronal degeneration. *Behav Brain Res*. 2011;221(2):555–63.

23. Laalou FZ, Carre AC, Forestier C, Sellal F, Langeron O, Pain L. Pathophysiology of post-operative cognitive dysfunction: Current hypotheses. *J Chir (Paris)*. 2008 Jul–Aug;145(4):323–30.

24. Pappa M, Theodosiadis N, Tsounis A, Sarafis P. Pathogenesis and treatment of post-operative cognitive dysfunction. *Electron Physician*. 2017 Feb;9(2):3768.

25. Benoist M. Natural history of the aging spine. *Eur Spine J*. 2003;12:S86–9.

26. Ferguson SJ, Steffen T. Biomechanics of the aging spine. *Eur Spine J*. 2003;12(Suppl. 2):S97–103.

27. Papadakis M, Sapkas G, Papadopoulos EC, Katonis P. Pathophysiology and biomechanics of the aging spine. *Open Orthop J*. 2011; 5:335–42.

28. Briggs AM, Greig AM, Wark JD, Fazzalari NL, Bennell KL. A review of anatomical and mechanical factors affecting vertebral body integrity. *Int J Med Sci*. 2004;1:170–80.

29. Ismail AA, Cooper C, Felsenberg D et al. Number and type of vertebral deformities: Epidemiological characteristics and relation to back pain and height loss. European Vertebral Osteoporosis Study Group. *Osteoporos Int*. 1999;9:206–13.

2

Neurophysiology: Age-related changes

DINU CHANDRAN, SMRITI BADHWAR, AND MANPREET KAUR

INTRODUCTION

The aging brain and cranium are known to undergo structural changes that can alter craniocerebral responses to both physiological and pharmacological stimuli. This chapter outlines fundamental concepts of cerebral physiology with special reference to variations and alterations in the geriatric population.

INTRACRANIAL COMPONENTS AND MONRO–KELLIE DOCTRINE

Skull is a non-expandable rigid semi-closed compartment housing three intracranial components: brain parenchyma (including interstitial fluid), blood, and cerebrospinal fluid (CSF). Quantitatively, 80% of the available intracranial volume (ICV) is occupied by brain parenchyma along with interstitial fluid, while CSF and blood occupy 10% each of the total ICV. The influence of the change in volume of one of these components on the volumes of the remaining components has been classically explained using the Monro–Kellie doctrine (1). The initial proposition of this doctrine by Alexander Monro in 1783 did not take into consideration the presence of CSF as an important intracranial component. Subsequent observations and evidence led to revision of the doctrine into its currently accepted form, stated as: "with an intact skull, the sum of the volumes of brain, blood and CSF is constant." Therefore, increase in volume of one of the components will be associated with a decrease in the volume of one or both of the other components (1,2). To understand the physiological implications of this doctrine, it is important to understand the quantitative relationship between the volumes of each component and the state of compressibility of each (Figure 2.1). Brain parenchyma is considered incompressible, and increase in volume of any intracranial component is accompanied by compensatory changes in CSF and/or blood volumes, in compliance with the Monro–Kellie doctrine.

The CSF is produced by the specialized capillary networks in cerebral ventricles known as the choroid plexus (CP) at a relatively constant rate of 0.35 mL/min in adults. In addition to CSF secretion, the CP-CSF system has been reported to play an important role in the development, homeostasis, and repair of the central nervous system. Aging is associated with a decline in all the functions of the CP-CSF system including CSF secretion and protein synthesis. The secretion rates in the elderly can decrease to 0.2 mL/min (3); however, some studies have also reported no reduction in CSF secretion with age (4). The total CSF volume amounts to 100–150 mL in adults, the majority of which stays

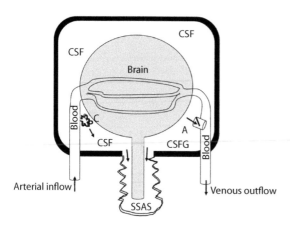

Figure 2.1 Schematic model depicting cranium and intracranial components. In steady state, arterial inflow is constantly balanced by venous outflow, keeping the total intracranial blood volume relatively constant. CSF is secreted from the choroid plexus (CP) and absorbed through the arachnoid granulations (AG) which act as one-way valves to the venous compartment. Spinal subarachnoid space (SSAS) acts as a high compliant space that can accommodate CSF translocated from the cranial compartment in response to rise in volume of any other intracranial component.

in the cerebral subarachnoid space and major cisterns of the brain. A relatively minor volume of CSF occupies the cerebral ventricles, spinal subarachnoid space, and spinal canal (4). Despite the reduction in CSF secretion, there is a net increase in CSF volume with age, accounting for 13%–33% of the total ICV as compared to just 7% in younger individuals (5,6). This increase in CSF volume has been attributed to a decrease in white matter from approximately 39% of ICV in young adults to 33% in the elderly (5). There is also an increase in the volume of the subarachnoid space with age (7).

CSF formation exists in dynamic equilibrium, with continuous absorption taking place through specialized structures called arachnoid villi and granulations. Arachnoid granulations are herniations of arachnoid membrane through the dura mater into cerebral venous sinuses. Arachnoid granulations operate as one-way valves, permitting bulk flow of all CSF constituents unidirectionally into the cerebral venous blood. The resistance to drainage of CSF increases with age, possibly due to calcification of the arachnoid villi, thickening of the arachnoid membrane (8), and central vascular hypertension (9). Despite this increase in

resistance, the intracranial pressure (ICP) does not change with age. ICP is a direct determinant of the cerebral perfusion pressure (CPP) and cerebral blood flow (CBF), making its monitoring vital for the assessment and management of various clinical neurosurgical and neurological conditions. At steady state, ICP has been shown to be determined by contributions from CSF and vascular components, as given by the relation:

$$ICP = CSF + Vascular\ component$$
$$ICP = (If \times Ro) + Pv$$

where If is the CSF formation rate, Ro is the CSF outflow resistance, and Pv is the vascular contribution to the ICP. It is implied from this mathematical relationship that any physiological or pathological factor that tends to increase the CSF production rate or outflow resistance will increase the ICP. The contribution of the vascular component to ICP is more complex and has not been modeled and expressed mathematically in a quantifiable manner. Since outflow resistance increases with age but CSF formation rate decreases, there is no net change in the ICP with age.

Every minute, the brain receives approximately 700 mL of blood, equivalent to double the total ICV. In steady state, the quantum of arterial inflow is constantly balanced by an equal amount of venous outflow, nullifying any significant change in total intracranial blood volume. Intracranial blood volume amounts to approximately 150 mL in adults. Forty-five percent of the blood volume stays in the microcirculation, and the remainder stays in the venous (40%) and arterial compartments (15%). The CBF is determined by CPP and cerebrovascular resistance (CVR) by the relationship:

$$CBF = \frac{CPP}{CVR},$$

where CPP = MAP − ICP, where MAP is the mean arterial blood pressure and ICP is the intracranial pressure.

$$CVR = \frac{8\eta l}{\pi r4},$$

where l is the length of the vessel, η is viscosity of blood, and r is the radius of the vessel. CBF is reported to decrease with age, while MAP increases with age (10).

MONITORING OF INTRACRANIAL PRESSURE

Clinically, ICP is monitored mostly by invasive methods. The methods can be classified based on the location of placement of the catheter or pressure transducer into (i) intraventricular, (ii) subdural/epidural, and (iii) intraparenchymal (1,11,12). The gold standard technique for measuring ICP involves placing an intraventricular catheter in the lateral ventricle connected to an external pressure transducer for continuous recording. Recording through ventricular catheters also permits therapeutic manipulation of the CSF pressure and prevents zero drifting of the pressure recording. With the advent of microtransducers that can be placed in any of the recording locations, the infection rates associated with the procedure have been reported to decrease (11). The prominent disadvantages of intraparenchymal recording have been reported to be the following:

- Zero drifting, which contributes to inaccuracy in ICP estimation with time.
- The limitation in deriving an estimate of real ICP based on the compartmentalized recording from a single parenchymal site.
- Noninvasive methods to measure ICP based on various imaging modalities, transcranial Doppler, and visual evoked potentials have been developed and tested, with limited success and accuracy so far.

Fluctuations in mean intracranial pressure

The technique of continuous ICP monitoring by using an intraventricular catheter was pioneered by Lundberg et al. in the 1960s. Based on systematic analysis of pressure recordings from series of patients, Lundberg et al. reported three characteristic fluctuations in mean ICP (1,12–14):

1. *A waves or plateau waves*: These waves are always of pathological origin and indicate significant reduction in the intracranial compliance (see "Intracranial compliance and its estimation" section). A waves are characterized by sudden and steep increases in the ICP to 50 mmHg or more from near-normal values. These fluctuations usually last for 5–20 minutes, followed by a sharp decline to the baseline values.

2. *B waves*: B waves are also considered pathologically significant and are associated with failing intracranial compensation to volume changes. B waves show rhythmic (0.5–2 Hz) oscillations in ICP rising steeply to 20–30 mmHg above baseline, followed by a sudden decline to baseline values. Unlike A waves, B waves do not show sustained periods of intracranial hypertension. The origin of B waves is probably linked to changes in cerebrovascular tone and cerebral blood volume.

3. *C waves*: C waves are reported to be of limited pathological significance. These are rhythmic oscillations in ICP, with frequencies ranging from 4 to 8 per minute, synchronous with the spontaneously occurring Traube–Hering–Mayer wave oscillations in arterial blood pressure. C waves have lower amplitude than B and A waves.

Intracranial pressure–volume relationship

Intracranial pressure–volume curves graphically depict the changes in ICP in response to changes in ICV. These graphical descriptions portray the role of compensatory ICV-buffering mechanisms and provide additional insights and quantifiable measures to predict the risk of intracranial hypertension with a progressive rise in ICV. The ICP–volume curve (Figure 2.2) shows an initial compensated phase, the earlier half of which (1) shows minimal rise in ICP with rise in ICV. The volume-buffering mechanisms described previously operate effectively during this phase, eliminating any change in ICP. The latter half (2) of the compensated phase shows marginal rise in ICP with rise in ICV; however, ICP is still within normal limits. More characteristic during this latter half of the compensated phase is the change in slope of the ICP–volume curve. The slope of the pressure volume curve that denotes change in ICP for unit change in ICV is defined as intracranial elastance ($\Delta P/\Delta V$). This slope has been wrongly expressed as compliance widely in literature, whereas in actual scientific parlance, compliance denotes the change in volume for unit change in pressure ($\Delta V/\Delta P$). Thus, compliance bears an inverse relationship with intracranial elastance. The latter half of the compensated phase shows a rise in intracranial elastance (fall in compliance) steeper than the rise

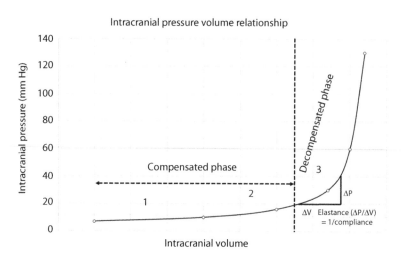

Figure 2.2 Intracranial pressure volume relationship with intracranial volume (ICV) in the X-axis and intracranial pressure (ICP) in the Y-axis. Phase 1 is characterized by negligible rise in ICP with rise in ICV, indicating a phase of complete compensation. Phase 2 is characterized by minimal rise in ICP (still within normal limits) and a more prominent rise in cranial elastance (fall in compliance), as indicated by the changing slope of the pressure volume curve. Phase 3 shows the decompensated phase, where a marked rise in ICP is observed with any further rise in ICV.

in ICP per se. The falling intracranial compliance is indicative of the impending failure of volume-buffering mechanisms operating already at physiological limits. Any rise in ICV beyond this point produces a sharp decline in intracranial compliance and a profound increase in ICP, characterizing the decompensated phase of the ICP–volume curve.

Intracranial compliance and its estimation

Experimental or clinical estimation of intracranial compliance necessitates recording of ICP responses to manipulation of ICV in order to generate the pressure–volume relationship. The procedure involves cannulation of the lateral ventricle, cisterna magna, or lumbar subarachnoid space to record neuraxis CSF pressure and produce increments or decrements in CSF volume by saline injection and CSF aspiration, respectively (15). The cannula at the external end is connected to a pressure transducer to record the changes in ICP. The volume manipulations are done using a syringe filled with sterile saline interposed between the cannula and the transducer. After recording the steady-state ICP after cannulation, volume manipulation is done initially by removing a specific

volume of CSF ($-\Delta V$) by aspiration. Removal of volume will lead to an immediate fall in ICP ($-\Delta P$), followed by a gradual recovery to the steady-state ICP values in 2–3 minutes. Similarly, a bolus injection of sterile saline will increase the CSF volume by ΔV and a consequent immediate rise in ICP(ΔP), followed by recovery to steady-state values in 2–3 minutes. A pressure–volume curve is thus plotted with volume increments or decrements in the X-axis and ICP values recorded immediately post-volume manipulation on the Y-axis (Figure 2.3a). It can be inferred from the pressure–volume curve that intracranial compliance (inverse of the slope) changes as a function of ICV. Intracranial compliance is higher on the horizontal portion of the pressure–volume curve than on its vertical limb. Plotting the ICP changes of the pressure–volume curve on a logarithmic scale (base 10) can transform the curve to a linear plot (Figure 2.3b). The slope of this line has been used as an estimate of craniospinal compliance, denoted as pressure–volume index (PVI). It is defined as the estimated volume (in mL) required to raise the ICP by a factor of 10.

In addition to the estimation of craniospinal compliance, the technique of bolus manipulation of ICV can also be used to estimate two important variables that determine the CSF pressure.

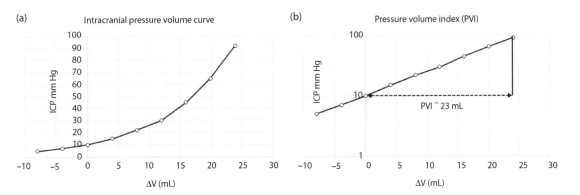

Figure 2.3 Determination of pressure–volume index (PVI). **(a)** Pressure volume curve derived by recording the ICP changes (Y-axis) to bolus volume manipulation (ΔV) of intracranial volume as represented in the X-axis. A logarithmic plotting of the ICP data transforms the curve into a linear plot **(b)** and can be used to derive the pressure–volume index (PVI).

The CSF pressure is determined by the product of CSF production rate (If) and resistance to CSF outflow (Ro). Following the removal of a CSF bolus, ICP shows an immediate fall, followed by gradual recovery toward baseline steady-state values. The rate of this pressure recovery is proportional to CSF production rate. Similarly, CSF outflow resistance can be estimated from the rate of pressure recovery observed after the immediate rise in ICP induced by bolus volume increment.

Usage of PVI in clinical practice to estimate craniospinal compliance has been limited by the need for bolus injections and removal of CSF. Another approach based on ICP waveform analysis has been proposed by Avezaat et al. (1,16) in 1979 to determine craniospinal compliance. The ICP waveform shows pulsatile changes synchronous with arterial pressure waveform. During each cardiac cycle, there is a pulsatile change in intracranial blood volume (ΔV), which might be equated with artificially induced volume increment used for deriving PVI. The pulse amplitude of ICP waveform (ΔP) thus represents the immediate pressure response to ICV increments synchronous with each cardiac cycle. The cardiac synchronous volume increments remain largely constant in a stable hemodynamic state uninfluenced by any changes in craniospinal elastance. The pulsatile changes in ICP waveform due to this volume increment are plotted against the conventional pressure–volume curve in Figure 2.4. Based on the graph, it can be inferred that the pulse amplitude of ICP waveform bears an inverse relationship with the craniospinal compliance and thus can be used as an estimate of the same.

CEREBRAL BLOOD FLOW

Adult healthy human brain on average receives 14% of the cardiac output every minute, which translates to approximately 50 mL/100 g/min. Gray matter, because of its higher metabolic demands, receives approximately four times higher blood flow (80 mL/100 g/min) than white matter (20 mL/100 g/min) in adults (17).

These values decrease by 0.5% per year with age (18). CBF values lower than 30 mL/100 g/min can lead to neurological symptoms, and those between 15 and 20 mL/100 g/min can lead to irreversible neuronal damage.

White matter volume reduces significantly with age, while the gray matter is reported to show a much lesser decrease with age (19). Both the CBF and the cerebral metabolic rate decrease with aging (19,20). However, some studies suggest that CBF does not change with age (21). Atrophic changes in the brain could explain some of the apparent reduction in the CBF and metabolic rate (22). However, CBF and metabolic rate in the frontal, parietal, and temporal areas decrease with aging independent of the reduction in brain volume (23). The decrease in CBF with age could be attributed to the associated changes in the vasculature characterized by decreased vascular compliance and endothelial dysfunction.

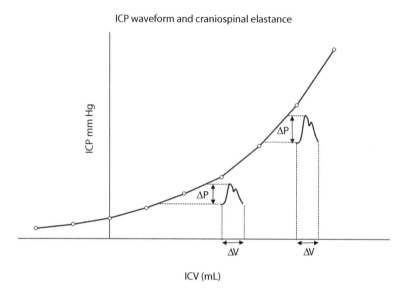

Figure 2.4 ICP waveform and craniospinal elastance. Depicts the changes in amplitude of ICP waveform with rise in ICV. ICP waveform amplitude increases with the fall in intracranial compliance (rise in slope of the pressure volume curve).

Cerebral blood flow and metabolic rate–flow metabolism coupling

Cerebral metabolic rate is a measure of the energy expenditure of brain computed from the amount of oxygen utilized by the brain (cerebral metabolic rate for oxygen [$CMRO_2$]) or from the amount of glucose metabolized by the brain (cerebral metabolic rate for glucose [CMRGlu]) in unit time. Amounts of oxygen utilized and glucose metabolized are quantified by measuring the arteriovenous concentration difference of the substance of interest and the CBF. Cerebral metabolism sustains the energy expended by the brain during the resting state to maintain the ionic gradients, biosynthetic functions, and other cellular housekeeping functions (basal need) as well as the additional energy expended for neural functioning and generation of electrical activity (functional need). Glucose is the metabolic fuel of choice for the brain. It derives 92% of its energy requirement through oxidative metabolism of glucose (17).

Flow metabolism coupling is the phenomenon by which CBF is tightly coupled to the metabolic demands of the brain, both regionally and globally (17). Increase in the metabolic rate due to synaptic transmission is temporally and spatially coupled to increase in blood flow to meet the enhanced demands for oxygen and glucose. Flow metabolism coupling being a dominant controller of CBF has been reported to be preserved during both sleep (24) and general anesthesia (25). Adenosine and nitric oxide (NO), two potent vasodilatory molecules, have been proposed as the chief molecular mediators of flow metabolism coupling. Increase in cerebral metabolism due to neuronal activation has been linked to increase in the concentration of these mediators in the local milieu, resulting in vasodilatation and increase in blood flow to the metabolically active region.

Hypothermia reduces $CMRO_2$ and consequently reduces CBF through flow metabolism coupling. Low temperature reduces energy expended by neurons for both basal and functional needs, producing significant reduction in $CMRO_2$ to 10% of normothermic values at temperatures as low as 15°C (17).

CBF and $CMRO_2$ have been shown to decrease significantly with age in the frontal and the insular cortices. In addition, $CMRO_2$ decreases significantly in other areas of the cortex (18).

CO_2-mediated vasoreactivity

Carbon dioxide (CO_2) is one of the most potent known physiological vasodilators of cerebral circulation. CO_2-mediated cerebrovascular reactivity is quantified as the change in CBF or blood flow velocities to spontaneous or imposed changes in arterial or end-tidal CO_2 concentrations. A rise in arterial or end-tidal CO_2 concentration is accompanied by an increase in CBF or flow velocities, and vice versa. The effect of rise in end-tidal or arterial concentration of CO_2 on CBF is almost instantaneous (within seconds) and takes approximately 2 minutes to stabilize. CO_2 rapidly diffuses across the blood–brain barrier and alters the pH of cerebral perivascular milieu, producing vasodilatation and increasing blood flow. The vasodilatory action of CO_2 on pial arterioles in anesthetized cats has been shown to be mediated through changes in extracellular pH, with CO_2 having no direct influence on vessel caliber (26). Similarly, in chronic hypocapnia and hypercapnia, CBF changes follow the adaptive changes in CSF pH rather than CO_2 concentrations (17). NO and prostaglandin E2 are considered to be the putative molecular mediators of CO_2-mediated vasoreactivity, even though the exact mechanisms of action are unknown (2,27).

The magnitude of CO_2-mediated CVR is different between the white and gray matter. White matter CVR is greater in the elderly compared to younger individuals, while the gray matter CVR is lower in the elderly population (28).

Cerebral blood flow responses to changes in partial pressure of oxygen

Unlike CO_2-mediated vasoreactivity, the influence of changes in arterial/tissue partial pressure of oxygen (PO_2) on CBF is modest and of limited clinical significance. Hypoxemia less than 50 mm Hg produces appreciable increase in CBF that tends to compensate for the reduced oxygen delivery to neurones produced by fall in arterial PO_2. The CBF responses to hypoxemia have a slower onset and a longer response time (approximately 6 minutes) to reach steady-state values in comparison with CO_2-mediated vasoreactivity (17). The cerebral vasodilatory response to hypoxemia has been mechanistically linked with metabolic shift to anaerobic glycolysis and consequent fall in extracellular pH due to the accumulation of lactic acid. In addition, adenosine has been implicated as a mediator of hypoxemia-induced vasodilatation (29) via its action through the opening of large-conductance calcium-activated potassium channels, leading to vascular smooth muscle relaxation. NO released by neuronal NO synthase is also proposed to play an important role in mediating the cerebrovascular response to hypoxemia (30,31).

Viscosity and cerebral blood flow

Blood flow in any vascular bed is inversely related to viscosity of blood, as given by Poiseuille's formula for computing vascular resistance: $R = 8\eta l / \pi r4$, where l is the length of the vessel, η is viscosity of blood, and r is the radius of the vessel. Viscosity of blood is primarily a function of hematocrit. Hemodilution increases CBF due to fall in viscosity and consequent reduction in resistance to blood flow, as depicted earlier. The CBF increases in anemia due to both reduction in viscosity and metabolically-induced vasodilation produced by decreased oxygen delivery to neuronal tissue (17).

CEREBRAL AUTOREGULATION

Autoregulation is a physiological regulatory phenomenon to ensure blood flow constancy to a vascular bed during changes in arterial blood pressure (32). It is present in most vascular beds but is particularly well developed in the brain.

Definition

Cerebral autoregulation is a homeostatic mechanism to regulate and maintain a fairly constant brain blood flow over wide ranges of arterial blood pressure; in other words, the perfusion pressure (33). The perfusion pressure of cerebral circulation is defined as the difference between mean arterial blood pressure (MAP) and the ICP. The quantitative relationship between CPP, CBF, and CVR is given as follows:

$$CBF = \frac{CPP}{CVR}$$

therefore,

$$CVR = \frac{CPP}{CBF}$$

where $CPP = MAP - ICP$, MAP is the mean arterial blood pressure, and ICP is the intracranial pressure.

Another approach of defining autoregulation is based on responses in the caliber of *resistance vessels* as occurrence of vasodilatation in response to decrease in CPP and vasoconstriction in response to increase in CPP (33). It can also be defined in terms of changes observed in CVR. A completely effective autoregulation implies that CBF remains constant and the CVR changes proportionally to changes in CPP. The definition of choice depends on the experimental model and the parameters of interest. The CBF responses may be more optimal to describe autoregulation during in vivo studies, whereas the caliber changes are good to define autoregulation in studies of isolated vessels. Cerebrovascular resistance seems a better parameter to understand the flow changes beyond the limits of autoregulation. The autoregulatory curve depicting the relationship between CBF, CVR, and CPP is shown in Figure 2.5. Cerebrovascular resistance reaches a minimum somewhat below the lower limit of autoregulation (LLA). At still lower pressures, there is a steep rise in CVR due to the collapse of vessels. At the other end, beyond the upper limit of autoregulation (ULA),

passive vasodilatation to high intravascular pressure results in a fall in CVR and a corresponding rise in CBF.

Importance

The brain has a high metabolic demand, accounting for 20% of the body's resting energy consumption despite weighing only 2% of the total body mass (32), and therefore requires adequate nutritional flow. This high perfusion demand means that the brain is very susceptible to ischemic injury. Conversely, disproportionately high CBF relative to metabolic need is also undesirable, as it can result in blood–brain barrier dysfunction, with plasma protein extravasation and transudation of fluid into the interstitium and pericapillary astrocytes. Such changes result in the development of hyperperfusion syndromes, which are characterized by debilitating neurological sequelae, including seizures, headaches, encephalopathy, and stroke (34). Therefore, it is vital to have stringent regulation of CBF to maintain normal brain function. Cerebral autoregulation is a protective mechanism that prevents brain ischemia during

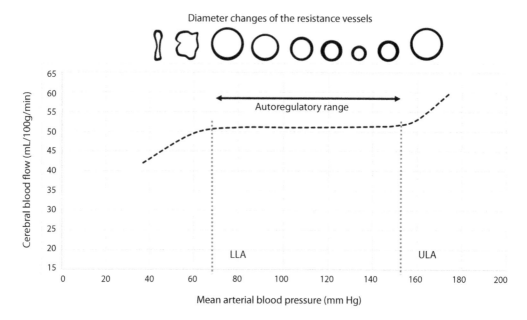

Figure 2.5 Autoregulatory curve of cerebral circulation. Autoregulatory curve of cerebral circulation with mean arterial pressure (MAP) plotted in the X-axis and cerebral blood flow in the Y-axis. Black vertical dotted lines indicate the lower (LLA) and upper limits (ULA) of autoregulation. The top panel pictorially depicts the diameter changes of resistance vessels with changes in MAP. Below, the LLA vessels collapse, while within the autoregulatory range a progressive decrease in diameter is observed with the rise in MAP. Vessels passively dilate beyond the ULA.

hypotension, and capillary damage and brain edema during hypertension. If autoregulation were not present, an otherwise-trivial fall in the pressure—for example, during sleep—might cause tissue ischemia and possibly cell damage. Likewise, a sudden rise in arterial pressure—for example, during any kind of exercise—in the absence of autoregulation would lead to passive vasodilatation of arterioles and capillaries and a potential for development of brain edema (35).

Blood pressure range and limits of autoregulation

In healthy adults, under normal conditions, these limits are MAP of 60 and 160 mmHg and CPP of 50 and 150 mmHg, respectively (32,33).

It is important to note that cerebral autoregulation responds not only to blood pressure changes but also to changes in ICP (36,37). In the upright position in a normal brain, ICP and central venous pressure (CVP) at the level of the head are negative and are therefore not accounted for.

Changes in MAP will thus largely govern the perfusion pressure, and hence CPP is roughly equivalent to MAP. The limits of autoregulation are not completely fixed and can be modulated, as they are under dynamic physiological control.

Mechanisms

The mechanisms of cerebral autoregulation may involve a combination of myogenic, neurogenic, and metabolic processes as well as endothelial cell–related factors.

Myogenic hypothesis

The myogenic theory states that the basal tone of the vascular smooth muscle is affected by change in perfusion or transmural pressure, and the small arteries and arterioles are constricting or dilating in response to increases or decreases in transmural pressure. The short latency and rapidity of autoregulatory response, which are initiated within a few seconds after a change in transmural pressure of the resistance vessels (26,38) and largely completed within 15–30 seconds, favor a myogenic response.

Experimentally, changes in transmural pressure correlate positively with changes in smooth muscle action potentials and membrane potentials, which

result in smooth muscle activation (26,39). Studies have shown that this smooth muscle activation is blocked by removal of calcium ions and addition of ethylene glycol tetra-acetic acid (40). Essentially, the stretching of vascular smooth muscles activates stretch-sensitive ion channels, which in turn initiate membrane depolarization through nonselective cation channels, resulting in the influx of calcium through voltage-gated calcium channels, and consequently, smooth muscle contraction (40,41). Some investigators believe that the myogenic mechanism sets the limits of autoregulation, whereas the metabolic mediators are responsible for cerebral autoregulation itself.

Metabolic hypothesis

The metabolic mechanism states that reduction in local blood flow results in the release of chemical factors that result in dilatation of cerebral blood vessels. That is, CBF constancy is maintained through release of the vasoactive mediators that couple the neuronal activity with blood flow. Regional CBF is then regulated by constriction and dilation of cerebral arterioles and by opening and closing of pre-capillary sphincters in the metarterioles, which are responsible for distribution of blood through the cerebrovascular bed. Putative mediators include CO_2, H^+, O_2, adenosine and adenine nucleotides, K^+, and Ca^{2+} (42). Among them, adenosine is the only mediator with experimental data to support.

Adenosine is a known vasodilator (43), and its level increases in the brain with moderate reduction in blood pressure. In moderate to severe hypotension, its level increases almost sixfold (44). Failure of adenosine antagonist caffeine to affect the pressure–flow relationship has been suggested as evidence contradicting the major role of adenosine in autoregulation (26,45,46). Although the rapidity of the autoregulatory responses has been considered to favor the myogenic hypothesis, the flow changes to metabolic demand also occur instantaneously.

In addition, NO has been shown to influence basal- and stimulus-mediated cerebrovascular tone. NO mediates its effect through cyclic guanosine monophosphate (cGMP) and a decrease in intracellular calcium. Other proposed substances include protein kinase C, melatonin, prostacyclin, activated potassium channels, and intracellular second messengers (47).

Neurogenic mechanism

The cerebral blood vessels, extraparenchymal and intraparenchymal, are innervated by nerves in a manner comparable to that of the blood vessels in the periphery (48). The nerves innervating the cerebral vessels contain transmitters of several chemical classes along with a variety of cognate receptors expressed on the vasculature. However, the exact role and mechanism of this innervation are still subjects of investigation. The neurotransmitters involved include acetylcholine (most abundant), norepinephrine, neuropeptide Y, cholecystokinin, vasoactive intestinal peptide, and calcitonin gene–related peptide (49). Stimulation and denervation of the sympathetic nerve supply marginally change CBF, even though they have a marked effect on cerebral blood volume, cerebral capacitance (50), ICP (51), and cerebrospinal fluid formation (52). Furthermore, sympathetic stimulation shifts the limits of autoregulation to higher pressures, resulting in rightward shift of the autoregulatory curve. This shields the brain against severe elevation of MAP by attenuating the consequent increase in blood flow (53–55).

Endothelial cell–related factors

Endothelial cell–related factors have also been implicated in autoregulation. Increments in flow without changes in transmural pressure in isolated vessels, both in situ and in vitro, induce vasodilatation, which is abolished by removal of endothelium (56,57). These observations suggest the release of a vasodilatory mediator by endothelium in response to increase in flow. Harder et al. (39) studied the role of endothelium in mediating or modulating the vascular responses to elevation of transmural pressure. With intact endothelium, high transmural pressure resulted in membrane depolarization, action potential generation, and vasoconstriction. Following disruption of endothelium by using collagenase or elastase, these responses were lost, whereas contractile response to high potassium and serotonin levels was preserved. This suggests the endothelial dependence of responses of isolated cerebral blood vessels to changes in transmural pressure. It is speculated that endothelial cells may serve as a transducer in the autoregulatory response to pressure.

Endothelium-derived relaxing factor (EDRF) has been identified as NO or an NO-containing substance produced in cerebral blood vessels. Its action is mediated by the activation of guanylate cyclase and formation of cGMP. An impaired endothelium-dependent response with decreased production of EDRF but increased release of EDRFs, such as endothelin and arachidonic acid, has been reported in subarachnoid hemorrhage.

Cerebral autoregulation in the geriatric population—clinical implications

CBF decreases with age, but there is no effect of increasing age on cerebral autoregulation. No changes in dynamic cerebral autoregulation (DCA) were observed in the elderly population (19). The autoregulatory index, which is a measure of DCA, was similar between younger and older individuals at rest, during a 30-minute 70° head-up tilt and after the tilt. While cerebral autoregulation was found to be less effective in the elderly under sevoflurane anesthesia as compared to young adults (58), the authors observed that the difference between the two age groups is less than the two standard deviations of interhemispheric difference, thereby suggesting that it may not be clinically relevant even though it achieves statistical significance. Cerebral autoregulation has also been found to be preserved in the elderly population by evaluating spontaneous (59) and induced (10,19) fluctuations in MAP.

Cerebral autoregulation is impaired in traumatic brain injury (TBI), depending on the severity of the disease (60,61). Progressive impaired autoregulatory response during the first 9 days after TBI mirrors worsening of the underlying injury, and worsening cerebral autoregulation may mirror worsening TBI. Impaired cerebral autoregulation would result in a passive relationship between MAP and CBF, implying that a fall in MAP would result in a decrease in CBF, making a subject susceptible to cerebral ischemia. Patients with intact autoregulation but reduced intracranial compliance may also be at risk of cerebral ischemia. In such a situation, a decrease in MAP causes cerebral vasodilation, increase in cerebral blood volume, and consequently an increase in ICP. Increase in ICP further decreases the CPP, leading to further cerebral vasodilation, ensuing in a vicious cycle called the vasodilator cascade. Poorer outcomes have been associated with patients >47 years of age with TBI (62).

Aging-induced variations in cranial and cerebral physiology require special consideration during anesthetic management of geriatric patients for various surgical interventions.

REFERENCES

1. Hawthorne C, Piper I. Monitoring of intracranial pressure in patients with traumatic brain injury. *Front Neurol.* 2014;5:121.
2. Wilson MH. Monro-Kellie 2.0: The dynamic vascular and venous pathophysiological components of intracranial pressure. *J Cereb Blood Flow Metab.* 2016 Aug;36(8):1338–50.
3. May C, Kaye JA, Atack JR, Schapiro MB, Friedland RP, Rapoport SI. Cerebrospinal fluid production is reduced in healthy aging. *Neurology.* 1990 Mar;40(3 Pt 1):500–3.
4. Gideon P, Thomsen C, Ståhlberg F, Henriksen O. Cerebrospinal fluid production and dynamics in normal aging: A MRI phase-mapping study. *Acta Neurol Scand.* 1994 May; 89(5):362–6.
5. Guttmann CR, Jolesz FA, Kikinis R et al. White matter changes with normal aging. *Neurology.* 1998 Apr;50(4):972–8.
6. Courchesne E, Chisum HJ, Townsend J et al. Normal brain development and aging: Quantitative analysis at in vivo MR imaging in healthy volunteers. *Radiology.* 2000 Sep; 216(3):672–82.
7. Narr KL, Sharma T, Woods RP et al. Increases in regional subarachnoid CSF without apparent cortical gray matter deficits in schizophrenia: Modulating effects of sex and age. *Am J Psychiatry.* 2003 Dec;160(12):2169–80.
8. Bellur SN, Chandra V, McDonald LW. Arachnoidal cell hyperplasia. Its relationship to aging and chronic renal failure. *Arch Pathol Lab Med.* 1980 Aug;104(8):414–6.
9. Rubenstein E. Relationship of senescence of cerebrospinal fluid circulatory system to dementias of the aged. *Lancet.* 1998 Jan 24; 351(9098):283–5.
10. Carey BJ, Eames PJ, Blake MJ, Panerai RB, Potter JF. Dynamic cerebral autoregulation is unaffected by aging. *Stroke.* 2000 Dec 1; 31(12):2895–900.
11. Czosnyka M, Pickard JD. Monitoring and interpretation of intracranial pressure. *J Neurol Neurosurg Psychiatry.* 2004 Jun;75(6):813–21.
12. Wiegand C, Richards P. Measurement of intracranial pressure in children: A critical review of current methods. *Dev Med Child Neurol.* 2007 Dec;49(12):935–41.
13. Dunn LT. Raised intracranial pressure. *J Neurol Neurosurg Psychiatry.* 2002 Sep;73(Suppl. 1): i23–7.
14. Lundberg N, Troupp H, Lorin H. Continuous recording of the ventricular-fluid pressure in patients with severe acute traumatic brain injury. A preliminary report. *J Neurosurg.* 1965 Jun;22(6):581–90.
15. Shapiro HM. Intracranial hypertension: Therapeutic and anesthetic considerations. *Anesthesiology.* 1975 Oct;43(4):445–71.
16. Avezaat CJ, van Eijndhoven JH, Wyper DJ. Cerebrospinal fluid pulse pressure and intracranial volume-pressure relationships. *J Neurol Neurosurg Psychiatry.* 1979 Aug; 42(8):687–700.
17. Vavilala MS, Lee LA, Lam AM. Cerebral blood flow and vascular physiology. *Anesthesiol Clin N Am.* 2002 Jun;20(2):247–64.
18. Leenders KL, Perani D, Lammertsma AA et al. Cerebral blood flow, blood volume and oxygen utilization. Normal values and effect of age. *Brain J Neurol.* 1990 Feb;113(Pt 1): 27–47.
19. Carey BJ, Panerai RB, Potter JF. Effect of aging on dynamic cerebral autoregulation during head-up tilt. *Stroke.* 2003 Aug;34(8): 1871–5.
20. Nobler MS, Mann JJ, Sackeim HA. Serotonin, cerebral blood flow, and cerebral metabolic rate in geriatric major depression and normal aging. *Brain Res Brain Res Rev.* 1999 Nov; 30(3):250–63.
21. Helenius J, Perkiö J, Soinne L et al. Cerebral hemodynamics in a healthy population measured by dynamic susceptibility contrast MR imaging. *Acta Radiol.* 2003 Sep;44(5): 538–46.
22. Yoshii F, Barker WW, Chang JY et al. Sensitivity of cerebral glucose metabolism to age, gender, brain volume, brain atrophy, and cerebrovascular risk factors. *J Cereb Blood Flow Metab.* 1988 Oct;8(5):654–61.
23. Grossman H, Harris G, Jacobson S, Folstein M. *Neuroimaging and the Psychiatry of Late*

Life. Cambridge: Cambridge University Press, 1997.

24. Madsen PL, Schmidt JF, Wildschiødtz G et al. Cerebral O2 metabolism and cerebral blood flow in humans during deep and rapid-eye-movement sleep. *J Appl Physiol (1985)*. 1991 Jun;70(6):2597–601.

25. Lam AM, Matta BF, Mayberg TS, Strebel S. Change in cerebral blood flow velocity with onset of EEG silence during inhalation anesthesia in humans: Evidence of flow-metabolism coupling? *J Cereb Blood Flow Metab*. 1995 Jul;15(4):714–7.

26. Kontos HA. Validity of cerebral arterial blood flow calculations from velocity measurements. *Stroke J Cereb Circ*. 1989 Jan;20(1):1–3.

27. Schmetterer L, Findl O, Strenn K et al. Role of NO in the O_2 and CO_2 responsiveness of cerebral and ocular circulation in humans. *Am J Physiol*. 1997 Dec;273(6 Pt 2):R2005–12.

28. Thomas BP, Liu P, Park DC, van Osch MJP, Lu H. Cerebrovascular reactivity in the brain white matter: Magnitude, temporal characteristics, and age effects. *J Cereb Blood Flow Metab*. 2014 Feb;34(2):242–7.

29. Morii S, Ngai AC, Ko KR, Winn HR. Role of adenosine in regulation of cerebral blood flow: Effects of theophylline during normoxia and hypoxia. *Am J Physiol*. 1987 Jul;253(1 Pt 2):H165–75.

30. Hudetz AG, Shen H, Kampine JP. Nitric oxide from neuronal NOS plays critical role in cerebral capillary flow response to hypoxia. *Am J Physiol*. 1998 Mar;274(3 Pt 2):H982–9.

31. Berger C, von Kummer R. Does NO regulate the cerebral blood flow response in hypoxia? *Acta Neurol Scand*. 1998 Feb;97(2):118–25.

32. Paulson OB, Strandgaard S, Edvinsson L. Cerebral autoregulation. *Cerebrovasc Brain Metab Rev*. 1990;2(2):161–92.

33. Lassen NA. Cerebral blood flow and oxygen consumption in man. *Physiol Rev*. 1959 Apr; 39(2):183–238.

34. van Mook WNKA, Rennenberg RJMW, Schurink GW et al. Cerebral hyperperfusion syndrome. *Lancet Neurol*. 2005 Dec;4(12): 877–88.

35. Strandgaard S, Paulson OB. Cerebral autoregulation. *Stroke*. 1984 Jun;15(3):413–6.

36. Häggendal E, Johansson B. Effects of arterial carbon dioxide tension and oxygen saturation on cerebral blood flow autoregulation in dogs. *Acta Physiol Scand Suppl*. 1965;258:27–53.

37. Sadoshima S, Thames M, Heistad D. Cerebral blood flow during elevation of intracranial pressure: Role of sympathetic nerves. *Am J Physiol*. 1981 Jul;241(1):H78–84.

38. Symon L, Held K, Dorsch NW. A study of regional autoregulation in the cerebral circulation to increased perfusion pressure in normocapnia and hypercapnia. *Stroke*. 1973 Apr;4(2):139–47.

39. Harder DR, Kauser K, Roman RJ, Lombard JH. Mechanisms of pressure-induced myogenic activation of cerebral and renal arteries: Role of the endothelium. *J Hypertens Suppl*. 1989 Sep;7(4):S11–5, discussion S16.

40. Hill MA, Davis MJ, Meininger GA, Potocnik SJ, Murphy TV. Arteriolar myogenic signalling mechanisms: Implications for local vascular function. *Clin Hemorheol Microcirc*. 2006;34(1–2):67–79.

41. Jackson WF. Ion channels and vascular tone. *Hypertension*. 2000 Jan;35(1 Pt 2):173–8.

42. Kuschinsky W, Wahl M. Local chemical and neurogenic regulation of cerebral vascular resistance. *Physiol Rev*. 1978 Jul;58(3): 656–89.

43. Wahl M, Kuschinsky W. The dilatatory action of adenosine on pial arteries of cats and its inhibition by theophylline. *Pflugers Arch*. 1976 Mar 11;362(1):55–9.

44. Winn HR, Welsh JE, Rubio R, Berne RM. Brain adenosine production in rat during sustained alteration in systemic blood pressure. *Am J Physiol*. 1980 Nov;239(5): H636–41.

45. Phillis JW. Adenosine in the control of the cerebral circulation. *Cerebrovasc Brain Metab Rev*. 1989;1(1):26–54.

46. Phillis JW, DeLong RE. The role of adenosine in cerebral vascular regulation during reductions in perfusion pressure. *J Pharm Pharmacol*. 1986 Jun;38(6):460–2.

47. Faraci FM, Sobey CG. Role of potassium channels in regulation of cerebral vascular tone. *J Cereb Blood Flow Metab*. 1998 Oct; 18(10):1047–63.

48. Edvinsson L. Neurogenic mechanisms in the cerebrovascular bed. Autonomic nerves, amine receptors and their effects on

cerebral blood flow. *Acta Physiol Scand Suppl.* 1975;427:1–35.

49. Zervas NT, Lavyne MH, Negoro M. Neuro-transmitters and the normal and ischemic cerebral circulation. *N Engl J Med.* 1975 Oct 16;293(16):812–6.

50. Edvinsson L, Nielsen KC, Owman C, West KA. Evidence of vasoconstrictor sympathetic nerves in brain vessels of mice. *Neurology.* 1973 Jan;23(1):73–7.

51. Edvinsson L, Owman C, West KA. Changes in continuously recorded intracranial pressure of conscious rabbits at different time-periods after superior cervical sympathectomy. *Acta Physiol Scand.* 1971 Sep;83(1):42–50.

52. Lindvall M, Edvinsson L, Owman C. Sympathetic nervous control of cerebrospinal fluid production from the choroid plexus. *Science.* 1978 Jul 14;201(4351):176–8.

53. Edvinsson L, Owman C, Siesjö B. Physiological role of cerebrovascular sympathetic nerves in the autoregulation of cerebral blood flow. *Brain Res.* 1976 Dec 3;117(3):519–23.

54. Mueller SM, Heistad DD, Marcus ML. Effect of sympathetic nerves on cerebral vessels during seizures. *Am J Physiol.* 1979 Aug; 237(2):H178–184.

55. D'Alecy LG, Rose CJ, Sellers SA. Sympathetic modulation of hypercapnic cerebral vasodilation in dogs. *Circ Res.* 1979 Dec;45(6):771–85.

56. Busse R, Trogisch G, Bassenge E. The role of endothelium in the control of vascular tone. *Basic Res Cardiol.* 1985 Oct;80(5): 475–90.

57. Holtz J, Förstermann U, Pohl U, Giesler M, Bassenge E. Flow-dependent, endothelium-mediated dilation of epicardial coronary arteries in conscious dogs: Effects of cyclooxygenase inhibition. *J Cardiovasc Pharmacol.* 1984 Dec;6(6):1161–9.

58. Burkhart CS, Rossi A, Dell-Kuster S et al. Effect of age on intraoperative cerebrovascular autoregulation and near-infrared spectroscopy-derived cerebral oxygenation. *Br J Anaesth.* 2011 Nov;107(5): 742–8.

59. Yam AT, Lang EW, Lagopoulos J et al. Cerebral autoregulation and ageing. *J Clin Neurosci.* 2005 Aug;12(6):643–6.

60. Bouma GJ, Muizelaar JP, Fatouros P. Pathogenesis of traumatic brain swelling: Role of cerebral blood volume. *Acta Neurochir Suppl.* 1998;71:272–5.

61. Stoyka WW, Schutz H. The cerebral response to sodium nitroprusside and trimethaphan controlled hypotension. *Can Anaesth Soc J.* 1975 May;22(3):275–83.

62. Petkus V, Krakauskaitė S, Preikšaitis A, Ročka S, Chomskis R, Ragauskas A. Association between the outcome of traumatic brain injury patients and cerebrovascular autoregulation, cerebral perfusion pressure, age, and injury grades. *Med Kaunas Lith.* 2016; 52(1):46–53.

3

Neuropharmacology: Age-related changes

KATLEEN WYATT CHESTER, OLIVIA JOHNSON MORGAN, AND KRUTI SHAH

INTRODUCTION

With the advancement of health-related research and technology, the proportion of persons 65 years and older is predicted to grow at a rate that exceeds persons younger than 65 between 2012 and 2050, according to the U.S Census Bureau (1). By 2050, the population of Americans ≥65 years is expected to increase to over 80 million, and one in four adults will be ≥85 years old (2). The increasing life expectancy and growing proportion of older patients can in part be credited to development of safer and more effective medications and procedures. Among these procedures, neurosurgical and neuroendovascular interventions have impacted the survival and functional status of the geriatric population.

With age as an independent risk factor for perioperative morbidity and mortality (3), it is important for providers to have a working knowledge of age-related changes in pharmacokinetics and pharmacodynamics of the geriatric patient requiring neuroanesthesia. Failures to age-adjust anesthetic doses (inhaled and intravenous) increase the risk of adverse events in the perioperative elderly patient (4,5). Unfortunately, the pharmacology of neuroanesthesia for older adults is not well researched. Neuroanesthetic decision-making for elderly patients requires thoughtful consideration of limited evidence combined with a risk–benefit evaluation including patient-specific factors such as baseline cognitive status and comorbidities. Neuroanesthetic challenges facing the clinician when caring for geriatric patients include polypharmacy, drug interactions, drug–disease interactions, alterations in typical response to perioperative medications, and postoperative cognitive dysfunction (POCD).

GENERAL CONCEPTS OF GERIATRIC PHARMACOTHERAPY

Clinical manifestations of normal aging include (6):

- Changes in the biochemical makeup of tissues
- Reduced capacity of body systems
- Reduced ability to adapt to physiologic stress
- Increased vulnerability to disease

As the body ages, there are physiologic changes to every organ system. General changes in the aging body include:

- Decreased total body water
- Decreased lean body mass
- Increased body fat
- Decreased albumin
- Increased alpha-1 acid glycoprotein

The organ systems involved in drug pharmacokinetics and pharmacodynamics that are affected by diseases of older age include the neurological, cardiovascular, gastrointestinal, genitourinary, endocrine, and renal systems (Table 3.1). Age-associated physiologic changes may result in reduced functional reserve capacity and reduced ability to maintain homeostasis. These alterations can make stressful situations such as surgical procedures more difficult for older patients, as they are more susceptible to decompensation (7).

When caring for older adults, it is important to consider the patient's overall health status, age, disease burden, and concurrent medications. Clinical pharmacists can assist with the care of complex older patients by assisting with comprehensive medication histories and evaluating the appropriateness of each medication using tools such as Beers criteria, START/STOPP criteria, and the medication appropriateness index (MAI) score (8–10). Pharmacists can review patient medication lists and provide recommendations on alternate therapy as patients transition through levels of care from the perioperative phase to inpatient units or even directly home or to a facility. Careful medication review with each transition of care is paramount for decreasing the risk of adverse drug events and polypharmacy. Many older patients are susceptible to polypharmacy, defined as the use of four or more medications or the use of multiple medications without indication. If older patients experience an adverse event, evaluation of current medications for possible cause and removing the offending agent is necessary before prescribing another medication to mitigate the adverse effect which leads prescribing cascade. Simplifying medication regimens for older adults increases compliance and reduces the risk of medication errors.

PRINCIPLES OF PHARMACOKINETICS IN OLDER ADULTS

Pharmacokinetics refers to disposition of a drug in the body and processes that impact the drug concentration. Absorption, distribution, metabolism, and excretion of medications are affected with the aging process and disease states associated with increasing age (Table 3.2).

Absorption is least affected by the natural changes that occur with aging since most drugs are absorbed via passive diffusion. For medications that undergo passive diffusion from the gastrointestinal tract, there is an increase in the rate of absorption but no change in the extent of absorption in elderly patients. As the body ages, decreased active transport in the gastrointestinal tract reduces absorption of vitamins such as iron, cyanocobalamin, and calcium. Medications administered via subcutaneous or intramuscular routes may have reduced absorption from impaired skin and muscle perfusion. Changes in absorption of topical medications have also been noted.

With age, body composition changes yielding decreased total body water and increased fat. The distribution of a drug is primarily dependent on volume of distribution and protein binding. The changes in the volume of distribution can have a direct impact on the dose that should be utilized. As mentioned previously, tissue perfusion may decrease with aging, which can slow drug distribution to fat and muscle. Lipophilic medications will have an increased volume of distribution in elderly patients and could potentially cause adverse effects due to prolonged half-life. Hydrophilic medications will have less distribution and result in higher plasma concentrations, which can also increase risk of adverse effects. Older adults with acute and chronic illnesses can have low albumin and high alpha1-acid glycoprotein. Low albumin may increase the free fraction of acidic drugs and high alpha1-acid glycoprotein may decrease free fraction of basic drugs; however, the area under the curve (AUC) is usually unchanged. There may be small increases in AUC from drugs administered intravenously that have high hepatic extraction ratio and extensive protein binding, such as phenytoin. P-glycoprotein, a membrane transporter protein throughout the body, including the

Table 3.1 Impact of age on organ systems of geriatric patients

| Organ system | Age-related changes and how they affect the body | | Other age-related changes |
	Decreased	Increased	
Neurological	• Size of hippocampus, frontal lobe, and temporal lobe • Number of receptors • Short term memory, coding, and retrieval and executive function	• Sensitivity of remaining receptors	• Altered sleep patterns
Cardiovascular	• Response to stress • Baroreceptor activity • Cardiac output • Heart rate	• Orthostatic hypotension • Systemic vascular resistance with loss of arterial elasticity and dysfunction of systems maintaining vascular tone	
Genitourinary	• Estrogen • Atrophy of vagina	• Prostatic hypertrophy with androgenic hormonal changes	• Detrusor hyperactivity may predispose to incontinence
Renal	• Glomerular filtration rate • Renal blood flow • Filtration factor • Tubular secretory function • Renal mass	• Serum blood urea nitrogen and serum creatinine with chronic kidney disease	
Gastrointestinal	• Hepatic size • Hepatic blood flow • Phase I metabolism • Motility of the large intestine • Vitamin absorption by active transport mechanisms • Splanchnic blood flow • Bowel surface area		
Endocrine	• Levels of estrogen, testosterone, TSH[a], and DHEA-S[b]		• Altered insulin signaling

Source: Hajjar ER et al. In: DiPiro JT et al. (eds) *Pharmacotherapy: A Pathophysiologic Approach.* 10th ed. New York, NY: McGraw-Hill Education; 2017, http://accesspharmacy.mhmedical.com/Content.aspx?bookid=1861&sectionid=146077984. Accessed March 30, 2019.

[a] TSH: thyroid stimulating hormone.
[b] DHEA-S: Dehydroepiandrosterone sulfate.

blood—brain barrier, has been minimally studied in elderly patients. The risk of toxicity related to its activity is unknown (11).

The major organ responsible for drug metabolism is the liver. Hepatic metabolism is dependent on liver perfusion, capacity, activity of hepatic enzymes, and protein binding, which can all be altered by the aging process. Metabolism of high extraction ratio drugs can be reduced secondary to reductions in liver size and hepatic blood flow of

Table 3.2 Age-related changes of pharmacokinetic phases

Pharmacokinetic phase	Pharmacokinetic parameters	Effects
Absorption	Passive diffusion remains intact	No change
	Reduced GI transit time	No clinically relevant change in extent of absorption although time for full absorption may be prolonged
	Reduced active transport and decreased bioavailability for some drugs	Reduced activity of some medications
	Reduced first-pass metabolism resulting in increased absorption of some high clearance drugs and decreased absorption of drugs from prodrugs	• Increased bioavailability of medications that undergo first-pass metabolism • Decrease bioavailability of active drug from parent drugs
Distribution	Increased total body water	Reduced volume of distribution and increased plasma concentrations of water-soluble drugs
	Increased total body fat composition	Increased volume of distribution and increased half-life of lipid-soluble drugs
	Decreased serum albumin	Increased free fraction of drug yielding increased drug activity
	Increased serum alpha-1-glycoprotein	Decreased free fraction of basic drugs that bind alpha-1-glycoprotein
	Increased permeability of blood brain barrier	Increased CNS concentrations of medications
Metabolism	Reduced activity of phase I hepatic metabolic pathways	Decreased clearance and increased half-life of drugs with poor hepatic extraction and high hepatic extraction ratios
Excretion	Reduced renal function	Decreased clearance and increased half-life of medications cleared renally

Source: Hajjar ER et al. In: DiPiro JT et al. (eds) *Pharmacotherapy: A Pathophysiologic Approach*. 10th ed. New York, NY: McGraw-Hill Education; 2017, http://accesspharmacy.mhmedical.com/Content.aspx?bookid=1861&sectionid=146077984. Accessed March 30, 2019.

20%–50% (12). Medications with high extraction ratios that have shown reduced hepatic clearance in adults include diltiazem, lidocaine, metoprolol, morphine, and verapamil (13). While phase I drug metabolism is reduced in older adults compared to younger patients, phase II hepatic metabolism remains intact. It stands that standard doses of medications undergoing phase I metabolism could result in prolonged duration of action. The effects of age-related changes in hepatic metabolism have been demonstrated with benzodiazepines. Diazepam and alprazolam undergo phase I metabolism to active metabolites, which may have longer duration of action in older patients, whereas lorazepam and oxazepam undergo phase II metabolism

to inactive metabolites and are preferred for older adults (14).

Of note, benzodiazepines in general should be avoided in older adults when possible, according to the Beers Criteria (8). Decreased first-pass metabolism can result in increased bioavailability of medications; however, the bioavailability of the active metabolite of prodrugs is reduced due to impaired hepatic conversion of the prodrug to its active form. Drugs and metabolites are excreted via urine, feces, bile, or lungs, but the primary route is renal excretion. Up to 30% reductions in kidney size have been demonstrated between 30 and 80 years of age (15). Interestingly, as many as one-third of older adults may have no reduction in renal clearance as measured by creatinine clearance. Declines in kidney function are more correlated with disease processes such as hypertension, diabetes, and heart disease. Serum creatinine is a marker of renal function but should not be used alone in elderly patients when evaluating renal function. Elderly patients with compromised renal function may appear to have a normal serum creatinine due to reduced muscle mass (16). The Cockcroft and Gault equation for estimating creatinine clearance (CrCl) in mL/min is commonly used for renal dose adjustments of medications (17). The Modified Diet in Renal Disease equation and the Chronic Kidney Disease Epidemiology Collaboration equations estimate glomerular filtration rate (18). Medications should be renally adjusted based on CrCl, as most studies use this marker for renal adjustments according to study protocol.

PRINCIPLES OF PHARMACODYNAMICS IN OLDER ADULTS

Despite widely available evidence describing the pharmacokinetics of the elderly population, less is known about the pharmacodynamic impacts of aging. Pharmacodynamics is the physiological and biochemical effect drugs have on the body. Aside from the concentration of a drug at the site of action explained by pharmacokinetics, the magnitude of a drug's effect can be attributed to pharmacodynamics. There are three mechanisms responsible for this property (19):

- Drug–receptor interactions
- Post-receptor cellular signaling
- The body's natural counterregulatory processes

Alterations of any of these pathways contribute to changes in medication response such as increased sensitivity, decreased effect, increased adverse effects, and reduced capacity to respond to adverse effects. Common pharmacodynamic concepts and terminology are provided in Table 3.3 (19). The pharmacodynamic impacts of aging extend to all organ systems.

Central nervous system

Age-related loss in brain mass impairs normal neuronal function in both excitatory and inhibitory neurotransmitter receptors. Most reported changes affect N-methyl-D-aspartate (NMDA), dopamine, and gamma aminobutyric acid (GABA) receptors, but changes in serotonin, adrenergic, and muscarinic receptors have also been reported. In particular, alterations in GABA receptors enhance sensitivity and the risk of adverse effects with certain sedatives (20).

Sensitivity to benzodiazepines increases up to threefold with aging due to altered GABA receptor composition and binding. These changes lead to increased sedation and slower response times that together contribute to fall-related injuries. In addition, the enhanced sensitivity of elderly patients to benzodiazepines plus the potential for additive effects of other medications can cause significant cognitive impairment (20). Receptor changes also influence elderly patients' dependence on benzodiazepines, placing them at greater risk of withdrawal. Withdrawal symptoms can include altered mental status, agitation, and seizures after abrupt discontinuation (21).

Geriatric patients are frequently prescribed neuroleptic and antipsychotic medications. At times these agents are prescribed for non-psychological disorders or underlying disease processes manifesting as psychological illness (21). In addition to sedation, elderly patients experience increased anticholinergic and extrapyramidal effects, orthostatic hypotension, and arrhythmias. Decreases in dopamine and dopaminergic receptors explain the increase in adverse effects compared to younger individuals (20). Furthermore, the antimuscarinic effects of neuroleptic medications increase agitation, confusion, delirium, and memory impairment. These cognitive effects are most frequent with tricyclic antidepressants (TCAs) and less likely with selective serotonin reuptake inhibitors (SSRIs) (21).

Pain is increasingly prevalent with age, and poor control can lead to an impaired quality of life. Despite importance of pain control, clinicians should be considerate of agent selection and dosing in the elderly. The World Health Organization (WHO) recommends prioritizing non-opioid analgesics before escalating to opioids, and providers should consider adjuvant agents when possible (21). At conventional doses, aging patients have increased sedation and respiratory depression to opioid agents, leading to fall injury and aspiration risk. Prescribing opioid therapy with lower initial doses and avoiding long-acting opioids for

Table 3.3 General pharmacodynamic concepts

Pharmacodynamic clinical concept	Definition
Agonist	• Drug that binds to receptor protein to produce a conformational change and elicit a cellular response. As a concentration increases, the response should also increase as more receptors are occupied. Maximal response occurs when all receptors are occupied.
Antagonist	• Drugs that bind receptors to prevent a cellular response. • **Competitive antagonists** which can be overcome by increasing the agonist dose. • **Noncompetitive antagonists** which cannot be overcome with increased agonist concentrations. Some noncompetitive antagonists are irreversible, and function cannot be restored until new receptors or enzymes are generated.
Partial agonist	• Drugs with the ability to activate a receptor but cannot produce a maximal cellular response despite all receptors being occupied.
Efficacy	• Extent to which a drug can produce a cellular response when all receptors are occupied. **Therapeutic efficacy** is the comparison drugs that affect the same biological system through different mechanisms.
Potency	• The amount of drug required to elicit a desired response. More potent drugs produce greater effects at smaller doses. Comparing potency of drugs can be done through comparing the concentration to produce half the maximum cellular response, ED_{50}.
Therapeutic index	• The range in drug concentration to which the efficacy and adverse effects are balanced.
Tachyphylaxis	• Rapid desensitization of an individual to a drug's effects.
Tolerance	• Gradual loss of response to a medication over days to weeks.

Source: Maxwell SRJ. *Medicine.* 2016;44(7):401–6.

opiate naïve patients is recommended. In switching agents, a 25%–50% dose-reduction allows for cross-tolerance and reduces the risk of adverse effects (22). Non-opioid agents also pose risks in older adults. Nonsteroidal anti-inflammatory drugs (NSAIDs) increase the risk of gastrointestinal bleeding and acute kidney injury in geriatric patients compared to younger individuals. More difficult to identify are the atypical effects of adjunctive antiepileptics used for pain control. A 50% dose reduction of antiepileptic drugs for pain is warranted to minimize adverse effects such as cognitive deficits, hematological abnormalities, and electrolyte imbalances. Dose adjustment should be based on clinical symptoms as not all effects are explained by serum drug concentrations (21).

Cardiovascular

Multifactorial changes within the cardiovascular system lead to impaired medication response in the elderly compared to younger individuals. Reduced compliance and elasticity of arteries leads to increased systolic blood pressure, decreased cardiac output, and decreased left ventricular ejection with left ventricular hypertrophy. This evidence would deem it reasonable to consider cardioprotective therapy in the elderly, but choice of agents should be carefully considered (23).

Beta blockers reduce morbidity and mortality in patients with cardiovascular disease. However, beta-adrenoceptor sensitivity and density decline with age. This decline, coupled with age-related cardiac changes, imparts more risk for beta blocker–induced adverse effects in elderly patients. Adverse effects of these agents include bradycardia, depression, cognitive impairment, and exacerbations of comorbid disease states. However, despite evidence for age-related risks, beta blockers are still recommended in heart failure, coronary artery disease, and acute coronary syndromes for the benefits on morbidity and mortality. Pharmacokinetic properties should be considered when prescribing a beta blocker in patients with hepatic, renal, or cognitive impairments. Doses should be started low and titrated conservatively (20,21).

Elderly patients experience greater response to calcium channel blockers than younger individuals. This effect is a class-wide effect among dihydropyridines (i.e., amlodipine, nifedipine, felodipine) and non-dihydropyridines (diltiazem, verapamil) through decreased baroreceptor response. Additionally, non-dihydropyridines have additive bradycardia and prolonged PR intervals through reduced sympathetic tone in the cardiac tissue or reduced muscarinic receptor activity. While smaller doses lead to an increased response, elderly patients have less compensatory response to this effect and doses should be titrated slowly (24). Less well understood is aging's effect on renin–angiotensin–aldosterone system (RAAS) blockers and diuretics. It is established that RAAS blocker concentrations in the body increase with age but lack in increased physiologic response due to decreased renin secretion. This leaves the elderly open to adverse effects such as acute kidney injury and hyperkalemia. Despite the adverse effects noted, elderly patients continue to benefit from RAAS blockers in a myriad of cardiovascular diseases (24). Diuretics remain beneficial in the elderly and are still considered a first-line therapy for hypertension. However, aging kidneys limit the amount of loop and thiazide diuretic concentrations that reach their sites of action in the nephron. While the lower concentrations of diuretics at their sites of action may yield decreased response, the age-related reductions in total body water and compensatory mechanisms contribute to increased risk for dehydration, electrolyte imbalances, and prerenal azotemia. Baseline patient-specific factors of nutritional status and pharmacokinetic properties should be evaluated when prescribing diuretic therapy (20,21).

Geriatric patients are frequently prescribed cholesterol-lowering therapy, particularly statins, for the primary and secondary prevention of cardiovascular disease. Cholesterol response with statin therapy is minimally impacted when comparing older and younger patients, but there is a dose-dependent increase in statin-associated myopathies and myalgias in the elderly. It is prudent to initiate a lower starting dose and to consider a patient's history of statin therapy and drug interactions.

Hepatic injury from statins is less common in the elderly, but serious hepatotoxicity remains possible. Discontinuation of statin therapy should be considered in the presence of severe adverse effects, but the risk of statin discontinuation syndrome should be weighed before discontinuing statin therapy for milder adverse effects (25).

Respiratory

Loss of elastic recoil and decreased gas exchange are the most common age-related respiratory changes, and geriatric patients are more susceptible to hypercapnia and hypoxia (26). In addition, the downregulated beta-adrenoceptors may impact beta agonist therapy in the setting of airway disease. Despite conflicting evidence that diminished effects of beta agonists may occur as individuals age, this effect cannot be attributed solely to receptor density. Impaired post-receptor cellular signaling leading to less activation of adenylate cyclase may be the cause of an attenuated response in the elderly. Ultimately, more comparative studies between older and younger individuals prescribed beta agonists are needed (20).

Endocrine

Geriatric patients have a high prevalence of metabolic and endocrine disorders, leading to increased morbidity. Hypothyroidism, osteoporosis, adrenal insufficiency, diabetes mellitus, and pituitary abnormalities are common diagnoses. One of the most complicated endocrine disorders in the elderly is diabetes mellitus, due to a decrease in glucose tolerance from reduced insulin secretion and sensitivity. These alterations lead to hyperglycemia in aging adults, even when adjusted for obesity and inactivity (21). However, inconsistent insulin resistance and lack of an adrenergic counter-response during hypoglycemia makes management difficult. The risk of adverse effects secondary to hypoglycemia is proportional to the intensity of glycemic control. Elderly patients with an A1c <7% are at increased risk of falls, cardiac ischemia, and hypoglycemia requiring emergent management. Frequency and severity of hypoglycemia can lead to irreversible dementia (20). As a result, more lenient goals are established for frail individuals and those with a shortened life expectancy (20,21,27).

Despite numerous agents to treat diabetes mellitus, studies targeting individuals >65 years old are scarce. Metformin is still considered first-line therapy for patients with type 2 diabetes, but subsequent or additive drugs should be used cautiously. Sulfonylureas, especially glyburide, have been implicated in increasing hypoglycemic episodes in the elderly secondary to decreased beta-adrenergic response leading to impaired detection of these events. Ultimately, further studies are needed to compare the pharmacodynamic and pharmacokinetic impact of diabetic medications for geriatric patients (27).

Hematology

The prevalence of medical conditions requiring antithrombotic therapy increases with age. There are exponential increases in the rate of atrial fibrillation as well as venous thromboembolism over the age of 70. Treatment of these conditions is challenging, given comorbidities, fall risk, and polypharmacy (28). An increased bleeding risk has been independently associated with age over 75 years old prescribed antithrombotic therapy. Thromboembolic and bleeding prediction tools should be used to help assess benefits versus risks when initiating antithrombotic therapy. Several pharmacodynamic factors including plasma protein concentrations can explain an altered response to anticoagulants with aging, but most mechanisms are unknown (29).

Vitamin K antagonists (VKAs) are the most recognized anticoagulant for having greater sensitivity in the geriatric patient due to pharmacodynamic changes. This is likely due to decreased dietary vitamin K intake, decreased production of vitamin K by the intestinal flora, and decreased synthesis of clotting factors from the liver or concomitant antiplatelet agents. Initial doses of VKAs in the elderly should be lower than what is usually recommended, and elderly female patients may need even lower doses due to risk of excessive anticoagulation compared to males. It is estimated that weekly warfarin doses to achieve therapeutic international normalized ratios (INRs) decline 0.4 mg/week per year of life. This finding was confirmed in previous studies that demonstrated an almost 50% reduction in weekly warfarin doses in older individuals compared to patients 20–59 years old (29). Numerous drug interactions can also impact the effectiveness and safety of VKAs.

In contrast to VKAs, newer direct oral anticoagulants (DOACs) inhibit specific targets in the coagulation cascade and do not require drug monitoring. In the major landmark trials that brought these drugs to market, <44% of enrolled patients ≥75 years old were included, and follow-up data regarding safety in the elderly is sparse (30). However, there is growing evidence to suggest that DOACs may have a better bleeding profile compared to VKAs, but age, body weight, and renal clearance should be considered when selecting an agent and initial dose (30).

Ultimately, aging is associated with modified pharmacodynamic pathways that affect responses to medications. While there are theoretical mechanisms for drug resistance and sensitivity, additional pharmacodynamic studies relating physiologic changes to drug response outside of pharmacokinetics are needed. With additional data and age-related trends, customizing medication management in the elderly will be safer and more effective.

SPECIFIC CONSIDERATIONS OF GERIATRIC NEUROANESTHESIA

Preoperative considerations

Older adults tend to have more comorbid conditions compared to younger individuals and are usually taking more medications. The majority of older patients are taking at least one medication, and 40% take at least five medications per week (31). As such, a careful and detailed medication history should be performed during the preoperative phase of care to identify and mitigate any potential perioperative drug interactions and medication risks, especially those that are unique to the geriatric population.

Medications for neurodegenerative disorders and antidepressants

It has long been known that older adults have higher risk for cardiovascular disease and cancer which could also affect younger patients, but patients of advanced age are also at risk for neurodegenerative diseases such as Parkinson disease (PD) and Alzheimer disease (AD), the most common causes of dementia in the elderly. Medications such as the acetylcholinesterase inhibitors used in the treatment of AD work centrally to inhibit the actions of acetylcholinesterase. In a dose-dependent manner, these medications improve cognition and function. In the anesthesia setting, these medications interact with neuromuscular blocking agents (NMBAs), increasing the duration of effect of succinylcholine by 50 min. The half-life of non-depolarizing NMBAs such as rocuronium may be prolonged from the down-regulation of acetylcholine receptors in the presence of the acetylcholinesterase inhibitors for the management of AD (32).

In PD, bromocriptine and levodopa/carbidopa, which modulate dopamine, can intensify hypotension induced by anesthetics (33). Serotonin syndrome characterized by hyperthermia, agitation, and rigidity is serious and potentially fatal condition resulting from the combination of serotonergic medications leading to excessive serotonergic activity in the body. An example of such a combination that should be avoided is selegeline, a monoamine oxidase inhibitor (MAOI) indicated for PD, prescribed concomitantly with meperidine, an opioid with serotonergic properties used for post-operative shivering. (33). MAOIs may also precipitate hypertensive crisis in combination with vasopressors such as ephedrine and phenylephrine (33). Despite these risks, it is recommended that medications for AD and PD should continue throughout the perioperative period, including during the operation itself via enteral feeding tube administration (33–36). Identifying the potential risks of this practice and careful monitoring are required.

Although tricyclic antidepressants (TCAs) should be avoided in elderly patients due to the risk of QRS prolongation and anticholinergic effects, circumstances exist when patients will present on these agents for conditions such as depression, neuropathy, or insomnia. TCAs in combination with anesthetic medications have been shown to provoke hypotension due to catecholamine depletion (33).

OPERATIVE CONSIDERATIONS

Induction of anesthesia

Agents used for induction typically include a high-dose opioid, a sedative, and a neuromuscular blocking agent. Lidocaine and beta blockers may be used adjunctively to blunt the adrenergic response during intubation. Hemodynamic fluctuations should be expected during intubation of the elderly patient so that measures can be taken to prevent adverse outcomes. In neurologically ill patients, careful attention to changes in heart rate and blood pressure during induction is paramount, as hypertension from a suboptimal medication approach can worsen or cause intracranial hemorrhage while hypotension can result in elevated intracranial pressure (ICP), reduced cerebral perfusion pressure (CPP), and ischemic insults. In the elderly, the onset of sedative and paralytic agents can be delayed due to age-related reductions in circulatory time (37). The optimal strategy or combination of medications for elderly patients undergoing neurosurgical procedures has not been identified (33). Instead, providers must carefully match patient- and procedure-specific characteristics to a customized induction strategy designed to mitigate the risk of adverse outcomes.

Maintenance of anesthesia

The maintenance of anesthesia follows similar principles in geriatric patients as the induction of anesthesia. The optimal agent(s) for the maintenance of anesthesia should be easily titrated, have favorable pharmacokinetic and pharmacodynamic properties, and be absent of adverse effects. Some medications may be safer to use in elderly patients for maintenance of anesthesia versus induction due to age-related changes in pharmacokinetic/pharmacodynamic (PK/PD) properties of the drugs.

Anesthetic strategies

The ideal neuroanesthetic strategy depends on the patient and the type of neurosurgical procedure. For example, the complexities of neuroanesthesia with awake anesthetic techniques vary considerably from emergent anesthetic techniques used during emergency surgeries for life-threatening brain injuries. Geriatric patients requiring neurosurgery pose additional challenges that must be addressed in any type of neuroanesthetic circumstance.

Awake neuroanesthetic techniques

Although the advancement of operative procedures in the elderly is evident with procedures such as deep brain stimulation for PD, craniotomies, and spine surgeries, progress has also been made in the use of awake anesthetic strategies. The advantages of awake procedures for geriatric patients include minimizing the risk of adverse side effects and drug interactions from exposure to anesthetics for deeper levels of sedation. Unfortunately, awake procedures pose great risk in patients with poor airways, cognition, or physiologic reserve, hence the need to diligently screen for older adults who would benefit from this anesthetic strategy. With these criteria, it remains that general anesthesia is employed for most elderly patients (33), and awake neuroanesthetic techniques should be considered for specific types of procedures and when deemed to be of minimal risk.

Scalp block by local anesthetics combined with intravenous sedation are the preferred medications for monitored anesthesia care (MAC) for awake neurosurgical procedures. Either consistently monitored anesthesia or an asleep-awake-asleep strategy may be used depending on the patient and type of neurosurgical procedure (38). Such procedures are viewed favorably for minimizing drug exposure, which benefits most patients, especially the elderly who are predisposed to adverse effects. During awake procedures, sedation and analgesia should be titrated to allow optimal conditions for cortical mapping and functional neurosurgery. In elderly patients, this includes maintaining the patient's mental status as close to baseline as possible while preventing the patient from moving during such delicate procedures.

THE IDEAL NEUROANESTHETIC APPROACH

In contrast to awake procedures, which are performed primarily electively and in patients who are hemodynamically stable at baseline, other neurosurgical procedures are emergent and involve critically ill patients. While these are extreme scenarios, the diversity of neurosurgical procedures requires detailed knowledge of anesthetic properties and a structured, patient-specific approach to each case. Although the ideal anesthetic technique for each type of neurosurgical case remains controversial, the ideal anesthetic agent should optimize cerebral hemodynamics by maintaining appropriate CPP, reducing ICP if already elevated, and lowering cerebral metabolic rate of oxygen consumption ($CMRO_2$). Each currently available

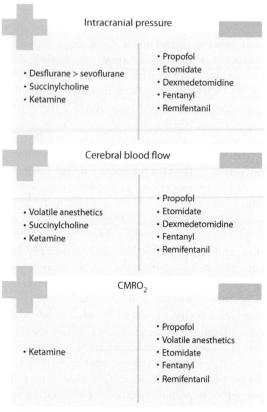

$CMRO_2$ = cerebral metabolic rate of oxygen consumption

Figure 3.1 Impact of paralytics and anesthetics on intracranial pressure, cerebral blood flow, and $CMRO_2$.

sedative impacts these cerebral parameters to varying degrees (Figure 3.1). In addition, the ideal neuroanesthetic agent(s) should preserve cerebral autoregulation while preventing secondary insults, and should allow for fast postoperative recovery (39,40). Due to limitations of volatile gases in this setting, a strategy known as total intravenous anesthesia (TIVA) is routinely utilized. Propofol with concomitant opioid administration is a common anesthetic combination for TIVA.

SELECT NEUROANESTHETIC AGENTS AND CONSIDERATIONS IN OLDER ADULT PATIENTS

Opioids

Traditional opioids modulate neurotransmission by activation of Mu receptors with varying Kappa receptor activity to reduce or eliminate pain by modulating neurotransmission. The synthetic opioids, fentanyl and remifentanil, are the most common intravenous opioids used during neurosurgical cases. These opioids minimally reduce cerebral blood flow (CBF) and ICP and tend to potentiate the effects of other anesthetic agents such as the volatile gases or propofol (40).

FENTANYL

Fentanyl can be administered as a bolus or infusion. Elderly patients generally experience a longer duration of action due to its lipophilic nature, higher volume of distribution, and longer clearance times. As with other anesthetics, dosing should be reduced by 50% in elderly patients to mitigate the risk of adverse effects, including hypotension and bradycardia with large doses.

REMIFENTANIL

Remifentanil is considered an ultra-short-acting opioid and is preferred by some for a smoother and faster wake-up time. In neurosurgical patients, wake-up times are important in rapidly obtaining postoperative neurologic examinations. The ultra-short-acting nature of remifentanil is a result of its degradation by blood and tissue esterases. Although reductions in esterases with age have been documented, the resulting 30% decline in remifentanil clearance between age 20 and 80 years of age is clinically irrelevant (41,42). In contrast, geriatric patients should be cautiously dosed with bolus doses, since the reduced Vd yields higher peak concentrations that could result in profound hypotension and bradycardia (41,42). EEG changes are typically seen at plasma concentrations in elderly patients that are half that of younger patients (41). As with other neuroanesthetic agents in elderly patients, the dose should be adjusted to 50% of standard dosing.

MORPHINE

Morphine is most commonly used in the postoperative setting for pain control. Judicious use in elderly patients is warranted. In older adults, morphine's volume of distribution is reduced by 50% in addition to reduced plasma clearance. The active morphine-3 and morphine-6 metabolites may accumulate in elderly patients with reduced renal function. Doses in this patient population should be reduced by at least 50% to account for pharmacokinetic changes in the elderly.

Sedatives

ETOMIDATE

Etomidate is routinely used as an anesthetic due to its rapid onset of action, producing sedation within 1 minute. After a single bolus dose of 0.3 mg/kg, patients generally recover within 5 minutes. Etomidate uniquely inhibits 11-beta-hydroxylase, thereby reducing plasma cortisol concentrations for up to 8 hours. In contrast to younger adult patients who experience no clinically significant cardiac effects from a bolus dose of etomidate, geriatric patients may experience decreases in heart rate, cardiac index, and mean arterial pressure (MAP). Geriatric patients with hypertension at baseline are particularly affected. Since older adult brains do not have a heightened sensitivity to etomidate, these effects on hemodynamics are likely the result of higher plasma concentrations after bolus administration due to reductions in volume of distribution and albumin-binding, which together significantly increase the free concentration of etomidate in the plasma compartment. The brains of older adults have not been shown to be more sensitive to etomidate (41,43). In addition to these hemodynamic effects, CBF decreases 20%–30% with etomidate and occurs with a proportional reduction in $CMRO_2$. ICPs are transiently reduced after etomidate induction. Use of etomidate for neuroanesthesia is primarily limited to induction doses versus continuous infusions or long-term use due to its effects on cortisol and since each milliliter of etomidate contains 35% propylene glycol v/v. Etomidate also causes pain on injection and myoclonus (44).

KETAMINE

Ketamine is a noncompetitive antagonist of the N-methyl-D-aspartate (NMDA) receptor antagonist. Ketamine increases CBF, $CMRO_2$, and ICP and should be avoided in patients with poor cerebral compliance or those who already suffer intracranial hypertension. Unlike GABAergic medications, ketamine has the potential to cause elevated heart rate, hypertension, and tachyarrhythmias. In rare cases, ketamine is associated with cardiovascular collapse as a result of catecholamine depletion in critically ill patients (45). Elderly patients with age-related reductions in cardiac reserve and comorbid cardiac conditions warrant careful consideration of the risks and benefits prior to using ketamine as an anesthetic agent. In addition, the response of an older adult to ketamine may be altered due significant reductions in NMDA receptor numbers and functionality along with heightened receptor sensitivity.

PROPOFOL

Propofol, a common highly lipophilic intravenous anesthetic, potentiates the actions of GABA type A receptors to exert its sedative effects, which have been found to be exaggerated in elderly patients at usual doses. These effects are a result of heightened sensitivity of the GABA type A receptors to the drug (41,46). Compared to younger patients, patients over the age of 60 years have been shown to have 20%–30% higher serum concentrations, especially after bolus induction doses (47). In fact, for induction of an elderly patient, it is recommended to use 50% of the standard induction dosing of 2–2.5 mg/kg to account for the decreased plasma compartment volume (47). In contrast, the 20%–40% increased total body fat of older adults yields longer durations of action of propofol compared to younger adults. It is well known that propofol causes dose-dependent reductions in blood pressure, and this effect is pronounced in elderly patients, mandating lower doses and slower administration rates. The potential for longer durations of effect from the increased volume of distribution combined with prolonged circulatory times could also prolong the duration of unwanted effects of propofol. Propofol is a preferred sedative in combination with fentanyl or remifentanil for TIVA in patients with increased ICP. Propofol compared to volatile gases achieves similar reductions in $CMRO_2$ at equal anesthetic depth but has the added benefit of also decreasing CBF.

DEXMEDETOMIDINE

Dexmedetomidine quickly produces light sedation by its action in the pontine locus coeruleus where it selectively activates central-alpha-2 receptors, thereby producing sedative effects quickly. Unlike other sedatives, dexmedetomidine does not impair the respiratory drive. Hemodynamically, this medication causes dose-dependent decreases in heart rate and blood pressure that are most pronounced with bolus doses. Although dexmedetomidine has mild analgesic effects and has been shown to be an opioid-sparing agent, it should not be used as monotherapy for analgesia. Since the actions

of dexmedetomidine are limited to the locus coeruleus, a noradrenergic nucleus near the 4th ventricle, it has no effects on electrophysiologic tests. Lacking electrophysiologic and respiratory effects, dexmedetomidine has gained much interest in functional neurosurgery and awake procedures (48). In addition, interest is growing for the use of dexmedetomidine as an adjuvant agent during particularly noxious parts of neurosurgical cases rather than increasing doses of the standard anesthetics in response to the patient's increasing heart rate and blood pressure.

VOLATILE GASES

The minimum alveolar requirement of volatile gases that prevents movement to noxious stimuli is inversely proportional to age so that the minimum alveolar concentrations in 80-year-old patients are 20% lower than patients half this age (41,49). The minimum alveolar concentration that produces unconsciousness follows a similar relationship to age. The physiology behind these age-related responses to volatile gases is not completely understood but likely involves altered functioning of neurotransmitter systems (41). Given that inhaled anesthetics are eliminated via the lungs, an inhaled anesthetic agent such as desflurane with low blood solubility could have advantages in elderly patients when inhaled anesthetics must be used. The low blood solubility of desflurane compared to other inhaled anesthetics allows for early recovery from anesthesia; however, in geriatric patients the difference in recovery time compared to isoflurane is controversial. Compared to propofol anesthesia, recovery times for desflurane is significantly faster in adult patients (49). Desflurane in particular is minimally metabolized to toxic metabolites, which is also favorable (49). Overall, inhaled anesthetics tend to have higher blood and tissue solubility in elderly patients due to higher percent body fat combined with lower minute ventilation, but this depends on the specific properties of the gas. Desflurane is limited in its use in high doses for induction of anesthesia due to significant cardiac adverse effects that could be exaggerated further in elderly patients with reduced cardiac reserve (49). Sevoflurane has been extensively used in neurosurgical patients. Neurosurgical studies have demonstrated that compared to sevoflurane, desflurane yields shorter times to extubation and recovery but similar perioperative complication rates, particularly in supratentorial craniotomy and resection procedures (50). Although volatile anesthetics reduce $CMRO_2$, they should be used cautiously in neurosurgical patients due to their dose-dependent, cerebral vasodilatory properties which increase CBF (Figure 3.1). These changes are more notable with isoflurane and desflurane, making sevoflurane a more attractive volatile anesthetic for neurosurgical cases. Studies have shown, however, less cerebral swelling with propofol anesthesia compared to inhaled anesthetics (50). None of these studies were specific to geriatric patients, although older adults were not excluded by trial design. In general, if volatile gases are used, it is recommended to limit MAC to 1–1.5 in patients with elevated ICPs to reduce MAC by 6.7% with each decade of life above 65 years of age (4).

NEUROMUSCULAR BLOCKING AGENTS

Anticipated actions of paralytic agents are also altered in geriatric patients. Elderly patients have fewer motor units and less muscle volume compared to adult patients. Older adults experience longer times to onset of paralysis from reduced cardiac output and blood flow to muscles (41). Great responses are seen with NMBAs that are hydrophilic, since the plasma compartment and total body water are reduced in this population (41). Clearance of the agents and duration of effects are prolonged from age-related changes of the renal and hepatic systems. Changes in blood flow to the liver combined with reduced renal function can alter vecuronium clearance by as much as 50% (41). The reduced clearance rates yield higher recovery indices in elderly patients. The recovery index is defined as the time from 75% block to 25% block. In elderly patients, these times can be increased as much as 200%. Vecuronium recovery times increased from 15 to 50 minutes and rocuronium times from 13 to 22 minutes from increasing age. Unlike vecuronium or rocuronium, cisatracurium is cleared by plasma esterases, and no appreciable differences in the actions of this paralytic have been noted in elderly patients (41).

Local anesthetics

Local anesthetics are administered via local skin infiltration or scalp block. Although patient age and weight does not predict systemic concentrations, caution should be exercised with use in the elderly. According to experts, the dose of lidocaine should be reduced due to impaired clearance and prolonged half-life, and it is likely that reduced dosing remains effective in the elderly (41,51). Local anesthetics are categorized into amides and esters based on structure. Amides are biotransformed in the liver, while esters are hydrolyzed by plasma esterases. Amides are susceptible to impaired clearance from reduced hepatic function of older patients. Simultaneously, older adults produce less albumin for local anesthetic protein binding. The result is higher unbound, active drug with the potential for local anesthetic toxicity (LAST). LAST is characterized by seizures, dysrhythmias, and cardiovascular collapse. Benzodiazepines and propofol have been used for seizure management in this setting; however, lipid rescue therapy may be considered for cardiovascular and CNS complications as well. High systemic concentrations above maximum thresholds are of increased concern in high-dose anesthetic combinations with epinephrine and geriatric patients with baseline cardiac history. Overall high-quality studies for safe practices of local anesthetic administration in elderly patients are lacking (52).

POSTOPERATIVE COGNITIVE DYSFUNCTION

Postoperative cognitive dysfunction (POCD) is defined as cognitive decline after surgery and anesthesia (33). Evidence suggests that POCD could develop from amyloid deposition and tau protein. In addition to surgery, other risk factors include age and history of stroke, while cerebral hypoperfusion, duration of anesthesia, and alterations in neurotransmitters increase risk as well. Elderly are more susceptible to POCD, which can present transiently with fluctuating symptoms or follow a more permanent and consistent pattern. Unfortunately, these changes significantly worsen recovery and increase hospital length of stay. Up to 40% of adults will experience some type of POCD postoperatively, with up to 10% of elderly patients having persistent dysfunction after 3 months (53). Preclinical data involving propofol and volatile anesthetics indicate that these agents may cause POCD; however, the evidence is controversial.

Bispectral index monitoring is of interest in the elderly population during surgical procedures, as it appears to result in lower total anesthetic doses and less incidence of POCD (33,54).

Some agents may harbor varying degrees of defense against POCD through neuroprotective properties. In cardiac and abdominal surgeries, ketamine has reduced the incidence of POCD. Likewise, ketamine infusions in elderly patients undergoing ophthalmic surgeries also reduced POCD. Mixed results have been noted with lidocaine and magnesium sulfate, while propofol and high-dose intraoperative dexamethasone have failed to show reductions in POCD. In fact, dexamethasone may increase POCD after surgery from increasing amyloid concentrations (33,55). It remains that none of these agents should be used with the intent of neuroprotection until more conclusive evidence becomes available.

CONCLUSIONS

The choice of neuroanesthetic strategy for older adults will depend on the surgical requirements, the patient's overall health and functional status, and properties of the anesthetic agents. Careful consideration of the goals of the neurosurgical procedure and the impact of anesthetics on cerebral dynamics is of paramount importance. Providers caring for geriatric patients requiring neurosurgical procedures must have a working knowledge of the age-related changes in the pharmacokinetic and pharmacodynamic properties of perioperative medications, as this patient population is more susceptible to serious adverse events.

REFERENCES

1. Welker KL, Mycyk MB. Pharmacology in the geriatric patient. *Emerg Med Clin North Am.* 2016;34(3):469–81.
2. Hajjar ER, Gray SL, Slattum PW Jr, Hersh LR, Naples JG, Hanlon JT. Geriatrics. In: DiPiro JT, Talbert RL, Yee GC, Matzke GR, Wells BG, Posey L (eds). *Pharmacotherapy: A Pathophysiologic Approach.* 10th ed. New York, NY: McGraw-Hill Education; 2017. http://accesspharmacy.mhmedical. com/Content.aspx?bookid=1861&sectio nid=146077984. Accessed March 30, 2019.
3. Griffiths R, Beech F, Brown A et al. Perioperative care of the elderly 2014: Association of Anaesthetists of Great Britain and Ireland. *Anaesthesia.* 2014;69(Suppl. 1):81–98.
4. Van Cleve WC, Nair BG, Rooke GA. Associations between age and dosing of volatile anesthetics in 2 academic hospitals. *Anesth Analg.* 2015;121(3):645–51.
5. Akhtar S, Liu J, Heng J, Dai F, Schonberger RB, Burg MM. Does intravenous induction dosing among patients undergoing gastrointestinal surgical procedures follow current recommendations: A study of contemporary practice. *J Clin Anesth.* 2016;33:208–15.
6. Cefalu CA. Theories and mechanisms of aging. *Clin Geriatr Med.* 2011;27(4):491–506.
7. Kane RL. *Essentials of Clinical Geriatrics.* New York: McGraw-Hill; 2013.
8. American Geriatrics Society Beers Criteria Update Expert Panel. American Geriatrics Society 2015 updated Beers Criteria for potentially inappropriate medication use in older adults. *J Am Geriatr Soc.* 2015;63(11): 2227–46.
9. Broeckling CD, Heuberger AL, Prenni JE. Large scale non-targeted metabolomic profiling of serum by ultra performance liquid chromatography-mass spectrometry (UPLC-MS). *J Vis Exp.* 2013;(73):e50242.
10. Samsa GP, Hanlon JT, Schmader KE et al. A summated score for the medication appropriateness index: Development and assessment of clinimetric properties including content validity. *J Clin Epidemiol.* 1994;47(8):891–6.
11. Brenner SS, Klotz U. P-glycoprotein function in the elderly. *Eur J Clin Pharmacol.* 2004; 60(2):97–102.
12. Corsonello A, Pedone C, Incalzi RA. Age-related pharmacokinetic and pharmacodynamic changes and related risk of adverse drug reactions. *Curr Med Chem.* 2010;17(6): 571–84.
13. McLachlan AJ, Pont LG. Drug metabolism in older people—A key consideration in achieving optimal outcomes with medicines. *J Gerontol A Biol Sci Med Sci.* 2012;67(2):175–80.
14. Chutka DS, Evans JM, Fleming KC, Mikkelson KG. Symposium on geriatrics—Part I: Drug prescribing for elderly patients. *Mayo Clin Proc.* 1995;70(7):685–93.

15. McLean AJ, Le Couteur DG. Aging biology and geriatric clinical pharmacology. *Pharmacol Rev*. 2004;56(2):163–84.

16. Swedko PJ, Clark HD, Paramsothy K, Akbari A. Serum creatinine is an inadequate screening test for renal failure in elderly patients. *Arch Intern Med*. 2003;163(3):356–60.

17. Cockcroft DW, Gault MH. Prediction of creatinine clearance from serum creatinine. *Nephron*. 1976;16(1):31–41.

18. Levey AS, Stevens LA, Schmid CH et al. A new equation to estimate glomerular filtration rate. *Ann Intern Med*. 2009;150(9):604–12.

19. Maxwell SRJ. Pharmacodynamics for the prescriber. *Medicine*. 2016;44(7):401–6.

20. Sera LC, McPherson ML. Pharmacokinetics and pharmacodynamic changes associated with aging and implications for drug therapy. *Clin Geriatr Med*. 2012;28(2):273–86.

21. Turnheim K. When drug therapy gets old: Pharmacokinetics and pharmacodynamics in the elderly. *Exp Gerontol*. 2003;38(8):843–53.

22. Naples JG, Gellad WF, Hanlon JT. The role of opioid analgesics in geriatric pain management. *Clin Geriatr Med*. 2016;32(4):725–35.

23. Mangoni AA, Jackson SH. Age-related changes in pharmacokinetics and pharmacodynamics: Basic principles and practical applications. *Br J Clin Pharmacol*. 2004;57(1):6–14.

24. Bowie MW, Slattum PW. Pharmacodynamics in older adults: A review. *Am J Geriatr Pharmacother*. 2007;5(3):263–303.

25. Ruscica M, Macchi C, Pavanello C, Corsini A, Sahebkar A, Sirtori CR. Appropriateness of statin prescription in the elderly. *Eur J Intern Med*. 2018;50:33–40.

26. Monarch S, Wren K. Geriatric anesthesia implications. *J Perianesth Nurs*. 2004;19(6):379–84.

27. Kezerle L, Shalev L, Barski L. Treating the elderly diabetic patient: Special considerations. *Diabetes Metab Syndr Obes*. 2014;7:391–400.

28. Robert-Ebadi H, Le Gal G, Carrier M et al. Differences in clinical presentation of pulmonary embolism in women and men. *J Thromb Haemost*. 2010;8(4):693–8.

29. Khoury G, Sheikh-Taha M. Effect of age and sex on warfarin dosing. *Clin Pharmacol*. 2014; 6:103–6.

30. Sadlon AH, Tsakiris DA. Direct oral anticoagulants in the elderly: Systematic review and meta-analysis of evidence, current and future directions. *Swiss Med Wkly*. 2016;146:w14356.

31. Barnett SR. Polypharmacy and perioperative medications in the elderly. *Anesthesiol Clin*. 2009;27(3):377–89, table of contents.

32. Kapoor MC. Alzheimer's disease, anesthesia and the cholinergic system. *J Anaesthesiol Clin Pharmacol*. 2011;27(2):155–8.

33. Berhouma M, Krolak-Salmon P. *Brain and Spine Surgery in the Elderly*. Cham, Switzerland: Springer; 2017.

34. Burton DA, Nicholson G, Hall GM. Anaesthesia in elderly patients with neurodegenerative disorders: Special considerations. *Drugs Aging*. 2004;21(4):229–42.

35. Inan G, Ozkose Satirlar Z. Alzheimer disease and anesthesia. *Turk J Med Sci*. 2015;45(5): 1026–33.

36. Nicholson G, Pereira AC, Hall GM. Parkinson's disease and anaesthesia. *Br J Anaesth*. 2002; 89(6):904–16.

37. Tripathy S. Geriatric neuroanesthesia. In: Prabhakar H (ed). *Essentials of Neuroanesthesia*. Saint Louis: Academic Press; 2017. pp. 653–9.

38. Skucas AP, Artru AA. Anesthetic complications of awake craniotomies for epilepsy surgery. *Anesth Analg*. 2006;102(3):882–7.

39. Hassan W, Nasir YM, Zaini RHM, Shukeri W. Target-controlled infusion propofol versus sevoflurane anaesthesia for emergency traumatic brain surgery: Comparison of the outcomes. *Malays J Med Sci*. 2017;24(5):73–82.

40. Cole CD, Gottfried ON, Gupta DK, Couldwell WT. Total intravenous anesthesia: Advantages for intracranial surgery. *Neurosurgery*. 2007;61 (5 Suppl. 2):369–77, discussion 77–8.

41. Rivera R, Antognini JF. Perioperative drug therapy in elderly patients. *Anesthesiology*. 2009;110(5):1176–81.

42. Minto CF, Schnider TW, Shafer SL. Pharmacokinetics and pharmacodynamics of remifentanil. II. Model application. *Anesthesiology*. 1997;86(1):24–33.

43. Arden JR, Holley FO, Stanski DR. Increased sensitivity to etomidate in the elderly: Initial distribution versus altered brain response. *Anesthesiology*. 1986;65(1):19–27.

44. Amidate™ [package insert]. Lake Forest, IL: Hospira, Inc.; 2017.

45. Koffman L, Yan Yiu H, Farrokh S, Lewin J 3rd, Geocadin R, Ziai W. Ketamine infusion for refractory status epilepticus: A case report of cardiac arrest. *J Clin Neurosci.* 2018;47:149–51.

46. Schnider TW, Minto CF, Shafer SL et al. The influence of age on propofol pharmacodynamics. *Anesthesiology.* 1999;90(6):1502–16.

47. Rana MV, Bonasera LK, Bordelon GJ. Pharmacologic considerations of anesthetic agents in geriatric patients. *Anesthesiol Clin.* 2017; 35(2):259–71.

48. Prontera A, Baroni S, Marudi A et al. Awake craniotomy anesthetic management using dexmedetomidine, propofol, and remifentanil. *Drug Des Devel Ther.* 2017;11:593–8.

49. Conzen P, Peter K. Inhalation anaesthesia at the extremes of age: Geriatric anaesthesia. *Anaesthesia.* 1995;50(Suppl.):29–33.

50. Magni G, Rosa IL, Melillo G, Savio A, Rosa G. A comparison between sevoflurane and desflurane anesthesia in patients undergoing craniotomy for supratentorial intracranial surgery. *Anesth Analg.* 2009;109(2):567–71.

51. Aronow WS, Frishman WH, Cheng-Lai A. Cardiovascular drug therapy in the elderly. *Cardiol Rev.* 2007;15(4):195–215.

52. Vasques F, Behr AU, Weinberg G, Ori C, Di Gregorio G. A review of local anesthetic systemic toxicity cases since publication of the American Society of Regional Anesthesia Recommendations: To whom it may concern. *Reg Anesth Pain Med.* 2015;40(6):698–705.

53. Coburn M, Fahlenkamp A, Zoremba N, Schaelte G. Postoperative cognitive dysfunction: Incidence and prophylaxis. *Anaesthesist.* 2010;59(2):177–84, quiz 85.

54. Chan MT, Cheng BC, Lee TM, Gin T, Group CT. BIS-guided anesthesia decreases postoperative delirium and cognitive decline. *J Neurosurg Anesthesiol.* 2013;25(1):33–42.

55. Ottens TH, Dieleman JM, Sauer AM et al. Effects of dexamethasone on cognitive decline after cardiac surgery: A randomized clinical trial. *Anesthesiology.* 2014;121(3): 492–500.

4

Preanesthetic evaluation

SUMMIT BLORIA AND ANKUR LUTHRA

INTRODUCTION

With aging of the world population (it is estimated that there will be 2 billion people older than 60 years on earth by 2050) (1), the number of geriatric patients undergoing neurosurgery is also constantly rising. This, in addition to the increased incidence of intracranial tumors with age, means that neuroanesthesiologists are likely to encounter a growing number of elderly patients being scheduled for neurosurgery in the future (2). These patients provide unique challenges to neuroanesthesiologists when they undergo neurosurgery, and as in routine anesthesia practice, a comprehensive preanesthetic checkup goes a long way in ensuring the best possible pre-, intra-, and postoperative care to elderly patients.

Although there is still some controversy about the exact age, most people accept the chronological age of 65 years as the definition of the "elderly" or older person. Aging has been defined as a universal and progressive physiologic process. It is characterized by diminishing end-organ reserve, lower functional capacity, progressive imbalance of homeostatic mechanisms, and an increasing incidence of pathologic processes (3). With aging, elderly patients are more susceptible to poor outcomes when they suffer from a disease as compared to young patients, because their homeostatic thresholds are narrower.

Limited direct scientific evidence exists regarding neuroanesthetic management of elderly patients, and many of the guidelines have been made employing findings of other non-cardiac surgeries in the elderly.

Preanesthetic evaluation is one of the most important components of patient care before administration of anesthesia. A preanesthetic evaluation helps develop rapport between the patient and anesthesiologist, as it is usually the first time the patient comes in contact with the anesthesiologist. Preanesthetic checkup is the process of clinical assessment that precedes the delivery of anesthesia care for surgery and for nonsurgical procedures. It helps to reduce anxiety levels in patients and leads to a shorter duration of hospitalization and reduced healthcare costs (4–7). It becomes more significant in cases of geriatric patients, who often have various preexisting diseases.

GOALS OF PREANESTHETIC EVALUATION

The goals of preanesthetic evaluation in geriatric neurosurgical patients remain the same as when caring for other neurosurgical patients, i.e.:

1. Evaluate the chief complaints of the patient, history of present illness, comorbidities of the patient, past history, personal history, drug history, history of any allergy, and family history.
2. Perform a general physical examination followed by examination of the major organ systems.
3. Order necessary laboratory investigations; interpret their results and order special tests whenever necessary.
4. Stratify the surgical and anesthesia risk on the basis of comorbidities present.
5. Optimize the status of patients so that they are in their best possible condition when they undergo surgery.
6. Formulate an anesthesia plan from the preoperative period to the intraoperative and postoperative period.
7. Explain to the patient and his/her relatives the present condition of the patient, the anesthetic plan, and the possible risks involved in the surgery including possible need of postoperative mechanical ventilation.

When caring for elderly neurosurgical patients, the following additional factors should be kept in mind:

1. Elderly patients are more predisposed to be suffering from various systemic diseases such as diabetes, hypertension, and cardiovascular diseases (8,9). The presence of these diseases should be ruled out before taking the patient for surgery.
2. These patients are often on a multitude of drugs (10). All drugs the patient is taking should be reviewed; the need to continue or discontinue any drug perioperatively should be discussed, and the possible interactions between these drugs and anesthetic drugs should be considered.
3. Aging is associated with a progressive fall in functional reserve. This implies increased neurosurgical mortality and morbidity, especially with increasing age (11,12).
4. Some elderly patients may not be able to give a full account of their medical history, so

Table 4.1 Indications for elderly patients undergoing neurosurgery

Chronic SDH
Occlusive cerebrovascular disease
Intracranial tumors
Spine surgery
Deep brain stimulation

involving the relatives/attendants during preanesthetic workup will be helpful.
5. The competence of the patient to give an informed consent and advance directives must be taken into account.

Some of the main indications for elderly patients for undergoing neurosurgery are listed in Table 4.1.

PATIENT-SPECIFIC CONSIDERATIONS

Airway issues in elderly neurosurgical patients

1. Elderly patients are considered difficult to ventilate. Atrophy of the facial muscles, including orbicularis oris, occurs with advancing age, leading to facial drooping at the corners of the mouth, which causes difficulty in attaining a tight bag mask seal during ventilation (13).
2. Note must be made of any missing or loose teeth during preanesthetic checkup. Missing teeth also contribute to difficulty in bag ventilation.
3. Inquiry about the presence of obstructive sleep apnea (OSA) is mandatory. The increased parapharyngeal fat accumulation due to aging that occurs even in non-obese subjects may lead to OSA (14). It also predisposes the patient to difficult intubation.
4. Examining the range of motion of neck is of vital importance. With normal aging, there has been demonstrated a decrease in elasticity of the atlanto-occipital ligaments (15). Also, after the age of 30 years, there is approximately 10° loss in the range of flexion and extension of the cervical spine after each decade.
5. For patients who may prove to be difficult to bag-mask ventilate, a specialized supralaryngeal device may be useful, and even preferable over bag mask. A difficult airway cart as well

as a backup plan must be readily available when caring for patients with possibility of a difficult airway.

Evaluation of cardiac risk in elderly neurosurgical patients

The risk stratification has traditionally been done with the *Revised Cardiac Risk Index* (RCRI), as for other non-cardiac surgeries. The RCRI employs the following six factors: high-risk surgery, cerebrovascular diseases, history of ischemic heart disease, congestive heart failure (CHF), diabetes or insulin, and presence of high creatinine levels to estimate the cardiac risk. Using these predictors, the estimated risk of cardiac death, nonfatal cardiac arrest, and nonfatal myocardial infarction (MI) following elective surgical procedures are 0.4% in cases where there is no risk factor out of the above, and 1.0% if there is one risk factor. The risk increases to 2.4% if there are two risk factors and to 5.4% if there are three or more risk factors (16).

The *Gupta MICA* model was introduced in 2011. This risk model predicts the risk of perioperative MI and cardiac arrest on the basis of following five factors: (i) abnormal creatinine, (ii) dependent functional status, (iii) type of surgery, (iv) American Society of Anaesthesiologists (ASA) class, and (v) increased age.

Recently, the *Geriatric-Sensitive Perioperative Cardiac Risk Index* (GSCRI) has been proposed as a significantly better predictor of cardiac risk in elderly patients undergoing noncardiac surgery compared to the RCRI and Gupta MICA model. The factors assessed in GSCRI are: (i) history of stroke, (ii) ASA class, (iii) type of surgery, (iv) functional status, (v) history of heart failure, (vi) abnormal creatinine, and (vii) diabetes mellitus.

Evaluating the patients for *hypertension* is vital, as the prevalence of hypertension increases with age. These patients have their cerebrovascular autoregulation curve shifted to the right, and this must be considered while planning anesthesia for these patients because such patients will tolerate any episode of hypotension very poorly. Hypertension is a risk factor for development of stroke, left ventricular hypertrophy, and ischemic heart disease, and these risks should be evaluated in patients who suffer from longstanding hypertension. In addition, reviewing the antihypertensive medications

the patient is taking and giving appropriate advice regarding continuing or stopping them perioperatively is a matter of significance for the attending anesthesiologist. All classes of antihypertensive medications are generally continued up to the morning of surgery except angiotensin receptor blockers or ACE inhibitors, where an individualized approach is to be followed. Elective surgeries should be postponed in cases of severe hypertension until blood pressure comes down to below 180/110 mmHg.

Evaluation of respiratory reserve in elderly neurosurgical patients

Old age is a definitive risk for development of postoperative pulmonary complications (POPC). POPC is defined as any pulmonary disease or dysfunction that is clinically significant or adversely affects the clinical course of the patient (17).

The elderly are more likely to suffer from COPD, and mortality and morbidity due to COPD are also greater in the elderly as compared to young adults (18,19).

Neurosurgery is considered a high-risk surgery for the elderly as far as development of postoperative pulmonary complications is concerned (20,21).

Any history of smoking should be documented, with documentation of "smoking pack years." Ideally cessation of smoking should occur 6–8 weeks prior to surgery.

Canet et al. suggested the following as independent risk factors for development of POPC: age, duration of surgery, preoperative decrease in oxygen saturation, preoperative anemia, respiratory infection in last month, duration of surgery, site of incision, and emergency surgery (22).

INDICATIONS FOR PREOPERATIVE PULMONARY TESTING

1. *Chest x-ray*: Recent chest x-ray (within 6 months) is warranted for patients aged more than 50 years with cardiopulmonary diseases who are undergoing major surgery (23).
2. *Arterial blood gas (ABG) analysis*: Not advised in all cases but should be done in patients suffering from severe respiratory diseases. In patients with severe COPD, $PaCO_2 > 45$ mmHg is one of the probable risk factors for POPC (24).

3. *Pulmonary function tests (PFTs)*: Not usually recommended in ASA 1 and 2 patients (NICE guidelines).

Prevention of postoperative pulmonary complications

1. Smoking cessation for 6–8 weeks prior to surgery
2. Inhaled bronchodilators and steroids for COPD
3. Treating respiratory tract infections with antibiotics
4. Chest physiotherapy

Preanesthetic evaluation in elderly neurosurgical patients with diabetes

Incidence of diabetes increases with age. In the United States, 25% of people above the age of 65 years have diabetes (25). In addition, many of these patients are on steroids. Hence, a fasting blood glucose level must be done in all these patients.

In diabetic patients, the possibility of chronic complications of diabetes, i.e. retinopathy, neuropathy and nephropathy, or any history of acute complications like DKA, should always be further evaluated.

Reviewing the recent trends of blood glucose and advising patients regarding discontinuation of hypoglycemic drugs perioperatively is important.

EVALUATION OF RENAL FUNCTION

Serum creatinine has been shown as a poor predictor of renal function in older individuals because decreased body mass keeps serum creatinine normal even with decreasing renal blood flow (26). The ability of kidneys to respond to abnormalities of volume and electrolyte abnormalities is also affected in geriatric patients. This must be kept in mind while selecting intraoperative drugs for these patients. Also, exposure of patients to sudden fluid overload intraoperatively should be prevented.

FRAILTY IN ELDERLY

Frailty is defined as multisystem loss of physiologic reserve which makes a person more vulnerable to disability during and after stress. The incidence of frailty in the community-dwelling population older than 65 years of age is approximately 6.9% (27).

Criteria used to define frailty are:

1. Weight loss criterion—loss of more than 10 lbs in 1 year
2. Exhaustion criterion—patient feeling exhausted moderate/most amount of time
3. Physical activity criterion—low physical activity
4. Walk time criterion—slow walkers are categorized as frail
5. Grip strength criterion—decreased grip strength is categorized as frail

Frailty is defined as a clinical syndrome when three or more of the frailty criteria are met.

Youngerman et al. demonstrated the positive correlation between frailty and poor outcomes in oncologic neurosurgery (28).

EVALUATION OF COGNITIVE FUNCTION

As aging occurs, changes take place in the brain leading to differences in thinking and behavior (29). Cognition is frequently impaired in elderly patients. Cognitive impairment has been defined as any impairment of intellectual abilities in an individual that results in the inability of that individual to manage his/her social or occupational activities. Cognition impairment has an age-related prevalence; approximately 5% of persons aged over 65 residing in the community will suffer from significant cognitive impairment; by the age of 80 years the figure exceeds 20% (30). Assessment of cognitive impairment is important because it facilitates the diagnosis of disorders that impair thinking and allows for more accurate estimates of functional ability to be made. Cognition has also been shown to predict mortality during hospital admissions (31). Some of the tests to determine and test the cognitive function are:

1. *Mini-Mental State Examination (MMSE)*: MMSE tests the following parameters: orientation, recall, attention and calculation, registration, language, and copying.
2. *Abbreviated Mental Test (AMT)*: A 10-item scale consisting of 10 questions. It includes components requiring intact short- and

long-term memory, attention, and orientation. A score of less than 8 is the usual cutoff and suggests a significant cognitive deficit (32).

3. *Six-Item Screener (SIS)*: The SIS is composed of three orientation questions (day, month, and year) and a three-item recall task derived from the MMSE. A score of less than 3 implies cognitive impairment.

4. *Short Orientation Memory-Concentration Test*: Includes one memory, two calculation, and three orientation questions. The total scoring based on the responses comes out between 0 and 28, with higher numbers representing greater cognitive impairment.

5. *Mini Cog Test*: A three-word recall test than can be done in minutes. Inability to recall any of the three words implies that the patient has cognitive dysfunction.

6. *Clock-Drawing Test*: The doctor tells the patient to draw a circle on a piece of paper and then draw the numbers on the clock. The patient is then instructed draw the hands of clock to represent a specific time—the time "10 past 11" is typically used. The patient is then scored using a three-point scale, with one mark for each: a correctly drawn circle; appropriately spaced numbers; and hands that show the right time.

These screening tests, however, are not able to distinguish between the various causes of cognitive impairment. The main causes of cognitive impairment are briefly discussed below.

Delirium: Loosely defined as an acute confusional state characterized by hyperactivity and excitement. Delirium is more common in the elderly. It can be an atypical presentation of a disease in the elderly. Because of the medical and financial implications of delirium, preoperatively predicting occurrence of postoperative delirium and taking steps to prevent its occurrence are important. Advanced age, visual impairment (visual acuity <20/70), severe illness (APACHE score >16), blood urea nitrogen-to-creatinine [BUN/Cr] ratio ≤18, and cognitive impairment (MMSE score <24) have been described as the risk factors for development of delirium (33).

Dementia: Dementia is common in the elderly. Dementia rises in prevalence from <1% of people aged <65 years to around 3%–11% of those aged >65 years, and to 33% of those aged >85 years (34,35). It has many causes, the major ones being Alzheimer's disease, Parkinson's disease, frontotemporal dementia (caused due to tau protein deposition in the frontal and temporal lobes of the brain), vascular dementia (caused due to reduced blood flow to brain) and rare causes such as Huntington disease, normal pressure hydrocephalus, etc.

Depression: Depression is common in the elderly. It occurs in around 8%–16% of the community-dwelling population over the age of 65 years, is an independent predictor of postoperative delirium, and predicts greater risk for major adverse cardiac events (36–38).

Preanesthetic evaluation in elderly patients undergoing specific neurosurgical procedures

1. *Supratentorial Tumors*: Patient history should focus on symptoms (headache, seizures, elevated intracranial pressure [ICP] features, any focal deficit) and their duration. Many patients will be on osmotic diuretics, antiepileptics, and steroids, which are continued until the day of surgery.

   At the bare minimum, physical examination should include a general physical examination, neurological examination, and CVS and respiratory system examination.

   Radiology should be reviewed for the site of tumor, size, vascularity, and any signs of elevated ICP. Other things to consider are approximate duration of surgery, need for arranging blood products, intraoperative position of the patient, and need for special monitoring (TEE, EEG, evoked potentials).

2. *Infratentorial Tumors*: Important points to consider in history are:
   a. Presence of any cerebellar signs such as hypotonia, dysdiadochokinesia, intention tremors, nystagmus, etc.
   b. Any signs/symptoms of elevated ICP (headache, vomiting, papilledema).
   c. Presence of any cranial nerve involvement.
   d. Rule out presence of patent foramen ovale (PFO) if sitting position is planned during surgery. Keep in mind that elderly patients

suffer from increased episodes of hypotension upon attaining sitting position.

   e. If a prone position is being planned, proper eye care, care of extremities, and pressure points should be planned. Note that the cardiovascular and respiratory effects of the prone position are exaggerated in the elderly population.

3. *Spontaneous Subarachnoid Hemorrhage (SAH)*: Classification of the SAH according to Hunt and Hess, World Federation of Neurosurgeons (WFNS), and modified Fischer classification (Table 4.2 through 4.4) is done for prediction of intraoperative and postoperative course and overall morbidity of the patient, which may already be compromised in the elderly patient.

   Some important points to be considered are:

   a. Advanced age predicts increased mortality and morbidity in aneurysmal SAH. However, elderly patients with subarachnoid hemorrhage can be treated successfully, and results are still improving.

   b. Evaluation of the systemic manifestations of SAH also predicts morbidity and increased hospital stay in these patients including examination of:

      – *Respiratory system*: Pulmonary edema, aspiration. PaO_2 decreases with increasing age.

      – *Cardiovascular system*: ECG changes, myocardial dysfunction, Takotsubo cardiomyopathy (SAH induced).

      – *Electrolyte changes*.

      – *Acute renal failure*: SAH patients are usually hypovolemic; this along with baseline-impaired renal function predisposes these patients to develop renal failure. In addition, hypovolemic patients have a worse prognosis.

   c. Communicate with the surgeon regarding the intraoperative positioning and any special considerations such as the need to administer adenosine, indo-cyanine green (ICG), etc.

Arteriovenous malformations

Surgical management of arteriovenous malformations (AVMs) in the elderly has shown acceptable clinical outcomes (39).

Previously AVMs in elderly were managed conservatively on the belief that the risk of bleeding

Table 4.2 Hunt and Hess classification

GRADE 0	Unruptured aneurysm
GRADE 1	Asymptomatic or minimal headache and slight nuchal rigidity
GRADE 2	Moderate to severe headache, nuchal rigidity, but no neurologic deficit other than cranial nerve palsy
GRADE 3	Drowsiness, confusion, or mild focal deficit
GRADE 4	Stupor, mild or severe hemiparesis, possible early decerebrate rigidity, vegetative disturbance
GRADE 5	Deep coma, decerebrate rigidity, moribund appearance

Table 4.3 World Federation of Neurosurgeons classification

GRADE 1	GCS 15	No motor deficit
GRADE 2	GCS 13–14	No motor deficit
GRADE 3	GCS 13–14	With motor deficit
GRADE 4	GCS 7–12	With/without motor deficit
GRADE 5	GCS 3–6	With/without motor deficit

Table 4.4 Fischer grades

GRADE 1	No blood detected
GRADE 2	Diffuse thin layer of subarachnoid blood (vertical layers <1 mm thick)
GRADE 3	Localized clot or thick layer of subarachnoid blood (vertical layers ≥1 mm thick)
GRADE 4	Intracerebral or intraventricular blood with diffuse or no subarachnoid blood

decreases after 40 years of age; however, now many authors have suggested that AVMs in the elderly may be at greater risk of rupture (40–42).

The Spetzler and Martin grading system is the most widely used grading system to stratify the surgical risk, using three factors: (i) size, (ii) involvement of eloquent area of the brain, and (iii) pattern of venous drainage to stratify the risk (43).

Deep brain stimulation

Deep brain stimulation (DBS) is an important tool for the treatment of patients with neurological disorders who have an abnormality of function that is not usually accompanied by gross structural or anatomical changes, such as Parkinson's disease (44).

The procedure consists of placement of electrodes into deep brain structures for microelectrode recordings and macrostimulation for clinical testing of the patient. The electrodes are then connected to an implanted pulse generator.

DBS has been employed in Parkinson's disease, essential tremor, dystonia, Tourette syndrome, depression, obsessive compulsive disorder, anorexia, etc.

DBS can be done under monitored anaesthesia care (MAC), sedation, or general anesthesia, depending on patient characteristics.

Each class of patients will have characteristic concerns:

- *Parkinson's disease*: Increased risk of aspiration pneumonia and laryngospasm due to pharyngeal, laryngeal dysfunction; autonomic dysfunction, orthostatic hypotension, hypovolemia; potential drug interactions and adverse effects with anti-Parkinson medications
- *Dystonia*: Difficult airway, difficult positioning, difficult communication with the patient
- *Seizures*: Drug interactions possible due to enzyme induction by antiepileptic agents

SPINE SURGERY

A recent multicentric analysis of lumbar decompression without fusion in elderly patients, specifically including patients older than 80 years, suggested that increased age is associated with more extensive operations. These patients also have increased rates of non-home discharge, longer hospital stays, and minor complications (45).

DECISIONS REGARDING MEDICATIONS

Elderly patients are often on many drugs because of their comorbidities (antihypertensives, analgesics, heart ailments, etc.). In addition, many medications need to be administered in view of their neurosurgical status (anticonvulsants, mannitol, diuretics, steroids, etc.).

- Generally, all antihypertensives are continued perioperatively, with the exception of ACE

inhibitors/angiotensin receptor blockers, which is still controversial.
- Low-dose aspirin and statins are usually continued perioperatively (46).
- Clopidogrel is to be stopped around 5–7 days prior to surgery.
- Appropriate bridging therapy with low molecular weight or unfractionated heparin needs to be administered based upon the characteristics of the patient and discretion of the attending cardiologist, who weighs the risk–benefit ratio of anticoagulation versus surgery.
- Oral hypoglycemic agents are stopped on the day of surgery.
- Steroids administered for vasogenic edema are continued.
- Anticonvulsants are continued perioperatively; one must keep in mind their ability to cause enzyme induction while planning the anesthetics to be employed during surgery.
- Antidepressants may be continued during the perioperative period because stopping them suddenly may increase symptoms of depression and confusion (47). Many authors advise replacing SSRIs with other antidepressants 2–3 weeks prior to surgery in view of their tendency to increase intraoperative blood loss.

The final decision regarding stopping or continuing any drug perioperatively should be patient specific and should be taken after gauging the risks and benefits and discussion with all the physicians involved in the patient's care.

NEUROTRAUMA

Age is a prognosticating factor in head injury, with the elderly having a poorer prognosis. Falls and motor vehicle accidents are the common causes of trauma in elderly. Mosenthal et al. reported that around 73% of the elderly coming in with head trauma suffered from a comorbidity (48). Another study found that 9% of older adult patients with traumatic brain injury (TBI) were on warfarin preinjury. This was found to be associated with more severe TBI and a higher rate of mortality in these patients (49).

One may have only a limited time for preanesthetic evaluation in the elderly patient with head trauma. The important issues are:

- Evaluating vitals and Glasgow Coma Scale (GCS). The ability of the cardiovascular system to respond to shock may be impaired in older adults (50). There may be no tachycardia even in hypovolemia.

- Ruling out cervical spine injury.
- Assessing Cerebral autoregulation which may be impaired in the elderly. Cerebral autoregulation may be impaired in the elderly.
- Evaluating for injuries of other systems.
- Taking a brief history of the comorbidities, medication history, reviewing blood investigations.
- A brief airway examination, including asking about loose or artificial dentures.
- Ensuring availability of blood products.
- Planning postoperative management of the patient.

CONCLUSION

Elderly patients undergoing neurosurgery are a high-risk subset of patients, and their perioperative management can have a profound effect on their final outcome. While performing preanesthetic evaluation, a set of patient-specific considerations must be considered in all elderly patients posted for neurosurgery. These include evaluation of comorbidities, cognitive dysfunction, and airway, and evaluation of the major body systems, followed by surgery-specific considerations, which vary with the planned procedure.

With a growing number of elderly patients expected to undergo neurosurgery, it is important that the exact nature of the complications these patients face are better understood. A properly planned preanesthetic evaluation marks the initiation of perioperative care for the neuroanesthesiologist, and when this initial step is properly undertaken, perioperative care of the patient can be carried out in a more effective manner. Hence, pre-anesthesia evaluation in the elderly should be more than just evaluating the airway and reviewing a few laboratory reports, but a comprehensive process which gives us an insight into the patient's present status and helps us to better plan the perioperative care.

REFERENCES

1. United Nations. World population prospects. Available at: http://www.un.org/esa/population/publications/wpp2000/chapter5.pdf
2. Johannesen TB, Angell-Andersen E, Tretli S, Langmark F, Lote K. Trends in incidence of brain and central nervous system tumours in Norway, 1970 to 1999. *Neuroepidemiology.* 2004;23:101–9.
3. Weinert BT, Timiras PS. Invited review: Theories of aging. *J Appl Physiol.* 2003;95(4): 1706–16.
4. Klopfenstein CE, Forster A, Van Gessel E. Anaesthetic assessment in an outpatient consultation clinic reduces preoperative anxiety. *Can J Anaesth.* 2000;47(6):511–5.
5. Wijeysundera DN, Austin PC, Beattie WS et al. A population based study of anaesthesia consultation before major non-cardiac surgery. *Arch Intern Med.* 2009;169:595–602.
6. Pollard JB, Garnerin P, Dalman RL. Use of outpatient preoperative evaluation to decrease length of stay for vascular surgery. *Anesth Analg.* 1997;85(6):1307–11.
7. Van Klei WA, Moons KG, Rutten CL et al. The effect of outpatient preoperative evaluation of hospital inpatients on cancellation of surgery and length of hospital stay. *Anesth Analg.* 2002;94:644–9.
8. Cigolle CT, Blaum CS, Halter JB. Diabetes and cardiovascular disease prevention in older adults. *Clin Geriatr Med.* 2009;25(4): 607–641.
9. Kirkman MS, Briscoe VJ, Clark N et al. Diabetes in older adults. *Diabetes Care.* 2012; 35(12):2650–2664.
10. Qato DM, Alexander GC, Conti RM, Johnson M, Schumm P, Lindau ST. Use of prescription and over-the-counter medications and dietary supplements among older adults in the United States. *JAMA.* 2008;300(24): 2867–2878.
11. Mihailidis HG, Manners S, Churilov L, Quan GMY. Is spinal surgery safe in octogenarians? *ANZ J Surg.* 2017;87(7–8):605–609.
12. LeBlanc J, de Guise E, Gosselin N, Feyz M. Comparison of functional outcome following acute care in young, middle-aged and elderly patients with traumatic brain injury. *Brain Inj.* 2006;20(8):779–790.
13. Penna V, Stark GB, Eisenhardt SU, Bannasch H, Iblher N. The aging lip: A comparative histological analysis of age-related changes in the upper lip complex. *Plast Reconstr Surg.* 2009;124(2):624–628.

14. Malhotra A, Huang Y, Fogel R et al. Aging influences on pharyngeal anatomy and physiology: The predisposition to pharyngeal collapse. *Am J Med.* 2006;119(1):72.e9–14.

15. Stewart RE. Craniofacial malformations. *Pediatr Clin North Am.* 1978;25:485–90.

16. Ford MK, Beattie WS, Wijeysundera DN. Systematic review: Prediction of perioperative cardiac complications and mortality by the revised cardiac risk index. *Ann Intern Med.* 2010;152(1):26–35.

17. Lawrence VA, Hilsenbeck SG, Mulrow CD, Dhanda R, Sapp J, Page CP. Incidence and hospital stay for cardiac and pulmonary complications after abdominal surgery. *J Gen Intern Med.* 1995;10(12):671–8.

18. Fuhrman C, Jougla E, Nicolau J, Eilstein D, Delmas MC. Deaths from chronic obstructive pulmonary disease in France, 1979–2002: A multiple cause analysis. *Thorax.* 2006;61(11): 930–4.

19. Day GE, Lanier AP. Alaska native mortality, 1979–1998. *Public Health Rep.* 2003;118(6): 518–30.

20. Polanczyk CA, Marcantonio E, Goldman L et al. Impact of age on perioperative complications and length of stay in patients undergoing noncardiac surgery. *Ann Intern Med.* 2001;134(8):637–643.

21. Manninen PH, Raman SK, Boyle K, el-Beheiry H. Early postoperative complications following neurosurgical procedures. *Can J Anaesth.* 1999;46:7–14.

22. Canet J, Gallart L, Gomar C, Paluzie G, Vallès J, Castillo J, Sabaté S, Mazo V, Briones Z, Sanchis J, ARISCAT Group. Prediction of postoperative pulmonary complications in a population-based surgical cohort. *Anesthesiology.* 2010;113(6):1338–1350.

23. Archer C, Levy AR, McGregor M. Value of routine preoperative chest x-rays: A meta-analysis. *Can J Anaesth.* 1993;40(11):1022–7.

24. Qaseem A, Snow V, Fitterman N et al. Risk assessment for and strategies to reduce perioperative pulmonary complications for patients undergoing non-cardiothoracic surgery: A guideline from the American College of Physicians. *Ann Intern Med.* 2006;144(8): 575–80.

25. Centre for Disease Control and Prevention. National Diabetes Fact Sheet: General Information and National Estimates on Diabetes in the United States, 2011. Atlanta, Georgia, U.S. Department of Health and Human Services, Centers for Disease Control and Prevention, 2011.

26. Musso CG, Oreopoulos DG. Aging and physiological changes of the kidneys including changes in glomerular filtration rate. *Nephron Physiol.* 2011;119(Suppl. 1):1–5.

27. Fried LP, Tangen CM, Walston J et al. Frailty in older adults: Evidence for a phenotype. *J Gerontol A Biol Sci Med Sci.* 2001;56(3): M146–56.

28. Youngerman BE, Neugut AI, Yang J, Hershman DL, Wright JD, Bruce JN. The modified frailty index and 30-day adverse events in oncologic neurosurgery. *J Neuro Oncol.* 2018;136(1): 197–206.

29. Howieson DB, Loring DW, Hannay HJ. Neurobehavioural variables and diagnostic issues. In: Lezak MD (ed). *Neuropsychological Assessment.* 4th ed. New York: Oxford University Press; 2004.

30. Schoenberg BS. Epidemiology of Alzheimer's disease and other dementing illnesses. *J Chron Dis.* 1986;39(12):1095–104.

31. Campbell SE, Seymour DG, Primrose WR et al. A multicentre European study of factors affecting the discharge destination of older people admitted to hospital: Analysis of in-hospital data from the ACME plus project. *Age Ageing.* 2005;34:467–475.

32. Jitapunkul S, Pillay I, Ebrahim S. The abbreviated mental test: Its use and validity. *Age Ageing.* 1991;20(5):332–6.

33. Inouye SK, Charpentier PA. Precipitating factors for delirium in hospitalized elderly persons: Predictive model and interrelationship with baseline vulnerability. *JAMA.* 1996; 275(11):852–857.

34. Lobo A, Launer LJ, Fratiglioni L et al. Prevalence of dementia and major subtypes in Europe: A collaborative study of population-based cohorts. *Neurology.* 2000;54(11 Suppl.):S4–9.

35. Rocca WA, Bonaiuto S, Lippi A et al. Prevalence of clinically diagnosed Alzheimer's disease and other dementing disorders: A door-to-door survey in Appignano, Macerata Province, Italy. *Neurology.* 1990;40(4): 626–31.

36. Ellison JM, Kyomen HH, Harper DG. Depression in later life: An overview with treatment recommendations. *Psychiatr Clin North Am.* 2012;35(1):203–229.

37. Greene NH, Attix DK, Weldon BC, Smith PJ, Mc Donagh DL, Monk TG. Measures of executive function and depression identify patients at risk for postoperative delirium. *Anesthesiology.* 2009;110(4):788–95.

38. Frasure-Smith N, Lesperance F. Depression and anxiety as predictors of 2-year cardiac events in patients with stable coronary artery disease. *Arch Gen Psychiatry.* 2008;65(1): 62–71.

39. Pabaney AH, Reinard KA, Kole MK, Seyfried DM, Malik GM. Management of arteriovenous malformations in the elderly: A single-center case series and analysis of outcomes. *J Neurosurg.* 2016;125(1):145–51.

40. Heros RC, Tu YK. Is surgical therapy needed for unruptured arteriovenous malformations? *Neurology.* 1987;37(2):279–86.

41. Brown RD Jr, Wiebers DO, Torner JC, O'Fallon WM. Frequency of intracranial hemorrhage as a presenting symptom and subtype analysis: A population-based study of intracranial vascular malformations in Olmsted Country, Minnesota. *J Neurosurg.* 1996; 85(1):29–32.

42. Crawford PM, West CR, Chadwick DW, Shaw MD. Arteriovenous malformations of the brain: Natural history in unoperated patients. *J Neurol Neurosurg Psychiatry.* 1986;49(1): 1–10.

43. Spetzler RF, Martin NA. A proposed grading system for arteriovenous malformations. *J Neurosurg October.* 1986;65(4):476–83.

44. Miocinovic S, Somayajula S, Chitnis S, Vitek JL. History, applications, and mechanisms of deep brain stimulation. *JAMA Neurol.* 2013; 70(2):163–71.

45. Murphy ME, Gilder H, Maloney PR et al. Lumbar decompression in the elderly: Increased age as a risk factor for complications and nonhome discharge. *J Neurosurg Spine.* 2017 Mar;26(3):353–62.

46. Rahman M, Donnangelo LL, Neal D, Mogali K, Decker M, Ahmed MM. Effects of perioperative acetyl salicylic acid (ASA) on clinical outcomes in patients undergoing craniotomy for brain tumor. *World Neurosurg.* 2015 July;84(1):41–7.

47. Kudoh A, Katagai H, Takazawa T. Antidepressant treatment for chronic depressed patients should not be discontinued prior to anesthesia. *Can J Anaesth.* 2002;49(2):132–6.

48. Mosenthal AC, Livingston DH, Lavery RF et al. The effect of age on functional outcome in mild traumatic brain injury: 6-month report of a prospective multicenter trial. *J Trauma.* 2004; 56(5):1042–8.

49. Lavoie A, Ratte S, Clas D et al. Preinjury warfarin use among elderly patients with closed head injuries in a trauma centre. *J Trauma.* 2004;56(4):802–7.

50. Thompson HJ, Bourbonniere M. Traumatic injury in the older adult from head to toe. *Crit Care Nurs Clin North Am.* 2006;18(3):419–31.

5

Neurosurgery: Supratentorial tumors

MONICA S. TANDON, KASHMIRI DOLEY, AND DALJIT SINGH

INTRODUCTION

Supratentorial tumors (STTs) are the most common intracranial neoplasms in geriatric patients (>65 years) (1–3). With the global increase in the average life expectancy over the past few decades, the geriatric population has experienced not only a discernible increase in incidence of these STTs, but also a marked rise in the proportion of the associated neurosurgical interventions (1,2). Until recently, the neurosurgical approach for these patients was largely conservative, possibly due to the fear of increased mortality. However, due to the marked advancements in neurodiagnostic, neuromonitoring, and neurosurgical techniques, "age" has almost ceased to be a limiting factor, and a more aggressive approach that involves more extensive tumor resection and also correlates with improved survival is being advocated for management of STTs in these "older adults." However, given their aging-related physiological changes, reduced functional reserve, presence of multiple comorbidities, and increased frailty (decreased ability to withstand as well as respond to the stresses of surgery and anesthesia), geriatric patients continue to have a higher incidence of perioperative adverse events as compared with the younger population. Neuroanesthetists can play a significant role in improving the perioperative outcome of these patients; this requires formulation of an appropriate anesthesia strategy that is based on a comprehensive understanding of the vulnerabilities of "aging" along with the surgical complexities of the supratentorial (ST) region. The initial sections of this chapter provide an overview of these fundamental concepts: physiology of aging, functional neuroanatomy of the ST region, and common STTs and their pertinent clinicopathological considerations in geriatric patients; the latter sections discuss the preoperative planning, principles of neuroanesthesia for STT surgery, and the postoperative management of these patients.

BASIC UNDERSTANDING OF GERIATRIC PHYSIOLOGY

The process of aging is progressive; it involves functional and structural degenerative changes in all the organ systems, which ultimately lead to a decline in the functional reserve of the geriatric population.

Older adults have a higher and more labile blood pressure (BP), a reduced tolerance and impaired ability to respond to intraoperative cardiac stresses and acute hemodynamic changes, along with an increased predisposition for developing myocardial ischemia, arrhythmias, and congestive cardiac failure (CCF) in the perioperative period. Several factors contribute to this precarious cardiovascular reserve: a relatively noncompliant heart with a lower stroke volume (abrupt and inappropriate changes in cardiac output with even small changes in venous return), advanced atherosclerosis, venous stiffening (impaired ability to maintain a constant preload), decreased beta-adrenergic responsiveness to hypotension and catecholamine stimulation (exogenous and endogenous), impaired baro-reflexes and vagal tone (lesser heart rate [HR] variability and ability to maintain a constant cardiac output), reduced responsiveness of the renin–angiotensin–aldosterone system, and the concomitant presence of hypertension, coronary artery disease (CAD), rhythm disorders, and CCF (4–6).

There is a progressive decrease in the arterial partial pressure of oxygen (PaO_2) with advancing age; this is attributed to the increased ventilation perfusion mismatch and anatomical shunt (reduced chest wall mechanics, decreased pulmonary compliance, diminished respiratory muscle force, impaired pulmonary gas exchange, atelectasis due to small airway closure, retained secretions due to decreased ciliary function, and an ineffective cough) (4,5,7). The ability to respond to hypoxia and hypercarbia diminishes, while the risk of aspiration and the incidence of concomitant pulmonary disorders increases (e.g., chronic obstructive airway disease). Hence, it is not surprising that age, per se, is a significant independent predictor of risk for perioperative pulmonary complications (7).

The age-related decrease in the renal (and hepatic) blood flow, glomerular filtration rate, and tubular function, combined with an altered autoregulation, predispose older patients to a higher risk of perioperative acute kidney injury, especially due to nephrotoxic drugs (4,5). Moreover, the impaired handling of sodium and the reduced ability to maximally concentrate and dilute urine increase the risk of both dehydration and fluid overload. Furthermore, these patients have a poor tolerance for both hypovolemia and hypervolemia (suboptimal cardiac and renal function; increased incidence of concomitant atherosclerosis, hypertension,

coronary, and renal disease); while the former predisposes to hypotension and systemic hypoperfusion, the latter can result in CCF (4–6).

Most importantly, the increased propensity for neuronal cell death (especially in prefrontal and medial temporal lobes), coupled with a precarious cerebral homeostasis (changes in cerebral vasculature lead to increased cerebral vascular resistance and reduced cerebral perfusion pressure [CPP]) and an increased blood–brain barrier permeability (increased inflammatory response and structural brain damage) significantly increase the vulnerability of the aging brain to even minor insults which would otherwise be of no consequence in a younger brain (4,5,8). Older patients also have a higher incidence of cognitive deficits than the younger population.

FUNCTIONAL NEUROANATOMY OF THE SUPRATENTORIAL REGION

The ST compartment primarily consists of the two cerebral hemispheres: diencephalon, basal ganglia (BG), ventricles, and the white matter (WM) tracts (Table 5.1). Anatomically, each cerebral hemisphere has five lobes—frontal, parietal, temporal, occipital, and insula. On basis of the cytoarchitecture (neuronal organization), the cerebral cortex is divided into 52 Brodmann areas; these areas closely correlate with the functional organization of the cerebral cortex. Functionally, the cerebral cortex is divided three categories: motor, sensory, and association areas (9).

Motor areas (in the frontal lobe)

The primary motor cortex (in precentral gyrus) controls the activity of the voluntary muscles of the contralateral part of the body by sending axons to motor neurons in the brain stem and spinal cord, which finally innervate these voluntary skeletal muscles. The Broca's area (in the inferior frontal lobe of the dominant hemisphere) and frontal eye fields are responsible for production and articulation of speech, and for movements of the eyes, respectively.

Sensory areas

The primary sensory areas (somatosensory cortex [parietal lobe], visual area [occipital lobe], auditory areas [temporal lobe, insular cortex]) receive

Table 5.1 Functional neuroanatomy of the brain and its correlation with the clinical manifestations of supratentorial tumors

Pertinent functional neuroanatomy	Clinical features of the supratentorial tumor
FRONTAL LOBE: Motor, cognitive, speech, and language functions	
1. Motor regions	Motor disturbances: Contralateral hemiparesis, hyperreflexia, extensor plantar response (Babinski); magnetic-like apractic gait in butterfly gliomas (disturbed balance; difficulty in initiating walking)
Primary motor cortex	
Area 4: Precentral gyrus	Intellectual impairment (early onset with bilateral gliomas)
Initiation of voluntary movement	Cognitive impairment (especially with bilateral tumors)
Premotor cortex	Inability to perform "executive" functions, e.g planning and executing tasks (bilateral tumors)
Area 6: Supplemental motor cortex (motor association cortex)	Impairment of initiative and spontaneity: Abulia/akinetic mutism
Coordination of complex movement (sensory guidance of movement and control of proximal and trunk muscles of the body)	Personality changes: Pseudodepressed (apathetic)/pseudopsychopathic (euphoric); loss of inhibition
Frontal eye fields	Aphasia (dominant frontal lobe involvement): Expressive/mixed receptive and expressive
Area 8: Involved in eye movements, visual reflexes	
2. Prefrontal cortex	
Areas 9, 10, 11: Cognition (biological intelligence reasoning and judgment, problem solving, emotion, complex thoughts)	
3. Speech and language (dominant hemisphere)	
Broca's area: Area 44 (posterior inferior frontal gyrus)	
Articulation and production of speech	
Production of language	
TEMPORAL LOBE: Receptive language areas, optic pathways, semantics, limbic structures (memory, olfaction, behaviour, emotion)	
Primary auditory cortex	Aphasia (mixed expressive and receptive); dysphasia (anomia) (dominant temporal lobe tumors)
Areas 41, 42: Detection and recognition of speech	Wernicke aphasia: Language disorder characterized by fluent speech, paraphasias—wrongly produced words, defects in comprehension of language
Auditory association areas	
Area 21: Middle temporal gyrus; complex processing of auditory information	Seizures: Partial complex (psychomotor) Hallucinations: Auditory, olfactory; déjà vu
Area 22: Wernickes speech area in posterior superior temporal gyrus of dominant cerebral hemisphere; comprehension of written and spoken language	Memory impairment Contralateral superior quadrantanopsia May remain relatively "silent," particularly if in nondominant hemisphere
Area 37: Fusiform gyrus (lexicosemantics—words with visual percepts)	

(Continued)

Table 5.1 (*Continued*) Functional neuroanatomy of the brain and its correlation with the clinical manifestations of supratentorial tumors

Pertinent functional neuroanatomy	Clinical features of the supratentorial tumor
PARIETAL LOBE: Somatosensory processes, integrative motor functions, language processing, visual-spatial recognition	
Somatosensory cortex (*postcentral gyrus*): Areas 1, 2, 3: Primary sensory areas for touch and kinesthesia.	Generalized convulsions or sensory focal seizures
Somatosensory association cortex (*Superior parietal lobule*)	Cutaneous tactile, pain, temperature senses intact, but stereognosis and cortical sensory modalities (position sense, two-point discrimination) impaired on contralateral body side
Areas 5, 7: Visual guidance for limb and head movements	Contralateral homonymous hemianopia (or inferior quadrantanopia), constructional apraxia, and anosognosia (nonrecognition of bodily defects)
Area 40: *Inferior parietal lobule* (*supramarginal and angular gyri.*) Language perception and processing; visual-spatial cognition, calculation, and reading ability	Speech disturbances; notably, receptive aphasia or mixed expressive-receptive aphasia, agraphia, and finger agnosia (tumor involves dominant hemisphere)
	Contralateral (visuospatial tasks, e.g inability to copy facial gestures or to draw a picture
	Contralateral ocular ataxia (inability to reach for objects using visual guidance)
OCCIPITAL LOBE: Processing of visual stimuli	
Area 17: Primary visual cortex Detection of simple visual stimuli	Contralateral visual field deficits (quadrantic defect/hemianopia with macular sparing)
Areas 18, 19: Visual association cortex Complex processing of visual information	Visual illusions/hallucinations/agnosias/anosognosia
INSULAR CORTEX: Role in consciousness	
Involved in perception, self-awareness, cognitive functioning, and interpersonal experience	Seizures
DIENCEPAHALON: Deep midline structure embedded in the cerebral cortex	
Thalamus	
Relay station for most somatic sensory pathways (except olfaction) and few motor pathways	Symptoms of hormone imbalance, including weight loss/gain
Integrating center for somatic sensory; visual; visceral; some motor impulses	Symptoms of salt and water imbalance, including retaining water, swelling, and frequent urination
Maintenance and regulation of consciousness	Changes in vision (thalamus and hypothalamus are close to the visual pathway system in the brain)
Role in emotional connotations and crude sensations	
Hypothalamus	
Control of endocrine, autonomic system, emotions, circadian rhythms	
Regulation of temperature, food intake, water intake, and balance	

(Continued)

Table 5.1 (*Continued*) Functional neuroanatomy of the brain and its correlation with the clinical manifestations of supratentorial tumors

Pertinent functional neuroanatomy	Clinical features of the supratentorial tumor
BASAL GANGLIA: Located at base of the forebrain	
Role in control of voluntary motor movements, procedural learning relating to routine behaviors, cognition, and emotional functions	Movement changes, such as involuntary or slowed movements
	Muscle spasms and muscle rigidity
	Tremor
	Uncontrollable, repeated movements, speech, or cries (tics) Problems finding words
CORPUS CALLOSUM	
Largest commissure	Disconnection/split brain syndrome
Two anterior parts—rostrum and genu	Word blindness
Central part—trunk	Difficulty to carry out intended action and movements (Bristow syndrome)
Posterior part—splenium	
Frontal and temporal lobe gliomas	
Risk of postoperative motor, language and visual deficits if eloquent areas are involved	
Risk of venous infarction during resection of tumors in proximity to the sylvian fissure due to injury to inferior anastomotic vein of Labbe which drains into the transverse sinus	
VENTRICULAR SYSTEM	
Cerebral hemispheres: Lateral ventricles	Symptoms of hydrocephalus due to obstruction of the ventricles by the tumor
Diencephalon: Third ventricle	
WHITE MATTER TRACTS: Association, projection, commissural fibers	
Association fibers: Interconnect different cortical areas of the same side	
Uncinate fasciculus: Temporal pole to motor speech area and orbital cortex	
Cingulum fasciculus: Cingulum gyrus to parahippocampal gyrus	
Superior longitudinal fasciculus: Frontal to occipital and temporal lobes	
Inferior longitudinal fasciculus: Temporal to occipital lobe	
Projection fibers: Connect the cerebral cortex to the deep nuclei, brainstem, cerebellum, spinal cord, e.g corticospinal tracts, corticobulbar tracts, medial lemniscus optic radiation	
Commissural fibers: Connect corresponding areas of the two hemispheres. e.g corpus callosum, anterior, posterior, hippocampal, habenular, hypothalamic commissure	

signals from the sensory nerves and tracts through the relay nuclei in the thalamus.

Association areas

The association areas (motor, sensory, auditory, and visual association areas) integrate the sensory information with the more complex emotional states, memories, learning, and rational thought processes.

White matter

The WM tracts (myelinated nerve fibers), occupy the deeper part of the cerebrum; they connect various parts of the cortex to one another (association fibers) and also to other parts of the central nervous system (CNS) (projection fibers, commissural fibers) (9). The corpus callosum (CC) is the largest WM tract; it connects the two cerebral hemispheres with each other and is a common route for the spread of glial tumors.

Eloquent cortex

Eloquent cortex primarily refers to the main areas involved in speech (Broca's and Wernicke's areas) and sensorimotor functions (primary motor cortex, primary somatosensory cortex) along with the underlying important WM tracts (corticospinal tracts, superior longitudinal fasciculus, arcuate fasciculus); primary visual cortex is also considered as an eloquent area. Resection of tumors that involve or are in close proximity to these regions is associated with a high risk of postoperative motor weakness and language dysfunction.

Diencephalon, basal ganglia, and the ventricular system

The diencephalon is a deep midline structure that is embedded in the cerebrum and is comprised of the thalamus, hypothalamus, subthalamus, and epithalamus. The BG are located at base of the forebrain, and have strong connections with the cerebral cortex, thalamus, and other brain areas. The ventricular system is comprised of two lateral ventricles (in the cerebral hemispheres) and the third ventricle (in the diencephalon). Tumors that grow in these regions are relatively deep-seated and usually have a difficult surgical access.

Skull base

The skull base forms the floor of the cranial cavity. It is composed of five bones (ethmoid, sphenoid, occipital; paired frontal and temporal bones) and is divided into three regions: the anterior, middle, and posterior cranial fossae. Classically, resection of skull base tumors requires surgical approaches that involve a large incision, along with significant exposure and retraction of the brain, which predisposes to a delayed postoperative neurological recovery. Moreover, the inherent vascularity of some of these tumors as well as their proximity to critical neurovascular structures further increases the complexity of neurosurgical and neuroanesthetic management.

Falx cerebri

The falx cerebri is a double fold of dura mater that descends through the interhemispheric fissure in the midline of the brain between the two cerebral hemispheres. Its superior and inferior margins contain the superior sagittal sinus (SSS) and inferior sagittal sinus, respectively; there is a potential risk of injury to these sinuses during resection of tumors that arise from the falx or grow in close proximity to the sinus (e.g., meningiomas).

COMMON SUPRATENTORIAL TUMORS IN GERIATRIC PATIENTS

Metastatic lesions account for most of the STTs in older patients (2,3). The most frequently observed primary ST neoplasms in these patients are diffuse high-grade gliomas (HGG; glioblastoma multiforme [GBM; WHO grade IV], anaplastic astrocytoma [WHO grade III]) and extra-axial meningiomas; among these, GBM (IDH wildtype, de novo) is the most common as well as the most malignant neoplasm (median age at diagnosis 62 years; clinical history 4 months; median survival time 15 months) (1,10–13). Pituitary adenomas, anaplastic oligodendrogliomas (WHO grade III), and occasionally primary central nervous system lymphomas (PCNSL) also occur in this age group (1,12,13). Low-grade gliomas (WHO grade II), are relatively uncommon but behave more aggressively in these patients as compared with the younger population, and hence are treated as anaplastic neoplasms rather than as low-grade tumors. The incidence of STTs increases with advancing age, except GBMs, which tend to decline after 85 years of age (12).

ST gliomas

ST gliomas typically arise in the subcortical WM tracts in the cerebral hemispheres, enlarge rapidly, and spread contiguously to other parts of the brain by infiltrating along the WM tracts, surrounding cortical neurons (satellitosis), subependymal zone, and cerebrospinal fluid (CSF) pathways (subarachnoid seeding) (14) (Figure 5.1).

Frontal and temporal lobes are more frequently affected (60%–80% of patients) than parietal and occipital lobes; the eloquent cortex is involved in 25%–60% patients (15). Multilobar involvement (45%) is also common, e.g. front-temporal gliomas due to tumor spread through the uncinate fasciculus. Temporal gliomas tend to invade the midbrain and pons; gliomas that arise in regions below the CC can invade basal structures (e.g., thalamus and peduncles) by infiltration of corticospinal tracts (13,14). Bilateral involvement is also observed in 25%–30% of patients, e.g., bilateral frontal lobe tumors or butterfly gliomas (infiltration of genu/body of CC), bilateral parietal or occipital lobe tumors (tumor spread through splenium of CC), bilateral thalamic gliomas (infiltration of interthalamic adhesions) (1,11,14,15).

MANAGEMENT AND PROGNOSIS

The preferred treatment for HGGs is maximal safe surgical resection (MSR) followed by radiochemotherapy (temozolide) (15–18). Curative resection is usually not feasible because of the diffusely infiltrative and invasive nature of these tumors; nevertheless, MSR has been shown to delay the progression of the tumor, improve the functional outcome, and prolong duration of survival even in patients who are more than 80 years of age (11,13,15,16). The surgical goal is gross total resection (GTR) (>99% tumor removal) while preserving maximal brain function. This may be difficult to achieve in patients with eloquent area gliomas; hence a subtotal resection (>90% tumor removal) is usually performed (11,15,16). A biopsy may be considered if MSR is not considered to be feasible.

The prognosis is usually poor; despite optimal treatment, patients with GBM do not survive for more than 2 years; survival time for patients with anaplastic gliomas is 2–5 years (10–13). The prognosis worsens with increasing age, poor functional status, tumor size >4 cms, tumor location (infiltration of splenium, BG, thalamus, midbrain), and subtotal tumor resection (1,11–13,16).

PERTINENT ANESTHETIC CONSIDERATIONS

Generally, gliomas are not very vascular; hence their resection is usually not associated with significant blood loss. Frontal lobe tumors that are anterior to the precentral gyrus are generally favorable for aggressive resection. However, resection of the eloquent area, insular, and other deep-seated gliomas may be technically challenging due to a difficult surgical access, high risk of neurological morbidity, or both (Table 5.2). Specialized neuromonitoring techniques may be used intraoperatively to facilitate a more extensive and safer resection; these techniques often require a modification of the conventional neuroanesthesia technique.

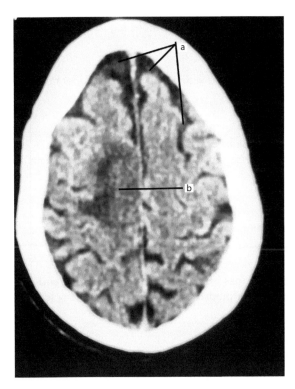

Figure 5.1 Contrast computerized tomography scan showing atrophic brain with wide sulci spaces filled with cerebrospinal fluid (a) with a large hypodense mass (glioma) (b) at motor area, with no mass effect due to atrophy of brain.

Table 5.2 Supratentorial gliomas: Pertinent considerations

Frontal and temporal lobe gliomas
Risk of postoperative motor, language and visual deficits if eloquent areas are involved
Risk of venous infarction during resection of tumors in proximity to the sylvian fissure due to injury to
  inferior anastomotic vein of Labbe which drains into the transverse sinus

Gliomas in the thalamus, hypothalamus, basal ganglia, corpus callosum, lateral ventricles
Deep-seated tumors with a difficult surgical access

Insular gliomas
Resection is technically challenging because of the depth of lesion and involvement/ proximity to
  critical neurovascular structures
(Insula is folded deep within the lateral sulcus; is shrouded by frontal, frontoparietal, and temporal
  opercula; and incorporates and is surrounded by several eloquent white-matter tracts and critically
  important vascular structures)
Surgical approaches: Transsylvian approach (splitting of the sylvian fissure widely to separate the
  opercula and sylvian vessels); transcortical approach (uses several frontal and/or temporal windows
  to access the tumor)
Key structures at risk during resection
Language, motor, limbic tracts
Language areas: Broca's area, Wernicke's area, arcuate fasciculus
Motor areas: Precentral gyrus, supplemental motor area, Corona radiata, internal capsule
White-matter tracts for higher language and limbic functions: Uncinate fasciculus, inferior
  occipitofrontal fasciculus
Blood vessels: Middle cerebral artery, middle cerebral vein, and their perforators, e.g lateral
  lenticulostriate vessels which supply the basal ganglia

Parietal lobe gliomas
Resection of gliomas involving the supramarginal gyrus associated with a high risk of postoperative
  language and visual deficits
Key vascular structures at risk during resection
Middle cerebral artery branches which originate from the sylvian fissure and supply this area
Superficial draining veins which drain into superior sagittal sinus or the middle cerebral vein
Superior anastomotic vein of Trolard, as it links the superior sagittal sinus to the middle cerebral vein

Cingulate gyrus gliomas
Difficult surgical access (deep seated)
(Cingulate gyrus: Perigenual/anterior [emotional control], midcingulate [motor control], posterior
  cingulate [visual-spatial function], and retrosplenial [memory access])
Surgical approaches: Transcortical; interhemispheric
Risk of supplementary motor area (SMA) syndrome
A constellation of impaired volitional movement without loss of muscle tone, hemineglect, and
  dyspraxia of the contralateral limbs; speech hesitancy or mutism (if dominant SMA cortex is
  affected)

HGGs tend to disrupt the blood–brain barrier, the regional autoregulation is usually impaired, and the brain parenchyma surrounding the tumor is relatively ischemic, possibly due to the compressive effect of the tumor. Furthermore, these tumors often have extensive peritumoral edema, which can persist or even rebound after surgical resection (wounded glioma syndrome). Meticulous perioperative hemodynamic management is vital; while hypertension can lead to an increase in tumor blood flow with consequent aggravation of the cerebral edema and an increased risk of intratumoral bleeding, hypotension can impair the cerebral perfusion of the surrounding brain.

ST meningiomas

Classically, these tumors arise from the arachnoid cap cells and grow slowly over time to produce circumscribed, non-infiltrating but highly vascularized lesions that displace the surrounding structures but do not invade them (19,20) (Figure 5.2). The majority of these tumors occur along the falx (including parasagittal), the sphenoid ridge and tuberculum sellae, or over the convexity; other common sites for their growth include the olfactory groove, lateral ventricle, tentorium, middle fossa, and the orbit. Parasagittal meningiomas can involve the eloquent cortex; falcine and parasagittal meningiomas tend to invade the SSS. Skull base meningiomas (clinoidal, tuberculum sellae, cavernous sinus, olfactory groove meningiomas) can involve (encase/adhere) the major arteries (internal carotid artery [ICA], middle cerebral artery [MCA], anterior cerebral artery [ACA]), the cavernous sinuses, and the cranial nerves (I–VI) in the anterior and middle cranial fossae.

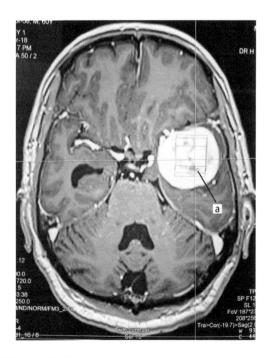

Figure 5.2 Contrast magnetic resonance imaging (MRI) T1 showing a well-marginated mass along sphenoid wing (a), brilliantly enhancing, suggestive of meningioma; no surrounding edema.

MANAGEMENT AND PROGNOSIS

Treatment options include observation, surgical resection, and stereotactic radiosurgery (SRS). Surgical resection is considered for patients who are either symptomatic or have large tumors, perilesional edema, and associated progressive symptoms. The ideal surgical goal is GTR of the tumor along with its dural attachment; however, this may be associated with greater morbidity if the meningioma is located in a critical location, if the dural involvement includes a wall of a patent dural sinus, and/or if the patient has a poor preoperative physical status (19–22). Considering that these tumors have slow growth rate, especially in older patients, and that the treatment is primarily aimed at preservation of neurological function and quality of life, a partial tumor resection is usually performed in these situations, followed by adjuvant radiotherapy/SRS. Meningiomas that are small or medium sized or have a difficult access (e.g., skull base meningiomas) can be treated with SRS (20,21). Management of skull base tumors may require a staged resection with the help of an interdisciplinary team (ear/nose/throat, maxillofacial, plastic, and neuro-ophthalmological surgeons).

ANESTHETIC CONSIDERATIONS

In addition to the risk of postoperative neurological deficits, the inherent vascularity of these lesions (highly vascularized lesions with peripheral feeding pedicles from local blood vessels) predisposes to significant perioperative blood losses (19) (Table 5.3). Resection of falcine and parasagittal meningiomas is associated with a high risk of venous infarction, severe blood loss, and venous air embolism (VAE) because of involvement of the SSS and the associated complex network of normal as well as abnormal collateral veins that develop over time. Venous infarction due to an inadvertent injury to the cortical veins that drain into the sinus, especially into its posterior two-thirds, can have catastrophic consequences, including venous congestion, severe cerebral edema, intracranial hypertension, intraparenchymal hemorrhage, seizures, and even cerebral herniation. Motor and language deficits can occur due to compromise of the veins that drain extensive eloquent areas of the brain to the venous sinuses; this is of particular concern when the sinus is occluded, because the brain may depend on these veins. Furthermore,

Table 5.3 Supratentorial meningiomas: Pertinent perioperative concerns

Convexity meningiomas
- Located on the surface of the cerebral hemisphere; can arise from any part of the cranial convexity
- Do not involve dural sinuses
- May cause compression of eloquent cortex
- Usually complete removal possible in most cases
- Preoperative embolization may be considered for meningiomas >5 cm with hypervascularity on magnetic resonance venography

Parasagittal and falcine meningioma
Risk of injury to:
- SSS: Blood loss; venous air embolism; venous infarct with intracranial hypertension
- Eloquent cortex motor strip (parasagittal)
- ACA and the draining veins; superior anastomotic vein of Trolard (drains into SSS)
- Risk of venous air embolism (SSS injury, semi-sitting position)
- Complete removal may not be possible if tumor invades the SSS

Sphenoidal meningioma
- *Anterior clinoidal/medial sphenoid wing meningiomas*
- Technically challenging
- Structures at risk: ICA, MCA, ACA, optic nerve, cavernous sinus
- May compress brainstem
- Deep portion of tumor has blood vessels from internal carotid artery; may invade lateral wall of cavernous sinus
- Complete removal may not be possible

Middle and lateral sphenoid wing meningioma
- More surgically accessible and resectable than clinoidal meningiomas
- Middle sphenoid wing meningiomas: Transsylvian approach associated with risk of injury to the sylvian veins

Olfactory groove meningiomas
- Structures at risk: ACA, optic chiasm
- Risk of CSF leak if dura is not closed in a watertight fashion
- External lumbar CSF drain may be placed to prevent or reduce brain retraction
- Frontotemporal (pterional) approach for small and medium-sized tumors; bifrontal craniotomy for large lesions

Tuberculum sellae meningiomas
- Structures at risk: ACA, ICA (may be encased/ displaced by tumor), cavernous sinus, optic nerve; small branches of ICA which supply the optic chiasm and optic nerves
- Hydrocephalus in cases of third ventricle compression
- Diabetes insipidus and hypopituitarism may occur postoperatively

Cavernous sinus meningiomas
- One of the most challenging tumors in regard to achieving radical surgical resection
- Can arise and remain within the sinus, extend outside the sinus and infiltrate its lateral wall, or growth inside and outside the sinus
- Structures at risk: Cavernous sinus, 3rd, 4th, 6th cranial nerve, ICA MCA, optic nerve

Abbreviations: SSS, superior sagittal sinus; ICA, internal carotid artery; MCA, middle cerebral artery; ACA, anterior cerebral artery; CSF, cerebrospinal fluid.

while preservation of the SSS takes precedence over a complete tumor resection, it also increases the risk of a postoperative hematoma due to bleeding from the tumor remnants that are adherent to the SSS. Sacrifice of the abnormal venous drainage through the bone that is resected for the craniotomy also predisposes to increased perioperative bleeding and VAE.

In view of these complications, the neuroanesthetist should review the neuroimaging studies (discussed later in the chapter) and take adequate measures for prompt detection and management of VAE and major blood losses during resection of these tumors. Preoperative tumor embolization, if feasible (for reducing the vascularity of tumors with a significant dural blood supply), helps to decrease the extent of intraoperative blood losses as well as the volume of lesion prior to the surgery.

ST metastasis

Most ST metastases originate from primary cancers of the lung (most common), breast, skin, kidney, and colon (23). These lesions can be solitary or multiple, and generally are well circumscribed and non-infiltrating in nature. Most of these tumors arise in the distribution of the MCA and within or near eloquent cortex, and are typically subcortical in location (usually gray matter—white matter interface).

MANAGEMENT

Treatment options include surgical resection by open craniotomy, SRS, and radiotherapy; GTR is usually feasible because of the non-infiltrating and well-defined nature of these lesions (22,23).

ANESTHETIC CONSIDERATIONS

Metastatic lesions are often associated with massive peritumoral vasogenic edema, which responds well to corticosteroid therapy; considerations pertaining to eloquent area tumors have been discussed in the previous sections.

Primary central nervous system lymphoma

Primary central nervous system lymphoma (PCNL) are a relatively uncommon form of extranodal non-Hodgkin lymphoma (Figure 5.3). They are highly aggressive, may be solitary or multiple, and are located superficially in the cortex or may have a deep periventricular location. Typically, they are composed of noncohesive neoplastic lymphocytes that diffusely infiltrate the neural parenchyma and the blood vessels. The prognosis is poor, with an average survival time of approximately a year, despite optimal therapy (1) Tumor resection offers no benefit, except in the rare circumstances of neurologic deterioration due to brain herniation (1). These patients usually undergo a diagnostic biopsy followed by chemoradiotherapy.

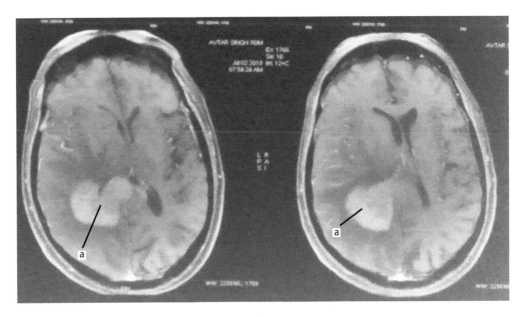

Figure 5.3 Magnetic resonance imaging (MRI) scan showing a paraventricular hyperintense lesion (a) with irregular margins, suggestive of lymphoma.

Pituitary adenomas

Pituitary adenomas are increasingly being diagnosed in geriatric patients. Patients usually present with galactorrhea or features of acromegaly. Nonsecreting tumors can grow silently for a long time and are usually diagnosed incidentally; management of these patients is described elsewhere in the book.

CLINICO-PATHOLOGICAL CONSIDERATIONS

The clinical manifestations depend primarily on the type, size, location, and rate of growth of the STT and the magnitude of rise in the intracranial pressure (ICP). The manifestations may be focal and/or generalized but are characteristically progressive in nature. Typically, the signs and symptoms progress insidiously over weeks to months in patients with malignant tumors (e.g., HGG) and over months to years in those with benign tumors (e.g., meningiomas). However, the presentation may sometimes be acute and apoplectic, often mimicking an acute stroke, and is usually due to an acute neurological deterioration caused by a life-threatening cerebral herniation, intra- or peritumoral hemorrhage, secondary vascular compromise, or due to epileptic seizures.

Focal manifestations include focal seizures (due to "irritation" of cortex by the underlying tumor) and progressive focal neurological deficits, such as weakness, sensory abnormalities, speech disturbances, and visual defects (tumors of eloquent cortex and subcortical nuclei); changes in mood, memory, or personality (anterior frontal or temporal lobe tumors); hemiparesis, hemisensory loss, and hemianopia (posterior frontal or parietal neoplasms); aphasia (left-sided sylvian fissure tumors); and visual deficits (occipital lobe tumors) (Table 5.1). Generalized manifestations occur due to "mass effect" by the tumor and include generalized convulsions and features of intracranial hypertension.

Several factors can modify the clinical manifestations of STTs in geriatric patients, which may cause a delay in the diagnosis of the disease.

Age-related atrophy of the brain and the reduced CSF production make the cranium more spacious; hence these tumors can grow for a long time without producing a significant increase in the ICP.

Further, patients with anterior frontal, anterior temporal, and skull base tumors, especially meningiomas and metastasis, are often asymptomatic or have very minimal neurological dysfunction despite the presence of a large intracranial mass. Sometimes nonspecific symptoms (e.g., confusion, forgetfulness, mental slowing, lethargy, apathy, memory deficits, personality changes, gait difficulties) are attributed to the normal aging process; however, history of a rapid neurocognitive decline (within 6 months) is highly suggestive of a STT and should prompt further diagnostic evaluation.

Ultimately, "mass effect" due to compression of the surrounding brain by the enlarging tumor, associated peritumoral cerebral edema, venous congestion due to occlusion of dural venous sinuses, and/or development of hydrocephalus (obstruction of CSF pathways by tumors within or adjacent to them) leads to an increase in the ICP. Once the limit of tolerance is reached, the ICP rises exponentially and leads to a much poorer clinical outcome. Rapid progression of symptoms over a short period of time indicates that the tumor and edema are expanding faster than the compensatory capacities of the brain, and the patient is at risk of developing an acute neurological deterioration. Presence of features such as alteration in mental status, headache, nausea, vomiting, papilledema, unilateral pupillary dilation, and oculomotor or abducens palsy are indicative of an increased ICP and the need for an immediate intervention; patients who prefer to keep their eyes closed or sleep are nearing a critical point on the volume pressure curve.

Intra- or peritumoral hemorrhage (particularly GBM, metastatic tumors) results in acute and marked increase in the ICP; life-threatening cerebral herniation can ensue when this rapidly expanding tumor mass forces the brain tissue from one intracranial compartment to another (through the relatively rigid dural openings between compartments), tearing the blood vessels and compressing the neuropil in the process. STTs usually cause cingulate (herniation of cingulate gyrus beneath the falx cerebri) or transtentorial herniation; tonsillar herniation (displacement of brain tissue through the foramen magnum) may also occur, though it is more common with posterior fossa lesions. Transtentorial herniation may be central (bilateral/symmetrical mass effect causes a downward shift of the diencephalon and upper brainstem, resulting in sequential failure of the diencephalon, midbrain, pons, and medulla) or uncal (unilateral mass effect which displaces the medial temporal lobe inferiorly and medially through the tentorial notch). A depressed level of consciousness, obtundation, lethargy, and irregular breathing are ominous signs which point toward a life-threatening neurosurgical emergency.

NEUROIMAGING OF STTs

While a computerized tomography (CT) scan is usually is the first line of imaging in an acute environment, contrast-enhanced magnetic resonance imaging (MRI) with T1-/T2-weighted and FLAIR sequences is the imaging modality of choice for diagnosis of most CNS tumors. T1 images usually are better at demonstrating anatomy and areas of contrast enhancement; T2 and FLAIR images are more sensitive for detecting edema and infiltrative tumor. Generally, an HGG appears as a contrast-enhancing mass, with a thick rind of enhancement, a central heterogeneous signal (necrosis, intratumoral hemorrhage), irregular or poorly defined margins, and surrounding vasogenic-type edema. On the other hand, an enhancing lesion that does not show necrosis but is infiltrative is suggestive of an anaplastic astrocytoma; absence of contrast enhancement and edema usually imply a low-grade astrocytoma.

A meningioma typically appears as a hypointense or isointense, homogenously enhancing, well circumscribed, extra-axial mass with a broad dural base, with a characteristic dural tail.

A PCNSL is characteristically identified as a T1 hypointense, T2 iso- to hyperintense mass with vivid homogeneous enhancement, restricted diffusion, relatively little associated vasogenic edema, and no central necrosis.

A metastatic lesion usually appears as a subcortical, well-defined enhancing lesion with surrounding vasogenic edema; hemorrhage be seen in metastatic melanoma, renal cell carcinoma, and thyroid neoplasms.

MR spectroscopy can help to assess the aggressiveness of a tumor; an increased choline and decreased N-acetylaspartate peak indicate increased cell turnover and hence a high probability of a malignant tumor; a concomitant lactate peak is indicative of anaerobic metabolism, commonly observed when a tumor outgrows its vascular supply and leads to necrosis.

PRE-NEUROSURGICAL PLANNING

The following section provides an overview of the pertinent components of pre-neurosurgical planning.

Surgical procedures, techniques, and timing of surgery

Most of the patients undergo a craniotomy and tumor resection; the craniotomy may be performed through an open, minimally invasive, or a stereotactic technique. A biopsy is usually reserved for patients in whom resection is not expected to be beneficial (e.g., PCNSL, for obtaining a histopathological diagnosis), or if their resection is associated with an unacceptable morbidity, e.g. patients with multiple metastasis, highly malignant tumors, deep-seated tumors—patients with a poor functional status. The biopsy may be performed through a burr hole (frame-based or frameless stereotactic; needle biopsy) or via a mini-craniotomy (direct open biopsy). A stereotactic biopsy is usually preferred over an open biopsy if the lesion is not associated with mass effect. Though it is relatively safe, there is a small, albeit definite, risk of hemorrhage, especially in patients with PCNSL (increased vessel fragility), or multifocal HGGs. It can be performed under general anesthesia (GA) or conscious sedation.

While most patients are operated on an elective basis, an emergency intervention may be required in those who develop an acute neurological deterioration (22). Patients with an obstructive hydrocephalus may undergo a temporary ventriculostomy or a ventriculoperitoneal (VP) shunt prior to the planned resection, or alternatively, may directly undergo a craniotomy and tumor resection, with the goal of relieving the hydrocephalus.

Surgical approaches and patient positioning

Neurosurgeons use either of the following surgical craniotomies (or their variants) for resection of STTs: pterional (frontosphenotemporal), temporal, subfrontal, bifrontal, parasagittal, parietal, and parieto-occipital (Figures 5.4–5.7). The common indications and potential concerns of these approaches are listed in Table 5.4.

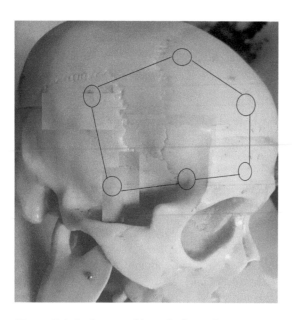

Figure 5.4 Surface marking of a large frontotemporal craniotomy, shown on a human skull model.

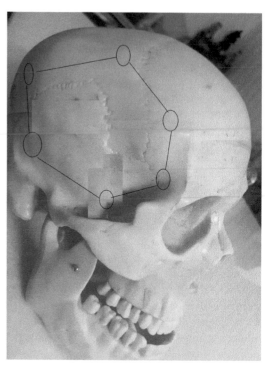

Figure 5.6 Surface marking of a temporoparietal craniotomy, shown on a human skull model.

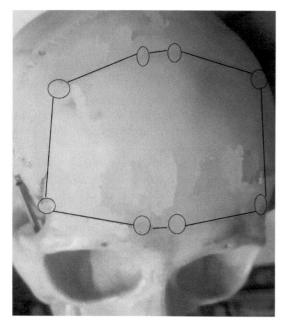

Figure 5.5 Surface marking of a bifrontal craniotomy, shown on a human skull model.

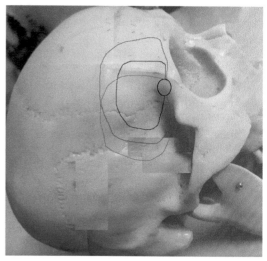

Figure 5.7 Surface marking of pterional (*black*); frontotemporal (*red*) and temporal (*blue*) craniotomy, shown on a human skull model.

Generally, craniotomies anterior to the coronal suture are performed in the supine position; lateral, semi-sitting, or prone positions are reserved for craniotomies posterior to the coronal suture (though supine may also be used). Meticulous attention should be given to proper positioning of these patients. An ideal position not only provides optimal surgical access to the tumor with minimal trespass of the normal brain, but also significantly improves the operating conditions (relaxed brain,

Table 5.4 Common surgical approaches for resection of supratentorial tumors: Positioning of the patient and pertinent concerns

Surgical approach variants / Common indications	Patient position / positioning of head and neck	Concerns and precautions
Pterional craniotomy (Frontosphenotemporal) **Variants** Frontotemporal craniotomy Cranio-orbito-zygomatic approach **Indications** *Pterional* Anterior and middle cranial fossa tumors, e.g, sphenoid wing, parasellar, and cavernous sinus meningioma *Frontotemporal craniotomy* Standard approach for intrinsic frontal and temporal lobe tumors; also used for suprasellar and anterior skull base tumors **Orbito-zygomatic approach** Lateral sphenoid wing meningiomas	*Standard supine position* Thorax elevated by 10°–15° (reverse Trendelenburg position) Head elevated above the level of the heart (to facilitate venous drainage); rotated approximately 45° toward the contralateral shoulder; slightly flexed laterally[a] Neck relaxed; extended so that the vertex is angled down 10°–30° (allows gravity to retract the frontal lobe off the anterior cranial fossa floor) Ipsilateral shoulder elevated with a shoulder roll in the long axis of the body) (facilitates head rotation toward the contralateral side) *At final position, malar eminence of the zygomatic bone should be the highest point in the operative field*	Breach of frontal sinus: CSF leak, pneumocephalus, and infection Epidural hematoma due to delayed bleeding from branch of superficial temporal artery
Temporal and subtemporal craniotomy **Indications** Middle cranial fossa tumors; best approach for temporal lobe tumors	*Lateral decubitus position* Patient placed on side opposite the operative site, with the sagittal plane parallel to the ground Head above the level of the heart (reverse Trendelenburg position) Neck laterally flexed, so that head is tilted slightly toward the floor and the dependent ear is brought toward the ipsilateral shoulder (allows gravity to facilitate gentle retraction of the temporal lobe) *Supine position* Similar to positioning for pterional craniotomy, except that head is turned to the contralateral side by approximately 90° for a subtemporal approach, and by 30°–75° for a temporal approach Large shoulder roll placed under ipsilateral shoulder	Temporal lobe venous infarcts or edema due to inadvertent injury to: Temporal veins draining into the sphenoparietal sinus (during dural opening) Injury to vein of Labbe (drains into temporal sinus) Subtemporal approach avoided for dominant hemisphere lesions

(Continued)

Table 5.4 (Continued) Common surgical approaches for resection of supratentorial tumors: Positioning of the patient and pertinent concerns

Surgical approach variants Common indications	Patient position positioning of head and neck	Concerns and precautions
Subfrontal and bifrontal craniotomy **Indications** Frontal lobe tumors Anterior cranial fossa tumors, e.g., olfactory groove meningiomas, tuberculum sellae meningiomas, hypothalamic and chiasmatic gliomas	*Supine position* Head and neck are elevated and extended so the ipsilateral brow is the most superior point on the operative field (allows the frontal lobe to fall away from the anterior cranial fossa) Unilateral approach: Head is in a neutral midline position along the long axis of the patient Bilateral approach: Head is rotated approximately 15° toward the contralateral shoulder	Breach of frontal sinus: CSF leak, pneumocephalus, and infection (if dura mater and frontal sinus are not properly closed) Superior sagittal sinus injury
Anterior and posterior parasagittal craniotomy *Parasagittal approach:* Third and lateral ventricular tumors Parasagittal and falcine meningiomas; midline gliomas	Frontal interhemispheric approach (lesions involving the SSS or deep to the anterior third of SSS): *Standard supine position* Head is elevated and flexed until the desired surgical site is comfortably within the surgeon's operative field, head is kept in a neutral midline position along the long axis of the patient Middle parietal interhemispheric approach (tumors in the area of the middle third of the SSS):	Injury to: Cortical veins that drain into sagittal sinus, especially those that drain into the posterior two thirds of the sagittal sinus
Interhemispheric approach: Tumors located within/ near to the falx, corpus callosum, medial frontal gyrus, cingulate gyrus, thalamus	*Standard supine position with flexion of head and neck* OR *Semi-sitting position* Posterior parasagittal approach (tumors in the area of posterior third of the SSS) *Supine: Greater degree of flexion required than the anterior parasagittal approach* OR *Park bench position (modification of the lateral position)* OR *Prone position (head elevated; neck flexed so that the craniotomy site at the highest point of the operative field)*	

(Continued)

Table 5.4 (*Continued*) Common surgical approaches for resection of supratentorial tumors: Positioning of the patient and pertinent concerns

Surgical approach variants Common indications	Patient position positioning of head and neck	Concerns and precautions
Parietal craniotomy	*Lateral position* Neck in long axis with spine Head turned facing floor so that craniotomy side is the highest point of the surgical field	Risk of injury to superior sagittal sinus and associated draining veins
Indications Tumors of the parietal region. Transcallosal approach for thalamic glioma Interhemispheric approach to lateral, third ventricular tumors	Cortical glioma: Ipsilateral side and shoulder up Interhemispheric lesions: Ipsilateral side down OR *Supine position with head turned to contralateral side* (as described above)	
Parietal-occipital	Parietal lobe tumors: *Lateral position* Head positioned so that the approach to the tumor is perpendicular to the floor	Risk of injury to superior sagittal sinus and associated draining veins
Indications Parietal-occipital tumors Intraventricular tumors in posterior horn of the ventricle Thalamic tumors	Lateral parietal tumors: Head is neutral with the long axis of the body Ventricular/periventricular tumors: Head bent toward the ipsilateral shoulder (so that superior parietal lobule is the highest point in the field) Occipital lobe tumors: *Lateral position with head turned toward the floor* OR *Prone position*	

[a]Head rotation can vary from 20°–60° depending on the target lesion.

which minimizes retraction of brain parenchyma; relatively clear and bloodless operating field; comfortable operating position for the surgeon) and reduces the chances of avoidable positioning-related complications.

The basic principles of head and neck positioning for these surgical approaches are described below. (Patient positioning is described in detail elsewhere in this book.)

An optimal surgical approach allows the most direct and maximal access to the STT. It is achieved when the head and neck of the patient are positioned such that the lesion lies at the highest point in the operative field, the trajectory to STT is perpendicular to the floor, and the exposed surface of the skull and an imaginary perimeter of the skull are parallel to the floor; generally, this requires a strategic combination of slight elevation, flexion/extension and lateral rotation of the head and neck (22).

Elevation of the head above the level of the heart (10°–15° of reverse Trendelenburg) facilitates cerebral venous drainage, decreases venous congestion, cerebral swelling, and ICP, and aids in providing a slack brain (24). Lateral rotation of the head and neck allows gravity to retract the normal brain away from the tumor and hence minimizes the need for retraction of the brain.

However, these maneuvers have associated risks. Compromise of the cerebral blood flow (CBF) can occur due to extreme rotation (compression of ipsilateral vertebral arteries), hyperflexion or hyperextension (compression of carotid arteries) of the head and neck; extreme lateral rotation and/or flexion of the neck can impair the venous return from the contralateral internal jugular vein (IJV), leading to venous congestion, rise in ICP, brain swelling, and increased surgical site bleeding. Importantly, these maneuvers require even more caution in older patients, who often have concomitant cervical spondylosis, vascular atherosclerosis, and/or osteoarthritis, and may not be able to tolerate even a modest degree of neck movement. Hence, preoperatively the neuroanesthetist must assess the mobility of the cervical spine and also review the width of the cervical canal from the neuroimaging studies in order to evaluate maximum range of head and neck movement that is safe for these patients; it may also be prudent to ask

for a Doppler ultrasound in patients with signs of vertebra-basilar insufficiency (vertigo on neck movement).

Generally, neck rotation in the range 0°–45° is usually well tolerated, as long as the neck remains supple. During flexion of the neck, at least two fingers' space should be ensured between the chin and the nearest bone (to avoid kinking of the tracheal tube and impairment of cerebral venous drainage).

Elevation of the ipsilateral shoulder (with a shoulder roll placed beneath it, on the longitudinal axis of the body) helps to achieve the desired position with less rotation of the neck and prevents compression of the IJV. Table 5.4 lists the various positions and the positioning of the head and neck used for the various surgical approaches for resection of STTs.

Adjuncts to safe tumor resection

One of the most important concerns with a neurosurgical intervention in geriatric patients is the risk of deterioration in their quality of life due to development of iatrogenic neurological deficits. This risk has been minimized in recent years with the use of advanced presurgical as well as intraoperative, neuroimaging, and neuromonitoring techniques, which enable the neurosurgeon to achieve a more extensive as well as safe resection of otherwise technically difficult tumors (Table 5.5).

PRE-NEUROSURGICAL TECHNIQUES

Functional MRI and diffusion tensor imaging with MRI tractography for eloquent cortex tumors

These techniques are useful for resection of tumors that lie within or are in spatial proximity to the eloquent cortex and subcortical areas, respectively.

A functional MRI (fMRI) is based on detection of changes in the cortical oxygen consumption while the patient performs a given task. It localizes the eloquent motor cortices as well as the language regions and can assess the extent to which they have been displaced by the STT. It also helps in evaluating whether an awake intraoperative language mapping procedure is likely to be beneficial, be of low yield, or is not needed at all, in patients with tumors in the language areas (25–27).

Table 5.5 Neuromonitoring and neuroimaging techniques to facilitate resection of supratentorial tumors

Pre-neurosurgical techniques
- *Functional MRI (fMRI) and diffusion tensor imaging (DTI) with MRI tractography: for eloquent cortex tumors*
  - fMRI: To identify primary motor cortex, Wernicke's area, Broca's area, primary visual cortex
  - DTI: To delineate a map of the main eloquent tracts and the subcortical connections between essential cortices, e.g corticospinal tracts, arcuate fasciculus, optic radiation
- *Angiography, computed tomography (CT) angiography, digital subtraction angiography (DSA) magnetic resonance angiography (MRA), and magnetic resonance venography (MRV)*
  - To define the relationship between the cerebral vasculature and the STT
- *Preoperative embolization of tumors with help of digital subtraction angiography*
  - To decrease the vascularity and size of meningiomas, prior to the surgery

Intraoperative techniques
- *Intraoperative ultrasound*
  - For rapid localization of the supratentorial tumor
- *Intraoperative neuroelectrophysiological monitoring*
  - Direct electrical cortical stimulation for intraoperative motor and speech mapping; awake craniotomy required for speech mapping
  - Monitoring of somatosensory-evoked potentials (SSEPs) and motor-evoked potential (MEPs) for identification of sensory and motor cortices, detection of encroachment on the cortical tracts during resection
- *Indocyanine green angiography*
  - For real-time evaluation of the relation of the blood vessels in proximity to the tumor
- *5-Aminolevulinic acid*
  - Fluorescent marker that accumulates in the glial tumor cells; allows a real-time evaluation of the extent of resection
- *Frameless stereotactic neuronavigation*
  - For real-time identification of the tumor, its relation to the critical neurovascular structures, along with evaluation of the extent of tumor resection
- *Intraoperative magnetic resonance imaging (MRI)*
  - Provides a real-time, updated MRI scan which may enable a more extensive tumor resection

Diffusion tensor imaging (DTI) is a form of diffusion-weighted MR imaging which can delineate a map of the main eloquent tracts, the subcortical connections between essential cortices, and can identify whether a WM tract is infiltrated, edematous, displaced, or interrupted by the STT. While a conventional MRI provides only anatomical information, DTI gives information about CNS connectivity, e.g. location of the arcuate fasciculus between the Broca's area and Wernicke's area (22,25–27). fMRI and DTI are often used complementarily to delineate a map of the main eloquent tracts; in addition, these data can also be used during the surgery to guide the extent of resection (EOR).

Angiography, magnetic resonance angiography, and magnetic resonance venography

These imaging modalities help to better define the relationship between the cerebral vasculature and the STT (22). They are especially useful for operative planning of meningioma surgeries. Magnetic resonance angiography (MRA) and angiography can visualize the relation of the tumor to the major blood vessels, their arterial feeders, and draining veins, displacement/encasement of these vessels by the tumor, occlusion of a sinus, collateralization in areas of sinus occlusion, and also determine whether there is a role for preoperative embolization. Magnetic resonance venography (MRV) primarily evaluates the venous system; it is very useful for determining which veins can be sacrificed and which major draining veins need to be left intact during the resection of the meningioma.

INTRAOPERATIVE NEUROMONITORING TECHNIQUES

Ultrasonography

Intraoperative ultrasound enables a rapid localization of the STT prior to the durotomy. It is also useful for evaluation of a brain shift or any other anatomic deformation experienced during resection of the STT.

Intraoperative neuroelectrophysiological monitoring (IONM)

Direct electrical cortical stimulation for central sulcus and language mapping

Direct electrical cortical stimulation (DES) is the gold-standard technique for assessing true eloquent cortical and subcortical sites during surgery (25). Direct motor cortex stimulation (posterior frontal lobe tumors) aids in identifying the edge of the tumor as it interfaces with the motor cortex. The alterations in the motor signals can be transient or permanent and are indicative of reversible and irreversible postoperative motor deficits, respectively; in addition, the extent of change correlates with the severity of the postoperative neurological deficits (28). Similarly, intraoperative speech mapping allows the neurosurgeon to maximally resect dominant temporal lobe tumors while minimizing the risk for a postoperative language deficit.

Intraoperative mapping of motor regions can be performed under GA or in an awake patient (under conscious sedation analgesia; however, speech mapping requires the patient to be awake, cooperative, and responsive during the mapping and hence requires an awake craniotomy. DES carries a risk of seizures, and the anesthetist should be prepared to manage them appropriately (ice-cold saline irrigation; escalating antiepileptic drug [AED] regimen).

Awake craniotomy

An awake craniotomy allows mapping of the language areas, the motor cortex, and the corticospinal tracts during resection of eloquent cortex tumors (29). It is useful for surface tumors (to determine which portions of the tumor are resectable) as well as for deep-seated lesions (to determine a safe trajectory to the lesion). In this technique, the patient is sedated during the craniotomy, is awoken for assessment of the speech and motor function during the cortical stimulation and mapping phase, and then re-sedated after the mapping, until the end of the surgery.

Monitoring of somatosensory evoked potential and motor evoked potential

Intraoperative somatosensory-evoked potential (SSEP) and motor-evoked potential (MEP) monitoring (cortical and subcortical) are also used to locate the sensory and motor cortices and warn the neurosurgeon of encroachment on the cortical tracts during resection.

Indocyanine green angiography and 5-aminolevulinic acid

Indocyanine green (ICG) angiography allows an intraoperative, real-time evaluation of the intradural vessels and venous sinuses and is especially useful during resection of parasagittal meningiomas (30). It has also been used during resection of insular gliomas, to identify and preserve the perforating branches of the MCA that course through the tumor (31). 5-aminolevulinic acid (5-ALA) is a fluorescent marker that accumulates in the glial tumor cells and is a good adjunct for a real-time evaluation of the EOR (26). It is administered orally in the preoperative period; intraoperatively, a special microscope is used to identify the fluorescent tumor tissue.

Frameless stereotactic neuronavigation

This technique involves the use of computers (graphic station software for intraoperative neuronavigation), preoperatively obtained neuroimaging (dedicated MRI or CT sequences; MRI or CT scans), and a frameless system (that uses facial bony landmarks or fiducial markers placed on the patient's scalp prior to the neuroimaging). During the surgery, the neuroimaging dataset is displayed on the navigational system, which creates an interface between this displayed neuroimaging and the patient's facial bony landmarks/fiducial markers and the displayed imaging (MRI or CT), to provide high-resolution three-dimensional images of the tumor and the brain (22,25,32). When the neurosurgeon places the probe on the patient, it is displayed on the system monitor in relation to the underlying brain anatomy and the tumor and provides a real-time feedback about the EOR. This technique enables the neurosurgeon to limit the size of the incision and the craniotomy, localize superficial tumors, determine the best trajectory to approach subcortical and deeply seated tumors, and minimize the tissue injury associated with brain dissection of normal brain tissue; it also assists in resection control (determining whether the intended resection has been accomplished).

Typically, routine enhanced MRI is the most common imaging modality used interactively in the operating room; however, data from multiple advanced imaging modalities, such as fMRI, DTI, positron emission tomography, and ultrasonography, can also be incorporated onto the navigation system to increase the likelihood of a successful operation. Incorporation of DTI fiber tracking into the image data set in particular has greatly enhanced the capability of neuronavigation; while the navigable anatomy was largely limited to cortical and periventricular regions previously, incorporation of DTI allows subcortical navigation also. This is especially valuable when used in combination with IONM; correlation of the anatomical data (provided by preoperative DTI dataset) with the functional data (obtained from the intraoperative neurophysiological mapping techniques) provides a more accurate feedback to the operating neurosurgeon regarding the vulnerable eloquent subcortical connections that need to be preserved during the resection (22,25,26).

A potential limitation with use of intraoperative neuronavigation is the alteration in the intraoperative anatomy because of brain shift (due to intraoperative fluid shifts and tumor resection), which reduces its accuracy after dural opening and may cause tumor remnants to be missed. Hence it is most useful when integrated with the conventional brain-mapping techniques (awake craniotomy, IONM) for resection of eloquent cortex tumors.

Intraoperative MRI

While conventional neuronavigation is based upon preoperative neuroimaging, an intraoperative MRI (iMRI) provides an updated MRI scan, obtained during surgery; this real-time guidance may enable a greater EOR. When used in combination with neuronavigation it can be utilized to identify the tumor remnants and can improve the accuracy of neuronavigation (22,26). However, it is more time consuming, more expensive, and its usefulness is limited by the quality of the images; its added benefit in terms of improved tumor resection and better outcomes still remains to be determined.

While the previously mentioned intraoperative techniques markedly improve the EOR, it is probably prudent to remember that they are best used as adjuvants, to complement the visual feedback that the surgeon is receiving from the gross appearance of the tumor.

PREOPERATIVE EVALUATION

Older patients have a higher incidence of adverse perioperative events than the younger population. Hence they merit a more extensive preoperative evaluation so that the risks pertaining to the surgery and the patient's morbidities can be assessed, and modifiable risk factors can be optimized prior to the surgery. Table 5.6 lists the pertinent components of the preoperative evaluation; a more detailed discussion on this topic is provided in the initial chapters of this book.

The American College of Surgeons National Surgical Quality Improvement Program (ACS NSQIP) and the American Geriatrics Society (AGS) have identified specific concerns that influence the perioperative morbidity of older patients and should be evaluated, and if feasible, optimized, prior to the surgery (33). These concerns include decreased functional performance, cognitive impairment, dementia, depression, systemic comorbidities (poor cardiac, pulmonary, and nutritional status), increased fragility (impaired physiological responses to perioperative stresses), alcohol and substance abuse/dependence, and an increased risk of postoperative delirium (33).

The functional performance of patients with brain tumors is usually assessed by the Karnofsky Performance Scale (KPS) (26). This is a 10-grade scale that categorizes these patients into three functional conditions: A, 100%–80% (patients who can work or maintain at home); B, 70%–50% (clinical status prevents patients from working); and C, 40%–0% (patients who are disabled); a lower score is associated with a poorer prognosis.

PREOPERATIVE OPTIMIZATION

Patients with a poor cardiac and/or pulmonary status should be referred to a specialist, and their

Table 5.6 Pertinent features of the preoperative evaluation of a geriatric patient with a supratentorial tumor

A. Evaluate the risks due to patient's premorbid condition
- *History and clinical examination*
  - Does the patient have features of raised ICP?
  - Headache, nausea, vomiting, blurring of vision, somnolence, low GCS, hypertension, bradycardia, and papilledema: Indicate low intracranial compliance
  - Pupillary asymmetry, hemiparesis, aphasia, deep shallow breathing: Indicate a decompensated state
  - Does the patient have seizures?
  - Assess the type (partial/generalized), frequency, duration of treatment, response to medication
  - Look for any focal neurological deficit: Motor, sensory, and cranial nerve deficit
  - Assess the cognitive ability and capacity to understand the anticipated surgery: Mini-Cog: 3-Item Recall and Clock Draw)/ Mini-Mental State Examination
  - Assess the functional status and ability to perform daily activities (functional status): KPS
  - Screen for depression: Patient Health Questionnaire-2 (PHQ-2)25; alcohol and substance abuse/ dependence (modified CAGE questionnaire [Cut down, Annoyed, Guilty, Eye-opener])
- *Review the systemic comorbidities*
  - Cardiac: METS (poor cardiorespiratory reserve if METS <4-inability to climb two flights of stairs); Revised Cardiac Risk Index; evaluation according to American Heart Association guidelines
  - Pulmonary evaluation: History of smoking, COAD, asthma, upper respiratory infections to identify risk factors for postoperative pulmonary complications
  - Renal disorders
  - Hepatic dysfunction, hypertension, diabetes mellitus
  - Assess the nutritional status: Mini Nutritional Assessment score
  - Identify risk factors for development of postoperative delirium
  - Determine the baseline frailty score: Hopkins frailty index/Canadian study of health and aging frailty index (modified frailty index)
  - Evaluate the hydration status
  - Evaluate ASA grade, Charlson Comorbidity Index
- *Assess the airway and range of head and neck movements; evaluate the neuroimaging studies for assessment of the cervical canal*
- *Review previous records*
  - Previous surgeries, anesthetic exposures, history of allergies
- *Current medications*
  - Steroid use; presence of side effects of steroids (hyperglycemia)
  - Diuretic use (associated hypovolemia, can be detrimental to patients with raised ICP)
  - Antiepileptic drugs
  - Past history of chemotherapy or radiation: Certain chemotherapeutic medications are associated with complications such as cardiomyopathy (doxorubicin) or inhibition of plasma cholinesterase activity (cyclophosphamide) and renal or hepatotoxicity
  - Antidepressants
  - Medications for comorbidities
- *Investigations*
  - Hematological: Hemoglobin, hematocrit, complete blood count
  - Coagulation profile: Prothrombin time, partial thromboplastin time, platelet count
  - Basic metabolic panel: Liver function tests including serum albumin, Kidney function tests (blood urea nitrogen, creatinine), serum electrolytes
  - Urine analysis
  - X-ray chest; baseline ABG, PFT (if indicated)
  - Electrocardiogram; Echocardiography, cardiopulmonary exercise testing (if indicated)

(Continued)

Table 5.6 (*Continued*) Pertinent features of the preoperative evaluation of a geriatric patient with a supratentorial tumor

B. Evaluate the risks due to primary surgical pathology and the proposed neurosurgical procedure

- *Review the neuroimaging studies*
  - CT scan, MRI (pre- and post-contrast T1-, T2-weighted images, flair sequences, diffusion and perfusion weighted MRI imaging)
    - *Location*: Intra-/extra-axial; specific lobe involvement (frontal, parietal, temporal, occipital); involvement of eloquent cortex (motor/sensory cortex, language cortex; deep midline gliomas: basal ganglia/internal capsule
    - *Size of the tumor* (largest diameter based on T1-contrast-weighted images)
    - *Extent of vasogenic brain edema* surrounding the tumor (on T2-weighted MRI scans)
    - *Extent of post-contrast tumor enhancement* (increased vascularity, invasiveness; indicative of extent of disruption of blood brain barrier)
    - *Intracranial mass effect*: Midline shift, ventricular enlargement/dilatation or compression; herniation (cingulated, temporal, uncal)
    - Relationship of the tumor to major blood vessels and draining sinuses
  - Advanced neuroimaging studies: Functional MRI, DTI, MRA, MRV
  - Complementary exams if necessary: CT of chest, abdomen, and pelvis, PET CT scan
- *Review details of the proposed surgical procedure*

Abbreviations: ICP, intracranial pressure; GCS, Glasgow Coma Scale; MET, metabolic equivalent; COAD, chronic obstructive airway disease; ABG, arterial blood gas; PFT, pulmonary function test; ASA, American Society of Anesthesia; MRI, magnetic resonance imaging; DTI, diffusion tractography; MRA, magnetic resonance angiography; MRV, magnetic resonance venography; CT, computerized tomography; KPS, Karnofsky Performance Score.

condition should be optimized prior to the surgery (if feasible); a psychiatric consultation should be considered for patients with cognitive impairment, dementia, or depression.

Perioperative corticosteroids

Corticosteroids limit peritumoral edema and improve intracranial compliance by decreasing tumor capillary permeability and tumor blood volume. They can provide temporary relief of the neurological deficits and symptoms related to the mass effect and cerebral edema, prior to the surgery (13,22,34). Dexamethasone has minimal mineralocorticoid activity and is usually preferred; the response to therapy usually begins within 24 hours, and maximum improvement is generally observed within 4 days of initiating treatment. Dexamethasone is often administered in the immediate postoperative period also, to limit postoperative edema from brain tissue manipulation.

The dose of dexamethasone is based on the amount of edema and mass effect, though the upper limit for short-term therapy has not been clearly established; however, a certain dose threshold must be exceeded before a decrease in intracranial hypertension is observed (13,22). Hence a higher dose is administered initially, which is then gradually tapered as neurological improvement occurs.

Typical doses are as follows:

- *Patients not previously on steroids:* Dexamethasone 10 mg IV followed by 4–6 mg every 6 hours until clinical improvement is observed (higher doses, up to 120 mg/day may be required in patients with severe vasogenic edema).
- *Patients already on steroids:* For acute deterioration, a dose of approximately double the usual dose may be administered.

The systemic side effects of steroids tend to be more severe in older patients, particularly when they are used for prolonged periods. Therefore their use should be limited to symptomatic patients, and for the shortest possible duration (34). Prophylactic H2 blockers or proton pump inhibitors are usually coadministered to prevent formation of gastrointestinal ulcers. Diabetic patients need particular attention; blood glucose must be monitored carefully, and insulin therapy may be required to control the hyperglycemia. In cases where corticosteroids are contraindicated (e.g., those with an active peptic ulcer, heart failure, or uncontrolled diabetes), diuretics such as acetazolamide or furosemide can be given to decrease the edema. Corticosteroids should also be avoided preoperatively in patients with a provisional diagnosis of lymphoma (rapid lymphodepletive effect causes problems in detection).

Perioperative AEDs

AEDs are given for management of seizures. Prophylactic administration of these drugs in patients with newly diagnosed brain tumors is not recommended; however, prophylactic preoperative AED administration may be indicated if the surgery involves a cortical incision; it can be tapered off after 1 week if no seizure episode occurs during this period (13,22,34–36).

Newer AEDs such as levetiracetam and lamotrigine are the preferred drugs for patients undergoing a craniotomy, especially for resection of a glioma. Since they have a more favorable profile (rapid titration to effective dose, mild adverse effects, low potential for interaction with chemotherapeutic agents, no induction of hepatic microsomal [P450] enzymes, no need for monitoring), they have largely replaced phenytoin (zero-order kinetics, narrow therapeutic index, significant bidirectional drug interactions, induction of cytochrome P450 enzymes may increase the metabolism of chemotherapeutic agents) as the AED of choice in these patients (34,36).

While older patients are more responsive to AEDs than the younger population, they are also more likely to experience the adverse effects of these drugs at much lower serum concentrations (especially imbalance and cognitive impairment). Hence close monitoring is vital, and levels below the usually effective range may be appropriate for these patients. A suggested dose regime is as follows:

- *In patients with history of seizures:*
  - *If patient on an AED*: Continue same dose
  - *If not on AED*: Load with levetiracetam 500 mg (or oral phenytoin [300 mg orally ever 4 hours × 3 doses; total 900 mg])

- *If no history of seizures:*
  - *If cortical incision planned*: Load with the previously mentioned dosages
  - *If cortical incision not planned*: AED usually not indicated

Venous thromboembolic event prophylaxis

These patients have a high risk of developing a venous thromboembolic event (VTE) in the perioperative period (old age, intracranial tumor, immobility due to paresis); the risk is as high as 20%–30% in patients with HGG (32). Hence VTE prophylaxis with intermittent pneumatic compression (IPC) devices should be started prior to the surgery. It is also prudent to stratify the risk of VTE with use of a scoring tool; The American College of Chest Physicians guidelines and the ACS NSQIP guidelines provide comprehensive information regarding prevention and treatment of VTE (5,33,37).

ANESTHETIC MANAGEMENT

Goals of the anesthetic management

The primary goals of the anesthetic management for these patients are:

- To maintain an optimal cerebral homeostasis: by maintenance of optimal CPP and cerebral oxygenation with stable hemodynamic, respiratory, and metabolic parameters.
- To provide optimal operating conditions for the surgeon (slack brain): by proper positioning of the patient (to facilitate cerebral venous drainage, gravity-assisted retraction of the brain parenchyma) and use of adequate measures to lower the ICP.
- To facilitate a smooth induction, and (if indicated) a smooth postoperative emergence and tracheal extubation to allow an early neurological assessment.
- To facilitate IONM.
- To anticipate and promptly manage potential intraoperative complications.

Anesthesia plan

In addition to the standard concerns pertaining to an STT craniotomy (Table 5.7), several other factors concerning the aging-related vulnerabilities and the altered pharmacology of the administered drugs increase the complexity of anesthetic management of older adults. Aging-related vulnerabilities include:

- Fragile physiological status
- Decreased cardiorespiratory functional reserve; alterations in renal and hepatic functions
- Increased frailty (decreased ability to withstand the stresses of surgery and GA)

Table 5.7 Standard perioperative considerations during supratentorial tumor surgeries

---

Diagnosis, site, size, morphology, invasiveness of the STT and its spatial relation to critical neurovascular structures in the brain
- *Intended surgical procedure and technique of surgery:*
  - Craniotomy and tumor excision/biopsy/ventriculoperitoneal (VP) shunt
  - Open/stereotactic surgery
- *Timing of the surgery:*
  - Elective
  - Expedited: Within days of decision to operate
  - Urgent: Within 24 hours of admission
  - Emergent: Within 2 hours of admission

Surgical approach to the tumor and position of the patient
- *Anesthesia technique:*
  - General anesthesia: For VP shunt, craniotomy
  - Monitored anesthesia care: For awake craniotomy, stereotactic surgery

Evaluation of the intracranial compliance (clinical and radiological features of raised intracranial pressure), to determine the extent of measures required to lower the ICP and provide a slack brain
- *Special perioperative requirements:*
  - Preoperative embolization of vascular tumors
  - Awake craniotomy for language mapping (intraoperative neurophysiological monitoring)
  - TIVA: For IONM
  - Avoidance of NDMRs: For MEP monitoring
  - VAE precautions (for surgeries in proximity to dural venous sinus; bifrontal craniotomy; semi-sitting position, or a marked elevation of the head during positioning)
  - Detection: Precordial Doppler/transesophageal echocardiography with end tidal CO_2 monitoring
  - Need for adjunctive measures for brain relaxation, e.g. placement of a CSF drain ventriculostomy catheter or lumbar drain

Anticipated surgical duration
- *Prevention and prompt management of perioperative complications:*
  - Sudden brain swelling
  - Significant blood loss: e.g. meningioma resection, venous dural sinus injury
  - Venous air embolism
  - Cardio respiratory instability: Due to severe blood loss, air embolism, decreased cardiorespiratory reserve, increased frailty, comorbidities
  - Neurological deficits due to iatrogenic injuries to critical neurovascular structures
- *Need for postoperative elective ventilation:*
  - Poor preoperative neurological status
  - Prolonged duration of surgery
  - Perioperative complication

Abbreviations: STT, supratentorial; VP, ventriculoperitoneal; TIVA, total intravenous anesthesia; IONM, intraoperative neuro electrophysiological monitoring; NDMRs, nondepolarizing muscle relaxants; MEP, motor-evoked potentials; CO_2, carbon dioxide.

- Multiple comorbidities: hypertension, diabetes mellitus, CAD, renal disorders, etc.
- Malnutrition
- Increased risk of postoperative cognitive dysfunction

No well-established recommendations regarding the perioperative management of geriatric neurosurgical patients exist; this is probably because this age group of patients has usually not been considered eligible for most of the clinical trials. Hence the anesthesia plan is largely based on a comprehensive understanding of the intricate interplay of all the above factors and their influence on the perioperative course; therefore, a meticulously planned, individualized management strategy, made with the collective consensus of a multidisciplinary team (neurosurgeon, neuroanesthetist, neurophysiologist, geriatric medicine specialist, oncologist), plays a vital role in the clinical outcome of these patients.

Anesthetic techniques

The majority of neurosurgical interventions for STTs (craniotomy, VP shunts) are performed under GA and controlled ventilation. Monitored anesthesia care may be required for patients undergoing an awake craniotomy for eloquent cortex tumors or a stereotactic biopsy; anesthetic management of these procedures is described elsewhere in the book.

Choice of anesthetic drugs

The most frequently used intravenous anesthetic agents are propofol and thiopentone; unfortunately, they also cause hypotension in elderly patients because of their negative inotropic and vasodilatory effects. Etomidate offers more hemodynamic stability; however, it is associated with risk of adrenal suppression. Dexmedetomidine, an α2-adrenoceptor agonist, provides sedation and analgesia without causing respiratory depression; it is increasingly being used for facilitating faster emergence and a shorter recovery time in neurosurgical patients, as well as for awake craniotomies (38).

The most commonly used inhalational agents are sevoflurane, isoflurane, and desflurane. Sevoflurane causes the least cerebral vasodilatation, with minimal disruption of the CBF–cerebral metabolism coupling at clinically relevant doses; it also has the least myocardial depressant, hypotensive, and arrhythmogenic effect among these agents. Desflurane has lower blood gas solubility; it can facilitate a faster recovery and earlier tracheal extubation in elderly neurosurgical patients (39). Nitrous oxide (N_2O) is preferably avoided as it causes cerebral vasodilatation, increases the CBF, cerebral metabolic rate of oxygen ($CMRO_2$), and ICP, impairs autoregulation, expands air bubbles, aggravates the extent of a VAE, and may also predispose to postoperative nausea and vomiting.

The decision to use an intravenous or inhalational anesthetic agent is largely based on the patient's neurological condition, planned IONM, and the proposed procedure. While both anesthetic agents decrease the $CMRO_2$, propofol is a vasoconstrictor which decreases the CBF, maintains the coupling between $CMRO_2$ and CBF, lowers the ICP, and preserves the cerebral autoregulation and carbon dioxide (CO_2) reactivity. On the other hand, inhaled anesthetics have a dose-dependent effect on the CBF. They cause a decrease in CBF when used in <1.0 minimum alveolar concentration (MAC) doses, and cerebral vasodilatation at higher concentrations, with an associated increase in CBF and an uncoupling between CBF and $CMRO_2$, but with some preservation of CO_2 reactivity; the cerebral vasodilatory effects tend to occur at lower concentrations in a diseased brain with preexisting intracranial hypertension. This "luxury perfusion" may increase the ICP and brain swelling in patients with an already reduced intracranial compliance. However, the cerebral vasodilatory effects can be avoided by hyperventilation to decrease the partial pressure of carbon dioxide ($PaCO_2$). In an open-label study which compared the effects of propofol-fentanyl, isoflurane-fentanyl, or sevoflurane-fentanyl anesthesia, in patients undergoing a STT resection surgery, the ICP was significantly lower, the CPP was higher, and the cerebral swelling after dural opening was also lower in patients who received propofol anesthesia (40).

Hence while intravenous agents are clearly a better choice in patients with marked intracranial hypertension, either of these agents can be used in patients with a normal intracranial compliance; in fact, low-dose inhaled agents are often used effectively as a part of balanced anesthesia to provide optimal operative conditions during craniotomy.

While inhalational agents cause suppression of MEPs and SSEPs (dose-related prolongation of latency and decrease in amplitude), "standard" doses of propofol, opioids, and dexmedetomidine (up to 0.6 ng/mL) typically have little effect on these evoked potentials (EPs). Hence total intravenous anesthesia (TIVA) with propofol/dexmedetomidine-opioid infusion is preferred over inhalational agents (though sensory recordings can also be obtained with <0.5 MAC doses of inhalational agents) if SSEP and MEP monitoring is being performed during the surgery.

Neuromuscular-blocking drugs and opioids have minimal direct effects on cerebrovascular physiology and ICP. Short-acting nondepolarizing muscle relaxants (NDMRs) (e.g., vecuronium, rocuronium, cisatracurium, atracurium) and opioids (fentanyl, remifentanil) are preferred during STT craniotomies of geriatric patients.

Older adults (>65 years) are particularly sensitive to opioid analgesics; use of these drugs is associated with a higher incidence of cognitive dysfunction or delirium, as well as a higher risk for hemodynamic and respiratory impairment; hence they should be used cautiously.

In addition, it is prudent to avoid or be careful with use of medications that have been classified as inappropriate for geriatric use by the American Geriatrics Society Beers Criteria; some of these include barbiturates, benzodiazepines, meperidine and non–Cox nonsteroidal anti-inflammatory drugs (NSAIDs) (41).

Doses of anesthetic drugs

The requirements of most anesthetic drugs decrease by 25%–75% in older patients (5,42). Their onset of action is delayed, and the duration of clinical effect is prolonged; furthermore, the vulnerability to adverse effects of drugs is increased, especially if patients are on multiple medications for various comorbidities. Several factors contribute to these aging-related pharmacological changes:

1. Increased drug potency due to:
   a. Increased free fraction of available drug due to alterations in drug pharmacokinetics and pharmacodynamics (altered volume of

distribution, slower drug metabolism and excretion due to alterations in cardiac output, and renal or hepatic clearance; changes in plasma proteins).
   b. Increased CNS sensitivity of the effect of anesthetic drugs.
2. Synergistic effect of multiple anesthetics, which become even more significant with increasing age; e.g., there is significant reduction in the dose requirement of propofol when midazolam pretreatment is added to standard propofol and fentanyl induction.
3. Multiple morbidities and increased frailty.

Hence it may be prudent to use lower doses of short-acting anesthetics, administered at longer intervals, to avoid the increased risk of prolonged anesthetic action and adverse events. Table 5.8 shows the clinical effect of aging-induced alterations in the pharmacology of commonly used anesthetic drugs and the recommended age appropriate adjustments in their dosages (5).

Preoperative preparation

MONITORING

HR, electrocardiography (ECG), arterial oxygen saturation (SaO_2), end tidal carbon dioxide ($EtCO_2$), invasive arterial BP (IABP) temperature, fluid intake, urine output, arterial blood gases (ABG), serum electrolytes, and glucose levels are routinely monitored during craniotomy. A preinduction arterial access is desirable, as elderly patients are likely to develop hemodynamic perturbations during anesthetic induction; it also enables an analysis of the ABG, hemoglobin, hematocrit, blood glucose, electrolytes, and osmolality (if mannitol or hypertonic saline is used). Serial ABGs should be performed, as the $EtCO_2$ may not correlate well with $PaCO_2$ due to more pronounced ventilation-perfusion mismatch in older patients.

A central venous line is highly recommended if significant intraoperative blood loss or hemodynamic instability is anticipated (e.g., for monitoring of central venous pressure [CVP], mixed venous oxygen saturation, administration of vasoactive drugs and fluids); it is also indicated for aspiration of the entrained air in patients with a risk of VAE (semi-sitting position surgery, risk of venous sinus injury). Occurrence of VAE is best detected

Table 5.8 Clinical effects of aging-related changes in pharmacology of anesthetic drugs and the recommended dose adjustments during anesthesia

Anesthetic agent	Clinical effect of aging-related changes in pharmacology	Recommended dose adjustment of the drug in geriatric patients
Propofol	↑ Blood concentration Delayed recovery	↓ Bolus dose and infusion rate by 40%–50%
Barbiturates	↑ Blood concentration Delayed recovery	↓ Bolus dose by 50% ↓ Infusion rate by 20%
Benzodiazepines	Increased and prolonged clinical effects	↓ Induction dose by 25%–75%
Etomidate	↑ Blood concentration	↓ Bolus dose by 50%
Inhalational agents	MAC ↓ with increasing age Delayed onset and prolonged duration of action	↓ MAC and end tidal concentration by 6% for each decade, after 40 years of age
Opioids	Delayed onset and prolonged duration of action Profound physiological response	↓ Bolus dose and infusion rate by 50%
Depolarizing NMBD	Prolonged clinical effects	Longer dose intervals
Depolarizing NMBD	Prolonged duration of action (atracurium: no change)	↓ Dose by 30% (except for atracurium and cisatracurium)

Abbreviations: MAC, minimum alveolar concentration; NMBD, neuromuscular blocking drug.

by precordial Doppler ultrasonography or transesophageal echocardiography, in combination with changes in the $EtCO_2$.

Temperature monitoring is particularly important, as elderly patients are prone to develop hypothermia due to altered thermoregulation from decreased muscle mass, metabolic rate, and vascular reactivity; it also enables a correct interpretation of IONM (5,43,44).

Monitoring of the depth of neuromuscular block (avoid hemiplegic extremities for monitoring neuromuscular blocking) and anesthetic depth (e.g., bispectral index, patient state index) are also desirable for a more precise titration of the anesthetic agent dosages, and to facilitate early postoperative recovery. SSEP and MEP monitoring are also commonly performed during STT craniotomies. Other monitoring techniques that may be used in specific situations include point-of-care viscoelastic assays (assessment of coagulation status and platelet function), jugular venous bulb oxygen saturation monitoring (global adequacy of cerebral perfusion), and transcranial Doppler ultrasonography (TCD) (assessment of cerebral perfusion; indirect estimation of ICP).

PREMEDICATION AND PRE-INDUCTION

Anticonvulsants, corticosteroids, antihypertensives, and cardiac medications are continued until the morning of surgery; anticoagulant and antiplatelet drugs may be withheld if possible preoperatively, after discussion with a cardiologist. Histamine (H2) blockers and gastric prokinetic agents are administered to counteract the decreased gastric emptying and the higher acid secretion associated with the elevated ICP and corticosteroid therapy; prophylactic 5HT 3 antagonists (e.g., ondansetron) are administered for prevention of nausea and vomiting; antibiotics are administered based on the institutional protocol, within 60 minutes before the surgical incision.

Sequential mechanical compression devices are applied to the lower extremities to reduce the risk of VTE. Normothermia is maintained with the use of forced-air warming blankets, warmed intravenous fluids, closed-circuit anesthesia, and appropriate adjustment of the operating room temperature.

Since these patients are at risk of hypotension during anesthetic induction (increased sensitivity to effect of anesthetic drugs, preoperative hypovolemia [dehydration due to concurrent administration of osmotic diuretics, decreased oral fluid intake, or both], poor cardiopulmonary reserve, concomitant antihypertensive therapy) it is prudent to preload these patients with an isotonic crystalloid (e.g., 0.9% NaCl) prior to induction of anesthesia.

Premedication is preferably avoided in patients with marked intracranial hypertension (risk of hypercarbia due to respiratory depression); small carefully titrated doses of benzodiazepines (e.g., midazolam 0.5–2 mg) and/or opioids (fentanyl 25–100 μg) can be administered in patients with a normal intracranial compliance, under the direct and continuous supervision of the anesthesiologist.

Anesthetic induction and maintenance

Anesthetic induction and tracheal intubation are usually achieved with combination of a sedative–hypnotic drug, intravenous opioid, and a short-acting NDMR, together with gentle hyperventilation administered until laryngoscopy is performed. A balanced technique is used for anesthetic maintenance, and usually includes a combination of an opioid and NDMR along with intravenous and/or inhalational agents. As previously mentioned, TIVA (usually with propofol and fentanyl/remifentanil) is preferred in patients with marked intracranial hypertension, and also when IONM is planned. MEP monitoring precludes the use of NDMRs (causes suppression of MEPs); in addition, a bite block should be placed to prevent tongue laceration during MEP monitoring.

It is imperative that the anesthetic induction and tracheal intubation are as smooth as possible, and without severe fluctuations in the BP. These patients can develop severe hypotension during induction; in addition, the prolonged drug circulation time tends to delay the onset of induction and muscle paralysis. Hence incremental, carefully titrated doses of induction drugs are recommended, to achieve the desired response. Hypotension is treated with a direct-acting vasoconstrictor, provided the patient does not have an incipient CCF.

Pressor responses occur during laryngoscopy and intubation, and are blunted with titrated doses of propofol (0.5 mg/kg), fentanyl (1–2 mg/kg) or remifentanil (0.25–1.0 mg/kg), beta blockers (esmolol [0.5–1 mg/kg] and labetalol [0.5–1 mg/kg]) or lignocaine (1–2 mg/kg) to avoid sudden deleterious spikes in the ICP. Cerebral vasodilating drugs such as nitroglycerin or nitroprusside should be avoided for lowering the BP, as they can increase the cerebral blood volume and the ICP.

Positioning and head fixation

Patients may be placed in the supine, lateral, semi-sitting, park bench, or prone positions, depending on the site and the surgical approach to the lesion. These patients are more vulnerable to peripheral nerve damage and pressure injuries from malpositioning than younger patients, due to their skin atrophy and decreased skin integrity (5). Hence it is important to ensure that their extremities are placed in an anatomically neutral position, there is no overstretching of any extremity or joint, and all pressure points are adequately padded. A combination of gel pads, foam cushions, pillows, and padded armrests are used for these purposes. Eyes should also be protected well to avoid any compression on the eyeballs. The specific precautions to be taken during the positioning of the head and the neck have been described previously in the section "Surgical approaches and patient positioning".

Immobility of the head is achieved with a skeletal pin fixation device (three or four pins), which is linked to the operating table with a Mayfield clamp; this clamp also allows for attachment of the stereotactic guidance system, as well as the magnetic coil for the intraoperative MRI. The insertion and tightening of the skeletal pins has a profoundly stimulating effect on the patient, which can result in a dramatic rise in the sympathetic outflow with associated arterial hypertension, tachycardia, and an increase in the ICP. Increasing the depth of anesthesia (propofol, fentanyl, or remifentanil bolus) or use of an antihypertensive agent, preferably in conjunction with a scalp block or local anesthetic (xylocaine) infiltration at the pin site, helps to reduce the hypertensive response to this highly noxious stimulus. On the other hand, a marked head-up or a semi-sitting position predisposes to postural hypotension, and should be promptly managed.

Intraoperative management

VENTILATION

Ventilatory parameters are adjusted to maintain normocapnia or mild hypocapnia (PaCO$_2$ 30–35 mmHg), mild hyperoxia, and low intrathoracic pressures (to improve cerebral venous return); positive end expiratory pressure, if required, should be used cautiously, as it may decrease the cardiac output and increase the ICP. The cerebral vasoconstriction achieved by the mild hyperventilation and the associated reduction in CBF, cerebral blood volume (CBV), and ICP aid in providing a lax brain. Excessive hyperventilation ($PaCO_2$ <30 mmHg) is detrimental, as the elderly brain is highly vulnerable to the cerebral ischemia caused by extreme cerebral vasoconstriction.

MAINTENANCE OF AN OPTIMAL CPP

These patients are likely to have impaired cerebral autoregulation; hence optimization of the hemodynamic parameters and avoidance of an increase in the ICP are vital for ensuring an adequate cerebral perfusion pressure (CPP = MAP – [ICP +CVP]; MAP: mean arterial pressure). This is achieved by maintaining high normotension (titrated administration of fluids, vasopressors, and/or inotropes, lowering the ICP (by pharmacological and nonpharmacological means), and preventing a rise in the CVP (by avoiding venous overload and obstruction of venous backflow). Though the hemodynamic goals may vary depending on the patient's intracranial pathology, comorbidities, and status of the cerebral autoregulation, generally the aim is to maintain the HR and BP within 20% of baseline awake normal values.

FLUID AND GLYCEMIC MANAGEMENT

Fluid management in older patients needs to be very meticulous; in fact, errors in fluid management are one of the most common causes of avoidable perioperative morbidity and mortality in these patients (45).

Both hypovolemia and hypervolemia are deleterious; hence the aim is to maintain normovolemia with isosmolar crystalloid solutions (e.g., 0.9% isotonic saline, plasmalyte). Colloid solutions can be administered for restoring the intravascular volume following diuresis or moderate blood loss. Hyperglycemia as well as hypo-osmolarity can worsen the cerebral edema, hence glucose-containing or hypo-osmolar solutions (e.g., lactated Ringer's solution, 254 mOsm/kg) should be avoided and the blood glucose should be maintained between 80 and 150 mg/dL.

Dynamic indices of fluid responsiveness (e.g., pulse pressure variation, stroke volume variation) are probably a better predictor of volume status than static markers like CVP and pulmonary capillary wedge pressure (46). In general, goal-directed (e.g., based on optimizing physiologic parameters) or restrictive fluid management strategies seems to improve outcome in elderly patients and may be preferred over fixed-volume strategies, which can cause fluid overload (5).

MEASURES TO REDUCE THE ICP AND PROVIDE OPTIMAL OPERATING CONDITIONS

A lower ICP not only improves the CPP but also helps to provide a slack brain with better maneuverability in deep and tiny corridors, decreased need for retraction of the brain parenchyma, and hence a reduced risk of retraction-induced ischemic brain injury.

Intraoperatively, both nonpharmacological and pharmacological measures are used for this purpose; these are listed in Table 5.9. Usually, the preoperative neurological evaluation (clinical evaluation, neuroimaging) provides a reasonable assessment of the intracranial compliance and the extent of ICP-lowering measures that would be required to provide optimal brain relaxation during the surgery; in addition, the neuroanesthesiologist can directly look at the surgical field to determine the need for additional ICP reduction measures.

Importantly, mannitol, hypertonic saline, or loop diuretics should be used cautiously, as they are entirely excreted in the urine. Elderly patients, especially those with a compromised renal function, hypovolemia, or both, are at risk of developing acute tubular necrosis with use of these drugs.

INTRAOPERATIVE COMPLICATIONS

Intracranial hypertension and fulminant brain swelling

On removal of bone flap, a tight or bulging dura can cause difficulties in the surgical access and increase the likelihood of ischemic brain injury. In addition, sudden brain swelling may occur during resection of the tumor, due to cerebral edema or bleeding inside the tumor. Rapid treatment is required; management is directed toward improving the CPP and reducing the ICP (Tables 5.9 and 5.10); a decompressive craniectomy may be the last resort in patients with refractory intracranial hypertension.

Severe blood loss, coagulopathy, and hemodynamic instability

Rapid and severe blood loss can occur during resection of vascular tumors (e.g., meningiomas)

Table 5.9 Measures to reduce the intracranial pressure and provide optimal operating conditions

Initial measures

Optimal positioning: mild head elevation (15°–30°), optimal neck positioning with no compression of the jugular veins (improves the cerebral venous drainage)

Mild to moderate hyperventilation (PaCO$_2$ 30–35 mmHg); mild hyperoxia (PaO$_2$ >100 mmHg); low airway pressures; minimal or no use of positive end-expiratory pressure

Ensure adequate cerebral perfusion pressure; maintain normovolemia, normotension, and normoglycemia, normothermia

Maintain an adequate depth of anesthesia (to prevent coughing and bucking on the endotracheal tube, which can result in an acute elevation in the ICP)

Corticosteroids (dexamethasone), to decrease the peritumoral vasogenic edema

Osmotic diuretics:

    Mannitol (0.25–1.00 g/Kg initial bolus followed by 0.25–0.50 g/Kg boluses as per requirement) or hypertonic saline (3%; 0.1–1.0 mL/kg/hour, to target a serum sodium level of 145–155 meq/L), 30 min before dural opening or furosemide (0.1–0.2 mg/kg IV), in elderly patients with a compromised cardiac function

(Initial target osmolarity: 300–320 mOsm per liter, serum sodium should not exceed 160 meq/L)

Additional measures in case of a tight brain, prior to dural opening

Brief period of hyperventilation just prior to the dural opening (to rapidly decrease the ICP and facilitate surgical exposure, prior to dural opening during craniotomy)

Addition of furosemide (0.1–0.2 mg/kg IV), in severe cases

Propofol bolus 0.5–1.0 mg/kg, if required (decreases CBF, CMRO$_2$, ICP)

Surgical drainage of cerebral spinal fluid.

Abbreviations: PaCO$_2$, partial pressure of arterial carbon dioxide; PaO$_2$, partial pressure of arterial oxygen; ICP, intracranial pressure; CBF, cerebral blood flow; CMRO$_2$, cerebral metabolic rate of oxygen.

Table 5.10 Management of intraoperative fulminant brain edema

Ensure proper positioning of head and neck, oxygenation, adequate anesthetic depth, normal airway pressures (no bronchospasm, kinking of the endotracheal tube)

Increase hyperventilation

Discontinue volatile agents and nitrous oxide; switch to total intravenous anesthesia (propofol, fentanyl/remifentanil)

Additonal bolus of mannitol (0.25–1.0 g/kg) or 3% NaCl (1–3 mL/kg) or furosemide (0.1–0.2 mg/kg)

Surgical drainage of CSF (external ventricular drain [catheter is inserted into the anterior horn of lateral ventricle and attached to an external drain])

Partial lobectomy/decompressive craniectomy: In cases of refractory intracranial hypertension

or due to an inadvertent dural venous sinus injury, and can result in profound anemia and hemodynamic instability, with significant worsening of the systemic and cerebral homeostasis. This can have an extremely detrimental effect on the perioperative outcome, especially in patients who have a precarious cardiovascular reserve.

The neuroanesthetist should be prepared to promptly detect and manage the blood losses and hemodynamic instability with administration of fluids (crystalloids, colloids), blood products (packed red blood cells, fresh frozen plasma, platelets, cryoprecipitate, etc.) and if required, direct-acting vasopressors (e.g., ephedrine, phenyl epinephrine) and inotropes. Because of the diminished responsiveness to adrenergic drugs, higher drug doses may be required to achieve the desired effect in elderly patients (6). Traditionally, a hemoglobin level of 10 g/dL was considered as the transfusion trigger; however, recent studies recommend that the decision to transfuse blood needs to be individualized; while transfusion is almost always required with a hemoglobin level of <8 g/dL and is rarely needed with hemoglobin levels >10 g/dL, the decision to transfuse blood with hemoglobin levels between 8 and 10 g/dL is usually made on the basis of several factors: overall fluid status, hemodynamic parameters, amount and speed of blood loss, patient's cardiac comorbidities and functional reserve, preoperative neurological condition, signs of inadequate perfusion and oxygenation of vital organs (tachycardia, hypotension, ST segment elevation or depression, onset of arrhythmias), and physiological end-points of oxygen delivery and oxygen requirements (lactate acidosis [lactate >2 mmol/L+ acidosis], decrease in central venous or mixed venous oxygen saturation to below 50% or 60%, respectively). Point-of-care assays (e.g., Sonoclot, Thromboelastogram, Rotem), which are based on intraoperative viscoelastic monitoring of coagulation, may be useful in guiding transfusion of the component therapy. In addition, prophylactic tranexamic acid, an antifibrinolytics drug (10 mg/kg IV bolus followed by 1 mg/kg/h during surgery) can be given to decrease the blood loss and perioperative transfusion requirements when an increased blood loss is anticipated in the perioperative period.

Venous air embolism

Management of VAE includes identification of the source of air and prevention of further air entry (notify the surgeon, flooding of the surgical field, closure of entrainment source, partial left lateral positioning with Trendelenburg tilt [Durant maneuver]), reduction of the volume of air entrained (aspiration of entrained air via multiorifice CVP catheter, discontinue N_2O; administer 100% oxygen), and management of the hemodynamic instability.

Postoperative management

EMERGENCE FROM ANESTHESIA: EARLY OR ELECTIVE DELAYED TRACHEAL EXTUBATION

An early postoperative emergence and tracheal extubation is feasible in most patients with a good preoperative status and an uneventful perioperative course. On the other hand, a planned delayed emergence and tracheal extubation may be a more prudent option in the following situations: preoperative impaired level of consciousness, difficult airway, poor functional performance score, severe

systemic comorbidities (especially cardiopulmonary impairment), a complicated intraoperative course (e.g., prolonged and extensive surgery [>6 hours], especially if associated with significant blood loss), hemodynamic instability, significant brain ischemia (e.g., extensive retractor pressure) and/or excessive brain swelling at closure, major GBM surgery, surgeries with a high risk of postoperative brain edema, and intracranial hypertension. These patients require mechanical ventilation in the intensive care unit; fentanyl/midazolam or propofol/dexmedetomidine infusion can be used for providing sedation during this period.

CONDUCT OF EMERGENCE AND TRACHEAL EXTUBATION

A rapid and smooth emergence with minimal hemodynamic perturbations and coughing/straining against the tracheal tube minimizes the risks of postoperative cerebral edema, intracranial hypertension, and intracranial hematoma. As noted earlier, use of carefully titrated doses of short-acting anesthetic agents is recommended; in particular, use of desflurane and dexmedetomidine is reported to facilitate a faster emergence, a shorter recovery time, and lesser cognitive dysfunction in neurosurgical patients (38,39).

The anesthetic depth is maintained until the pins are removed and dressing is secured, after which the anesthetic agents are gradually weaned, reversal agents are administered (if required), and a trial of spontaneous ventilation is given to determine the adequacy of ventilation and oxygenation. Coughing and straining on the tracheal tube are prevented by administration of a bolus of lidocaine (75–100 µg) or fentanyl (25–50 µg). Carefully titrated doses of labetalol (10–25 mg) or esmolol (25–50 mg) are given for treatment of emergence hypertension (systolic BP >140–160 mmHg).

Tracheal extubation is performed when the patient is fully awake, responsive to verbal commands, with stable hemodynamic and respiratory parameters, no new postoperative deficits, and adequate airway reflexes and muscle strength.

FAILURE TO EMERGE FROM ANESTHESIA

While mild cognitive impairment and lethargy is not uncommon in geriatric patients in the immediate postoperative period, failure to awaken within 30 minutes of cessation of anesthetic drugs should prompt a search for other potential causes of a delayed emergence. A depressed level of consciousness in these patients usually indicates residual anesthesia, most commonly due to an opioid overdose (bilaterally constricted pupils), but it can also be due to other causes, such as an intracranial hematoma, cerebral edema, nonconvulsive status epilepticus, hypoglycemia, electrolyte disturbances, hypothermia, pneumocephalus, vascular occlusion, and ischemia. Subfrontal, especially a bifrontal, craniotomy can also result in a delayed emergence ("frontal lobey" phenomenon due to excessive retraction of frontal lobes).

If an opioid overdose is suspected, carefully titrated small doses of naloxone or naltrexone can be administered to reverse the opioid effect. After nonsurgical causes have been excluded (electrolyte, glucose, temperature, ABG analysis), a brain scan should be performed to detect a hematoma, cerebral edema, or pneumocephalus; if it is negative, a spot EEG may be used to detect seizure activity, and MRI can be obtained to detect ischemic stroke; emergency measures may be required to lower the ICP if the neurological examination is indicative of severe intracranial hypertension and impending cerebral herniation. An intracranial hematoma may require an emergent surgical evacuation if it is causing a significant mass effect.

NEUROINTENSIVE CARE MANAGEMENT

Patients are usually transferred to the neurointensive care unit for postoperative observation, where they are closely monitored for adequacy of oxygenation and ventilation, hemodynamic stability, neurological recovery (especially level of consciousness, pupillary responses, motor examination, features of elevated ICP), pain control, fluid status, electrolytes (sodium, potassium), and glucose levels, and for occurrence of any postoperative complications. AEDs, corticosteroids, H2 blockers, osmotic diuretics, antibiotics, and thromboprophylaxis are continued in the immediate postoperative period, and gradually tapered off over the next few days. AED levels should be checked, as they are often in the subtherapeutic range because of the induced diuresis in the intraoperative

period. Meticulous care is taken to provide relief of postcraniotomy pain, prophylaxis of postoperative nausea and vomiting (PONV), and VTE, and to maintain the fluid and electrolyte balance.

Postcraniotomy pain relief

A multimodal approach using a combination of simple primary non-opioid analgesics (acetaminophen), a scalp nerve block or bupivacaine infiltration of the wound, and if required, small, carefully titrated does of opioids (fentanyl) is recommended for postoperative pain relief.

High-dose opioids are preferably avoided because of the increased sensitivity of older patients to opioids; moreover, the often disturbed cerebral autoregulation in the postoperative period, coupled with the opioid induced hypotension, respiratory depression, and CO_2 retention, can lead to rise an undesirable rise in ICP and decrease in the CPP. Furthermore, the sedation caused by these drugs may interfere with the neurological evaluation (5,41).

While use of NSAIDs has been restricted because of the fear of an intracranial hematoma (due to their antiplatelet activity), this is yet to be proven. While these drugs can be used for providing postcraniotomy analgesia, use of nonselective NSAIDs is not recommended (due to higher risk of gastrointestinal bleeding or peptic ulcer disease, especially with concomitant administration of parenteral corticosteroids, anticoagulants, or antiplatelet agents) (41).

PONV

5-HT3 receptor antagonists, such as ondansetron (4 mg IV) and granisetron (1 mg IV), are most commonly used for prophylaxis of PONV (caution: QT prolongation, serotonin syndrome); administration of dexamethasone also helps to reduce PONV (5,41).

Thromboprophylaxis

Mechanical thromboprophylaxis with intermittent pneumatic compression devices is continued in the postoperative period; early mobilization and maintenance of adequate hydration is encouraged. Considering the high risk of VTE in these patients, it may also be prudent to add pharmacological prophylaxis (with unfractionated heparin or low molecular weight heparin) once adequate hemostasis has been established (24–48 hours after surgery), after discussion with the neurosurgeon (32).

Occurrence of extremity pain or swelling should prompt an early Doppler ultrasound evaluation to detect DVT; chest CT should be done if the patient develops respiratory symptoms or pleuritic pain suggestive of pulmonary embolism.

Postoperative complications

Postoperative complications after STT surgeries may be neurological (neurological deterioration, neurological deficits, seizures), systemic (e.g., myocardial infarction, pulmonary thromboembolism, urinary tract infections, pneumonia, electrolyte disturbances—especially hyponatremia) and/ or regional (surgical site infection/abscess, etc.). The incidence of these complications is higher in patients who have a low preoperative KPS score, severe intraoperative blood losses, high tumor severity score (combining tumor location, mass effect, and midline shift), prolonged duration of surgery, or preexisting comorbidities (1,47). The following sections provide an overview of the pertinent neurological complications that can complicate the postoperative course of these patients.

NEUROLOGICAL COMPLICATIONS

Postoperative neurological complications are usually a consequence of direct injury to the brain tissue or cerebral vessels, brain edema, ICH, seizures, ischemia (reversible and irreversible); rarely, vasospasm may contribute to neurological deficit, especially if the surgery involves manipulation of arterial vessels, e.g. during a transsylvian approach to an insular glioma.

Edema and herniation

Significant postoperative brain edema can occur due to several reasons: presence of extensive preoperative edema, direct brain tissue manipulation/excessive retraction during the surgery, subtotal resection of malignant gliomas (effect of edema exerted from the residual tumor and necrosis on adjacent normal brain tissue), surgery of deep intrinsic tumors in which only minimal resection was possible, and after resection of highly infiltrating tumors that involve a large amount of WM. Maximal postoperative swelling usually occurs within one to the first

five days after the surgery, however it may also manifest earlier, in the immediate postoperative period, in patients with high-grade gliomas; though rare, this "wounded glioma syndrome" can evolve rapidly and result in acute brain herniation.

Intracranial hematoma

An intraparenchymal hematoma usually occurs due to a suboptimal hemostasis within the tumor bed or in association with a subtotal tumor resection (residual tumor predisposes to edema as well as hemorrhage: wounded glioma syndrome). Patients usually manifest with focal neurological changes, seizures, and/or deterioration in the level of consciousness.

Venous infarct

Neurological deterioration can also occur due to development of venous infarct (e.g., due to compromise of vein of Labbé, vein of Trolard, or of any large cortical vein draining into the sagittal sinus). Typically, the signs and symptoms manifest 2–3 days after the surgery as the venous congestion develops within the drainage field of the compromised vein and results in increased pressure and infarction; e.g., compromise of vein of Labbé can lead to a swollen temporal lobe, with a risk of cerebral herniation. These patients need aggressive medical measures to control the intracranial hypertension; an anterior temporal lobectomy may be required in patients with refractory intracranial hypertension.

CONCLUSION

Geriatric patients are at a high risk of complications during the postoperative period. Meticulous care, intensive monitoring, including the use of ICP and transcranial Doppler ultrasonography, prompt detection, and aggressive management of these postoperative complications is the key to a good clinical outcome in this vulnerable group of patients.

REFERENCES

1. Seddighi A, Vaezi M, Seddighi1 AS. et al. Brain tumors in elderly. *Intl Clin Neurosci J.* 2015;2(2):55–65.
2. Flowers A. Brain tumors in the older person. *Cancer Control.* 2000;7(6):523–38.

3. Atlas SW. Adult supratentorial tumors. *Semin Roentgenol.* 1990;25(2):130–54.

4. Alvis BD, Hughes CG. Physiology considerations in the geriatric patient. *Anesthesiol Clin.* 2015;33(3):447–56.

5. Mohanty S, Rosenthal RA, Russell MM, Neuman MD, Ko CY, Esnaola NF. Optimal perioperative management of the geriatric patient: A best practices guideline from the ACS NSQIP/American Geriatrics Society 2016. *J Am Coll Surg.* 2016;222(5):930–47.

6. Akhtar S, Rooke GA. Cardiovascular ageing. In: Dodds C, Kumar CM, Veering BT (eds). *Oxford Textbook of Anesthesia for the Elderly Patient.* 1st ed. United Kingdom: Oxford University Press; 2014. pp. 41–52.

7. Canet J, Sanchis J. Respiratory ageing. In: Dodds C, Kumar CM, Veering BT (eds). *Oxford Textbook of Anesthesia for the Elderly Patient.* 1st ed. United Kingdom: Oxford University Press; 2014. pp. 53–8.

8. Prakash A, Krishnan K. Ageing at system level: neurological ageing. In: Dodds C, Kumar CM, Veering BT (eds). *Oxford Textbook of Anesthesia for the Elderly Patient.* 1st ed. United Kingdom: Oxford University Press; 2014. pp. 37–40.

9. Gupta D. Neuroanatomy. In: Prabhakar H (ed). *Essentials of Neuroanesthesia.* 1st ed. United Kingdom: Elsevier; 2017. pp. 3–40.

10. Louis DN, Perry A, Reifenberger G et al. The 2016 World Health Organization classification of tumors of the central nervous system: A summary. *Acta Neuropathol.* 2016;131(6): 803–20.

11. Chaichana KL, Garzon-Muvdi T, Parker S et al. Supratentorial glioblastoma multiforme: The role of surgical resection versus biopsy among older patients. *Ann Surg Oncol.* 2011;18(1):239–45.

12. Fisher JL, Wrensch M, Wiemels JL, Schwartzbaum JA. Epidemiology of brain tumors. In: Win HR (ed). *Youmans Neurological Surgery.* 6th ed. Philadelphia PA: Elsevier Saunders; 2011. pp. 1179–87.

13. Hinojosa AQ, Kosztowski T, Brem H. Malignant gliomas: Anaplastic astrocytoma, glioblastoma multiforme, gliosarcoma. In: Win HR (ed). *Youmans Neurological Surgery.* 6th ed. Philadelphia PA: Elsevier Saunders; 2011. pp. 1327–40.

14. Lee I, Rosenblum ML. Invasion in malignant glioma. In: Win HR (ed). *Youmans Neurological Surgery.* 6th ed. Philadelphia PA: Elsevier Saunders; 2011. pp. 1141–50.

15. Babu R, Komisarow JM, Agarwal VJ et al. Glioblastoma in the elderly: The effect of aggressive and modern therapies on survival. *J Neurosurg.* 2016;124(4):998–1007.

16. Okada M, Miyake K, Tamiya T. Glioblastoma treatment in the elderly. *Neurol Med Chir (Tokyo).* 2017;57(12):667–76.

17. Almenawer SA, Badhiwala JH, Alhazzani W et al. Biopsy versus partial versus gross total resection in older patients with high-grade glioma: A systematic review and meta-analysis. *Neuro Oncol.* 2015;17:868–81.

18. Noorbakhsh A, Tang JA, Marcus LP et al. Gross-total resection outcomes in an elderly population with glioblastoma: A SEER-based analysis. *J Neurosurg.* 2014;120:31–9.

19. Al-Mefty O, Abdulrauf SI, Haddad GF. Meningiomas. In: Win HR (ed). *Youmans Neurological Surgery.* 6th ed. Philadelphia PA: Elsevier Saunders; 2011. pp. 1426–49.

20. Tin-Chung Poon M, Hing-Kai Fung L, Kan-Suen Pu J, Ka-Kit Leung G. Outcome of elderly patients undergoing intracranial meningioma resection – A systematic review and meta-analysis. *Br J Neurosurg.* 2014;28:3, 303–9.

21. Chen ZY Zheng CH, Tang Li et al. Intracranial meningioma surgery in the elderly (over 65 years): Prognostic factors and outcome. *Acta Neurochir (Wien).* 2015;157:1549–57.

22. Weingart JD, Brem H. Basic principles of cranial surgery for brain tumors. In: Win HR (ed). *Youmans Neurological Surgery.* 6th ed. Philadelphia PA: Elsevier Saunders; 2011. pp. 1261–6.

23. Lang FF, Chang EL, Suki D, Wildrick DM, Sawaya R. Metastatic brain tumors. In: Win HR (ed). *Youmans Neurological Surgery.* 6th ed. Philadelphia PA: Elsevier Saunders; 2011. pp. 1410–25.

24. Rozet I, Vavilala MS. Risks and benefits of patient positioning during neurosurgical care. *Anesthesiol Clin.* 2007;25(3):631–53.

25. Castellano A, Cirillo S, Bello L, Riva M, Falini A. Functional MRI for surgery of gliomas. *Curr Treat Options Neurol.* 2017;19(10):34.

26. Young RM, Jamshidi A, Davis G, Sherman JH. Current trends in the surgical management and treatment of adult glioblastoma. *Ann Transl Med.* 2015;3(9):121.

27. Garrett MC, Pouratian N, Liau LM. Use of language mapping to aid in resection of gliomas in eloquent brain regions. *Neurosurg Clin N Am.* 2012;23(3):497–506.

28. Koht A, Sloan TB. Evoked response monitoring. In: Prabhakar H (ed). *Neuromonitoring Techniques: Quick Guide for Clinicians and Residents.* 1st ed. United Kingdom: Elsevier; 2018. pp. 148–77.

29. Chacko AG, Thomas SG, Babu KS et al. Awake craniotomy and electrophysiological mapping for eloquent area tumours. *Clin Neurol Neurosurg.* 2013;115(3):329–34.

30. Della Puppa A, Rustemi O, Gioffrè G et al. Application of indocyanine green video angiography in parasagittal meningioma surgery. *Neurosurg Focus.* 2014;36:E13.

31. Shah A, Rangarajan V, Kaswa A, Jain S, Goel A. Indocyanine green as an adjunct for resection of insular gliomas. *Asian J Neurosurg.* 2016; 11(3):276–81.

32. Warnick RE. Surgical complications of brain tumors and their avoidance. In: Win HR (ed). *Youmans Neurological Surgery.* 6th ed. Philadelphia PA: Elsevier Saunders; 2011. pp. 1285–92.

33. Chow WB, Rosenthal RA, Merkow RP, Ko CY, Esnaola NF. Optimal preoperative assessment of the geriatric surgical patient: A best practices guideline from the American College of Surgeons National Surgical Quality Improvement Program and the American Geriatrics Society. *J Am Coll Surg.* 2012;215(4):453–66.

34. Gállego Pérez-Larraya J, Delattre JY. Management of elderly patients with gliomas. *Oncologist.* 2014;19:1258–67.

35. Glantz MJ, Cole BF, Forsyth PA et al. Practice parameter: Anticonvulsant prophylaxis in patients with newly diagnosed brain tumors. Report of the Quality Standards Subcommittee of the American Academy of Neurology. *Neurology.* 2000;54(10):1886–93.

36. Sayegh ET, Fakurnejad S, Oh T, Bloch O, Parsa AT. Anticonvulsant prophylaxis for brain tumor surgery: Determining the current best available evidence. *J Neurosurg.* 2014;121(5):1139–47.

37. Gould MK, Garcia DA, Wren SM et al. Prevention of VTE in nonorthopaedic surgical patients: Antithrombotic therapy and prevention of thrombosis. 9th ed. American College of Chest Physicians Evidence-Based Clinical Practice Guidelines. *Chest J.* 2012; 141(2_suppl):e227S–77S.

38. Soliman RN, Hassan AR, Rashwan AM et al. Prospective, randomized study to assess the role of dexmedetomidine in patients with supratentorial tumors undergoing craniotomy under general anaesthesia. *Middle East J Anesthesiol.* 2011;21(3):325–33.

39. Iannuzzi E, Iannuzzi M, Viola G, Cerulli A, Cirillo V, Chiefari M. Desflurane and sevoflurane in elderly patients during general anesthesia: A double blind comparison. *Minerva Anestesiol.* 2005;71:147–55.

40. Petersen KD, Landsfeldt U, Cold GE et al. Intracranial pressure and cerebral hemodynamic in patients with cerebral tumors: A randomized prospective study of patients subjected to craniotomy in propofol-fentanyl, isoflurane-fentanyl, or sevoflurane-fentanyl anesthesia. *Anesthesiology.* 2003;98(2): 329–36.

41. The American Geriatrics Society 2012. Beers Criteria Update Expert Panel. American Geriatrics Society updated Beers Criteria for potentially inappropriate medication use in older adults. *J Am Geriatr Soc Apr* 2012; 60(4):616–31.

42. Akhtar S, Ramani R. Geriatric pharmacology. *Anaesthesiology Clin.* 2015;33(3):457–69.

43. LacKamp A, Seiber F. Physiologic response to anesthesia in the elderly. In: Rosenthal R, Zenilman M, Katlic M (eds). *Principles and Practice of Geriatric Surgery.* New York: Springer; 2011. p. 300.

44. Esnaola NF, Cole DJ. Perioperative normothermia during major surgery: Is it important? *Adv Surg.* 2011;45:249–63.

45. Powell-Tuck J, Gosling P, Lobo D et al. British Consensus Guidelines on Intravenous

Fluid Therapy for Adult Surgical patients. 2008.

46. Marik PE, Cavallazzi R, Vasu T, Hirani A. Dynamic changes in arterial waveform derived variables and fluid responsiveness in mechanically ventilated patients: A systematic review of the literature. *Crit Care Med.* 2009;37(9):2642–7.

47. Asano K, Nakano T, Takeda T, Ohkuma H. Risk factors for postoperative systemic complications in elderly patients with brain tumors. *J Neurosurg.* 2009;111:258–64.

6

Neurosurgery: Posterior fossa surgery

NIDHI GUPTA

INTRODUCTION

With an increase in the life expectancy of people, the number of elderly patients presenting to medical services has increased dramatically in recent years. Furthermore, the incidence of intracranial tumors in this patient population is increasing day by day, partly due to incidental diagnoses of asymptomatic tumors associated with widespread use of cranial imaging (1).

Geriatric patients represent a complex subset of patients in view of their ageing physiology, multiple comorbidities, polypharmacy, cognitive dysfunction, geriatric syndromes (including frailty) and unpredictable life expectancy (2). Consequently, surgical options in this patient population have historically been fraught with an increased risk of perioperative morbidity and mortality. However, relief of debilitating or life-threatening neurological symptoms is also important to attain a better quality of life or to maintain an acceptable level of functioning in patients suffering from posterior fossa pathology. Moreover, development of newer minimally invasive neurosurgical techniques, better neurocritical care and advancing technology in the field of neuroanesthesia has led to refinement of neurosurgical practice in recent times. All these aspects have led to an increase in the number and variety of cases that are now being considered amenable to surgical management in geriatric population, with considerable ease and safety.

The existing literature on the appropriate neuroanaesthetic management of elderly patients planned for posterior fossa surgery is scarce. In general, posterior fossa surgery is associated with unique perioperative considerations such as varied surgical positioning and their associated complications, lengthy surgical procedures, intraoperative cardiovascular changes, potential for brainstem injury with consequent respiratory problems and sudden neurological deterioration in event of postoperative hematoma or acute obstructive hydrocephalus (3). Advancing age further adds to the complexity of this surgery, thus posing significant challenges to the attending neuroanaesthesiologists. The purpose of this chapter is to review the age-appropriate changes in the management of elderly patients scheduled to undergo posterior fossa surgery.

RELEVANT ANATOMY

The posterior cranial fossa is bordered anteriorly and laterally by the superior border of the petrous temporal bone, anteriorly and medially by the dorsum sellae of sphenoid bone, superiorly by the tentorium cerebelli (a wide tent-shaped fold of the dura which lies between the occipital lobe superiorly and the cerebellum inferiorly) and inferiorly by the foramen magnum. It primarily houses the brainstem (midbrain, pons and upper medulla), cerebellar hemispheres (essential for motor coordination) and the vertebrobasilar vascular system.

Brainstem is located ventrally to cerebellum and contains third to twelfth cranial nerve (CN) nuclei (essential for control of respiration and cardiovascular system) along with the numerous ascending and descending tracts. Hence, any small lesion or injury to the brainstem can damage multiple nuclei and tracts within, resulting in significant cardiovascular and neurological compromise. Similarly, because of close proximity, cerebellar pathologies including edema, haematoma or tumor can potentially compress and injure the brainstem.

During posterior fossa craniotomies, the intraoperative risk of bleeding and venous air embolism (VAE) is high in view of multiple large venous sinuses contained within the tentorial dural fold. Furthermore, the cerebrospinal fluid (CSF) pathway is very narrow through this region and any obstructive pathology may lead to acute hydrocephalus, which may manifest as a life-threatening increase in intracranial pressure (ICP).

POSTERIOR FOSSA LESIONS AND THEIR PRESENTING FEATURES IN ELDERLY

Cerebellopontine angle (CPA) tumours, located in the space between the cerebellum and pons, are the most common neoplasms in the posterior fossa of an adult patient, accounting for approximately 5%–10% of intracranial tumours (4). A significant fraction of CPA tumours are acoustic neuromas, a benign slow growing tumour arising from the Schwann cells of the vestibulocochlear nerve (CN VIII), usually starting in the internal auditory canal and growing outward into the posterior fossa, eventually compressing the brainstem. Elderly patients may present with progressive hearing loss (100%), tinnitus (35%), vertigo (15%), headache (45%) and unsteadiness (95%) due to compression of intracranial structures (5). In addition, the proximity of the eighth CN to the seventh and fifth CN's may lead to the tumours manifesting as ipsilateral facial palsy and facial numbness or tingling (65%). Compared to their younger counterparts, geriatric patients aged 70 years or older are over nine times more likely to experience subjective imbalance or unsteadiness (5). Similarly, fatigue and alteration in taste and lacrimation are seen more commonly in elderly patients. Headache is a less frequently reported symptom in elderly than the young patients.

Elderly patients diagnosed with acoustic neuromas are usually managed either conservatively (consisting of observation and routine radiographic monitoring of tumor size progression and new symptom development) or by radiosurgery (6). However, microsurgical resection is indicated in up to 50% of patients with refractory symptoms or in the setting of progressive neurological deterioration with brainstem compression associated with large tumors (1,5). In an analysis of the 2002–2010 National Inpatient Sample (NIS) database from United States, Sylvester et al. found that the elderly acoustic neuroma surgery patients were significantly more likely to be female with multiple comorbidities (hypertension, diabetes mellitus and chronic pulmonary disease) and required nonelective admission (7). During preoperative evaluation of these patients, it is important to remember that auditory function is often impaired, mostly due to age related presbyacousia. Hence, formal audiometric evaluation should be performed in case of an elderly patient with diminished hearing, since hearing aids may help several geriatric syndromes like gait disorders, falls, cognitive disturbances, and depression. Information obtained from a detailed patient history as well as formal evaluations (such as the Weber and Rinne tests) may help differentiate between sensorineural and conductive patterns of hearing loss. Furthermore, studies have found that elderly patients continue to have poor balance function even postoperatively (5,8). Apparently elderly patients have poorer functional and vestibular reserves than younger patients and other concomitant age-related issues affecting the global body balance, such as poorer visual acuity, diminished proprioception or cerebellar function, and a higher incidence of contralateral vestibular hypofunction. This may result in greater sensitivity to any vestibular insult associated with surgical resection of tumor, thus prolonging recovery and hospital stay. Hence, appropriate preoperative counselling and postoperative care planning should be done. Furthermore, though surgery remains an important curative treatment modality in the elderly, increased risks of surgery, must be thoroughly weighed against risks of conservative management, when counselling the geriatric patients (7).

Brainstem gliomas (BSG) are uncommon tumors in adults, constituting only 2% of all brain tumors. The most frequent presenting symptom is headache, which can be a manifestation of hydrocephalus. CN deficits primarily affecting the lower cranial nerves (LCN) and long-tract findings (spasticity of the limbs with extensor plantar reflexes) are also common. "Crossed" deficits, is another hallmark of brainstem pathology, characterized by facial signs and symptoms contralateral to arm and/or leg signs and symptom (9). Malignant high-grade BSG are rare in elderly with an overall poorer prognosis. Babu et al. reported seven elderly patients with malignant BSG, with a median age at onset of 65 years (10). Majority of patients in this cohort were male and Caucasian. Tumors were most commonly located in the pons (85.7%), with one tumor located in the tectal plate. The most common symptoms included facial weakness, blurry vision, headache, and extremity weakness. Majority of patients had a cranial neuropathy, with the most common CN affected on neurological examination being CN III, IV, and VI, found in 42.9% of patients. No palsies of CN I, V, IX, X, and XII were seen. Compared to younger patients, these tumors appear to be more aggressive with rapid tumor growth and infiltration in elderly patients as nearly 71.4% of patients had supratentorial extension of tumor and only two weeks of symptoms prior to surgery. Authors, thus recommended aggressive chemoradiotherapy which may result in improved survival in elderly patients while surgical resection may be considered for select patients in which the tumor is mostly exophytic (near the brainstem surface) and easily accessible or for tumors resulting in significant mass effect and obstructive hydrocephalus.

Brainstem cavernoma are another rare entity in elderly population and are most frequently found in pons (11). Patients often present with sudden bleeding/rebleeding episodes causing severe neurological deficits including ataxia, dysarthria, hemiplegia, quadriplegia and disturbances in consciousness. Apart from age related neurosurgical concerns in elderly, surgical excision of these cavernomas is in general difficult in view of their location and bleeding risk. However, compared to their young counterparts, elderly patients undergo rapid neurological deterioration in the event of rebleeding, leading to worsened outcomes. Thus, radical resection of the cavernoma in patients with severe symptoms, especially in those with multiple rebleeding events, may be recommended even in elderly patients, to remove the mass effect on brainstem and prevent further bleeding episodes (11). Surgery is best advised during the subacute phase of bleed, that is, when the hematoma is liquefied, to allow maximum removal of the hematoma with a minimal brainstem damage, thus facilitating neurological recovery (11,12).

Tumours in the region of the fourth ventricle usually present with signs and symptoms of acute hydrocephalus, including headache, nausea or vomiting. Lethargy and altered consciousness may be the initial symptoms of increased ICP in elderly. Bradycardia and hypertension may coexist, in part due to the local compression of vital cardiovascular centres within the brainstem.

Extra-axial tumours involving the posterior fossa consist mainly of meningiomas and neuromas encasing CN. Meningiomas are benign tumors for which surgery can potentially achieve excellent long-term outcome as long as the risks of surgery are acceptable. Other treatment options include waiting with close observation and radiosurgery. Surgical option, however, appears logical in view of slow but sustained growth pattern observed during serial radiological follow up. Nakamura et al. recommend surgery for elderly patients in good general medical condition (American Society of Anesthesiologists [ASA] Class 1–3) harbouring CPA meningiomas of even small or medium size, when the tumour has become symptomatic (13). Though recent literature suggests a comparable 1-year mortality rate following meningioma resection in the elderly compared to younger patients with acceptable outcomes (14) patients with severe systemic disease (ASA Class 4 or 5) and meningiomas located at the base of the skull, especially the posterior fossa, have been reported to have poorer outcomes in view of poor tolerance of even transient postoperative LCN deficits (15). Hence, surgical decision should be made on an individual basis taking pre-operative physical status, comorbidities and tumour location into account.

Cerebellar ischemic stroke and spontaneous cerebellar hemorrhage are another common entity causing major morbidity in the elderly population. Emergent surgical decompression is recommended by the American Stroke Association in patients with evidence of brainstem compression, hydrocephalus or clinical deterioration (16). However, emergency posterior fossa decompressive surgery for cerebellar infarctions or hematomas surgery in elderly patients has been found to be associated with a significant increase in hospital stay and mortality (17). Hence, appropriate counselling of family members should be done to help make an informed decision.

ANESTHETIC CONSIDERATIONS DURING POSTERIOR FOSSA CRANIOTOMY

Preoperative evaluation

The basic principles of pre-anaesthetic evaluation for any neurosurgical procedure should be followed, including a detailed medical history, clinical examination and investigations (3). Of note, history suggestive of any motor or sensory deficits, specific LCN involvement (such as impaired gag reflex or a weak cough), previous neurosurgical procedures and prior stoke or transient ischemic attack should be recorded. Localizing signs for the brainstem and cerebellar signs (ataxia, nystagmus, etc.) should be elicited. Imaging of the brain should be reviewed for the location and size of the pathology to assess the best surgical approach and appropriate patient-positioning, proximity of the lesion to sinuses and major blood vessels and to look for signs of hydrocephalus or raised ICP.

With normal aging, the maximal physiologic body reserves decline, thus limiting the ability of elderly patients to respond to the stress of major surgery. Thus, careful evaluation of the cardiovascular, respiratory, neurological, renal, haematological/immunological and musculoskeletal systems is of paramount importance in elderly patients undergoing major neurosurgical procedures. Moreover, elderly patients may present with several pre-existing comorbidities, including diabetes, cardiovascular disease, chronic obstructive pulmonary disease (COPD), renal insufficiency, thyroid disorders, thromboembolic disorders, cognitive decline, undernutrition, sarcopenia, malignancies, chronic smoking and alcoholism. Hence, one of the main goals of preoperative evaluation in elderly patients is identification, risk stratification and optimization of co-existing medical problems.

Preoperative evaluation of elderly patients posted for elective posterior fossa surgery should be done few days prior to surgery to allow preoperative optimization and pharmacological manipulation of chronic co-morbidities. Even for an emergency surgery, preoperative optimization should begin as early as possible to achieve best possible postoperative outcomes.

Dehydration and the electrolyte abnormalities may be present in presence of preoperative diabetes insipidus, nausea and vomiting due to raised ICP, inadequate oral intake in patients with altered consciousness or administration of osmotic diuretics and radiological contrast agents. Since, hypovolaemia may be difficult to recognize in elderly patients in absence of reactive tachycardia, it should be proactively identified and corrected preoperatively. Fluid resuscitation must be carried out carefully to avoid fluid overload in view of volume intolerance. Elderly patients with comorbidities are frequently on multiple medications, including antihypertensives and cardioprotective medications (β-blockers, statins, antiplatelet medication in patients with coronary artery stent *in situ*), oral hypoglycaemics, insulin and/or renal dialysis. Hence, the neuroanaesthesiologist must formulate the best drug plan perioperatively, in close consultation with a geriatrician and the neurosurgeon. Of note, medications with significant vasodilatory and bleeding potential (e.g., angiotensin-converting enzyme inhibitors, angiotensin receptor blockers, non-steroidal anti-inflammatory drugs and antiplatelets) should be withheld prior to surgery, as per the recent guidelines (18,19).

The overall anaesthetic risk should be assessed based on the severity of the patient's medical condition and invasiveness of proposed procedure. Since, majority of neurosurgical procedures in the elderly are of intermediate to higher risk, it seems rational to obtain a 12-lead electrocardiography (ECG) and 2-D echocardiography prior to surgery to obtain a baseline for comparison. Exercise tolerance is probably a better predictor of cardiorespiratory complications than laboratory testing. Hence, stress testing should be reserved for patients with known or suspected cardiac disease or a history of lower functional reserve (as measured by metabolic equivalents).

Routine preoperative chest x-rays do not add any meaningful information to the preoperative clinical examination of patients, although abnormalities are found more frequently in patients older than 70. Chest x-ray is, however, indicated in symptomatic patients, those with suspected but undiagnosed pulmonary disease and in patients undergoing higher risk non-thoracic procedures. Furthermore, after posterior fossa surgery, elderly patients are less tolerant to postoperative LCN deficits with a higher risk of aspiration and postoperative pneumonia (13). Hence, a preoperative chest X ray may help to estimate the existing lung condition and help decide regarding early tracheostomy in the event of LCN injury. Preoperative lung expansion techniques including deep breathing maneuvers, incentive spirometry and chest physiotherapy helps to optimize respiratory reserves and should be a part of preoperative preparation of elderly patients.

The pre-operative assessment should also include consideration of the suitability of the patient for the proposed position during surgery. A clear communication should be made with the neurosurgeon regarding the planned surgical procedure and proposed patient position, explaining whether it is appropriate for the pathophysiological status of the patient or to suggest a suitable alternative. Patients should be screened for any co-existing cranio-vertebral junctional abnormalities or carotid artery disease through dynamic cervical spine imaging and Doppler study of neck vessels to look out for carotid insufficiency. Cervical spine instability or restricted neck mobility may result in an increased risk of difficulty in securing the airway and difficulty in patient positioning. Similarly, carotid artery stenosis may lead to cerebral hypoperfusion in elderly when extreme neck flexion is performed (20). For patients planned for surgery in semi-sitting position, a contrast-enhanced transcranial Doppler or a bubble contrast transthoracic echocardiography (TEE) study should be performed to detect the presence of a right-to-left shunt through a patent foramen ovale (PFO). If a PFO is detected, its endoscopic closure should be attempted preoperatively, as per the institutional protocols (21).

In the end, a detailed written informed consent explaining the existing neurological condition of patient, co-existing medical comorbidities along with their stratified risk, risks and benefits of having or not having surgery, how the proposed intervention might affect the quantity or quality of a patient's remaining life, possibility of need for post-operative ventilation or tracheostomy and extended intensive care unit (ICU) stay should be obtained from the patient or family members.

Induction and maintenance

The basic anaesthetic goals during anesthetic induction and maintenance in elderly patients undergoing posterior fossa surgery includes:

- Attaining optimal anaesthetic depth during induction to avoid hypotension as well as prevent sympathetic response to laryngoscopy
- Ensuring adequate cerebral oxygenation
- Avoiding any increase in ICP
- Careful patient positioning, thus avoiding or minimizing the possibility of positioning related complications
- Anesthetic modifications for facilitating intraoperative neurophysiological monitoring (IONM)
- Prevention, early identification and effective management of intraoperative complications such as VAE and haemodynamic instability
- Smooth and rapid emergence

Appropriate non-invasive monitoring (pulse oximetry, non-invasive blood pressure and ECG) should be started prior to induction. In patients with signs of increased ICP or significant cardiac illness, establishing invasive arterial blood pressure (ABP) monitoring prior to induction enables prompt detection and treatment of any haemodynamic instability. Induction is achieved by administering an appropriate dose of an induction agent, an opiate and a muscle relaxant, taking into account the haemodynamic status and pharmacological considerations in elderly (22). With aging, there is decreased baroreceptor sensitivity, which impairs the ability to compensate for even short-term changes in blood pressure by an increase in heart rate. Hence, slow titration of both induction and maintenance anesthetics to the desired effect is of paramount importance to maintain stable haemodynamics. In patients with significant cardiovascular comorbidity, anaesthesia-induced decrease in systemic vascular resistance (SVR) may be prevented by phenylephrine, an alpha-1-agonist, to maintain normal vascular tone.

After induction of anaesthesia, endotracheal intubation is usually performed with an appropriate-sized reinforced cuffed endotracheal tube. Further monitoring devices such as a temperature probe, urinary catheter, and central venous catheters are sited after induction of anaesthesia. Head pin application is a potent stimulant and should be performed after infiltration of a local anaesthetic agent and a bolus of a short-acting opiate. Anaesthesia may be maintained with either volatile agents or intravenous agents. All volatile anesthetics engender myocardial depression, increases myocardial sensitivity to catecholamies, and causes significant vasodilatation. As elderly patients are unable to effectively compensate for the vasodilatory effects of the volatile anesthetics, there may be significant hemodynamic instability (23). Furthermore, volatile anesthetics may have a long and unpredictable duration of action in elderly compared to younger patients, thus delaying emergence (22). Use of nitrous oxide (N_2O) is controversial in posterior fossa craniotomies as it has been implicated in increasing the risk and severity of VAE, postoperative nausea and vomiting (PONV) and tension pneumocephalus (24). Though recent literature lends support to the use of N_2O in neurologically and cardiovascularly "at risk" patients undergoing major non-cardiac surgery (25,26); considering high-risk of PONV after posterior fossa craniotomy and poor tolerance of adverse effects of VAE, avoidance of N_2O appears reasonable in elderly patients with pre-existing poor pulmonary function (27). Recent literature also suggests total intravenous anesthesia (TIVA) as the most commonly employed technique for anaesthetic maintenance during posterior fossa craniotomy as rapid emergence may be facilitated by using short-acting drugs such as propofol and remifentanil (28). In addition, TIVA facilitates IONM, commonly employed during posterior fossa craniotomy.

Intraoperative monitoring

Elderly patients undergoing posterior fossa surgery should undergo uninterrupted monitoring of ECG, pulse oximetry, capnography, and invasive ABP, throughout the course of the surgery, including during patient positioning. Additional monitors include measuring hourly urine output and fluid intake, oesophageal temperature monitoring and neuromuscular monitoring. Special monitoring during posterior fossa surgery includes monitoring for VAE and neurophysiological monitoring because of high-risk of VAE and neurological injury. Continuous invasive ABP monitoring is

quintessential in view of associated cardiac comorbidities and high incidence of intraoperative haemodynamic instability associated with posterior fossa surgery. ABP monitoring further allows repeated assessment of arterial blood gases, haemoglobin concentration and blood glucose, thus assisting to optimize ventilatory and glycaemic control and blood transfusion. During semisitting craniotomies, the arterial line transducer should be located and zeroed at the level of tragus to estimate accurate cerebral perfusion pressure (CPP).

Cardiac output (CO) monitors have a limited evidence in elderly population and may be less accurate, owing to poorly compliant vessels (2). However, in patients with significant cardiovascular morbidity and/or planned for surgery in semisitting position, less invasive CO monitors (e.g. PiCCO system [Pulsion Medical Systems, Munich, Germany and Philips Medical Systems], Vigileo FloTrac monitor [Edwards LifeSciences, Irvine, CA], LiDCO monitor [LiDCO, Cambridge, UK]) may be contemplated to guide intraoperative fluid and inotrope management.

In addition to its role in detecting VAE, TEE is also used as a real-time dynamic monitor for timely evaluation of myocardial function and hemodynamics in high-risk surgical patients (29). Considering the utility of TEE in elderly patients, Suriani et al. have recommended its use, suggesting that it may have a significant impact on intraoperative management of patients older than 66 years of age. However, older age has been associated with a potentially higher risk of postoperative dysphagia, bleeding complications, systemic hypotension and serious gastrointestinal injury with the use of intraoperative TEE (30,31). Moreover, TEE is an extremely sensitive monitor of VAE (discussed below in VAE monitoring section), is relatively contraindicated in patients with restricted cervical spine mobility and associated with tongue swelling after neurosurgery in sitting or prone positioning (31). Hence, the decision to use intraoperative TEE as a physiologic cardiac monitor or for monitoring TEE should be individualized based on the patient's physiological status, risk of VAE and risk-benefit analysis.

Studies have shown that central venous monitoring has poor correlation with blood volume and is a poor marker of fluid responsiveness, especially in elderly patients with poorly compliant vessels (32). Hence, central venous catheterisation should be contemplated only if the sitting position is planned (to aspirate air bubbles in case of VAE) and for vasoactive drug support in patients at risk of significant intra- and postoperative haemodynamic instability. When used during semi-sitting position craniotomies, care should be taken to position the catheter tip at the atriocaval junction, using either ECG guided technique or TEE (33).

Depth of anesthesia monitoring using processed electroencephalographic monitors such as Bispectral Index Monitors (BIS) or entropy is recommended to prevent relative anesthetic overdose and to reduce postoperative delirium (PD) in elderly patients (2,34). Neuromuscular monitoring should be routinely used in elderly patients undergoing neurosurgical procedures with muscle relaxation because of high-risk of unpredictably prolonged neuromuscular blockade.

DETECTION OF VAE

Currently, there are several monitors available which can detect VAE, each having its own advantages and disadvantages, and with varying sensitivity and specificity (3). Among all devices, TEE is the most sensitive for the diagnosis for VAE (0.02 mL of air kg^{-1}) and is currently the gold standard modality (33). However, TEE is too sensitive and even detects clinically non-relevant VAE episodes, leading to its overestimation in patients undergoing sitting/semisitting position craniotomies, without any clinical relevance (35–37). Bubble contrast TEE using agitated saline is an accepted gold standard modality to detect right-to-left shunt across a PFO (38). In addition, TEE allows accurate measurement of PFO size and morphologic details, and also assists in PFO closure device deployment.

Precordial Doppler (PCD) ultrasound is a sensitive non- invasive tool for the diagnosis of VAE (0.05 mL of air kg^{-1}). However, proper positioning of the probe over the anterior chest wall is crucial for it to receive signals from air bubbles traversing the right side of the heart. The probe is usually placed at the superior venae cava - right atrial junction on the chest wall (which corresponds with the third or fourth intercostal space), just to the right of the sternum. Schubert et al. however, found left parasternal placement of probe (3rd–6th intercostal space) more reliable for optimal detection of VAE during craniotomy than the right parasternal border placement (39). After final patient positioning, a bubble test using small bolus of agitated saline (10 mL of normal saline mixed with 0.25 mL of air) through the right atrial catheter should be performed for assessing the correct position of probe. Once a PFO is ruled out by preoperative TEE, combined use of a PCD and capnography (End-tidal carbon dioxide (EtCO$_2$) monitoring) represents the usual standard of care for VAE monitoring during most posterior fossa surgeries. The major disadvantage with the use of this modality is the interference encountered with the use of cautery during surgery.

EtCO$_2$ monitoring is convenient and available on most anaesthetic machines. A sudden change of 3–5 mmHg EtCO$_2$, without a change in minute volume ventilation, is an efficient indicator of clinically significant VAE. End-tidal nitrogen detection is more sensitive than EtCO$_2$ as the warning appears approximately 60–90 s before the reduction of EtCO$_2$. Pulmonary artery catheters can detect rises in right heart pressures. However, it is the most invasive modality and less sensitive than PCD as well. Pulse oximetry and ECG changes are unreliable and very late markers of air embolism.

NEUROPHYSIOLOGICAL MONITORING

During posterior fossa surgery, the brainstem and CN's are very sensitive to any kind of direct or indirect manipulation including surgical dissection, mechanical forces (such as stretching, compression, irrigation and bone drilling) and use of bipolar electrocauterization, thus leading to major neurological morbidity. Hence, with the increase in the general safety profile of these surgeries, current focus is on minimizing the neurological morbidity, most importantly hearing loss and facial paresis.

IONM techniques can identify and assess the integrity of CN, their nuclei and corticospinal or corticobulbar pathways. Hence, continuous IONM during surgery helps to preserve CNs by allowing timely changes in the surgical strategy (e.g., reduction of traction/pressure, stopping the surgical resection, rinsing of the surgical field with saline or increasing the blood pressure) (40). Techniques commonly used to monitor integrity of neural structures during posterior fossa neurosurgery includes early brainstem auditory evoked potentials (BAEPs), free-running electromyography (EMG), direct CN stimulation and long-tract monitoring with somatosensory evoked potentials (SEPs) and motor evoked potentials (MEPs).

MEP/SEP monitoring also provides information on the depth of anesthesia and therefore facilitates interpretations of CN (especially BAEP) monitoring changes. With IONM during posterior fossa surgery, Slotty et al. have reported sensitivity and specificity of 98% and 77%, respectively, for detecting CN deficits and 95% and 85%, respectively, for long-tract deficits (40). Among infratentorial pathology, brainstem lesions (especially brainstem cavernomas), and petroclival lesions (meningiomas and chordomas) are closely associated with concurrent CN IONM and SEP/MEP alterations.

Positioning of the patient in the sitting or prone position requires marked neck flexion. Overstretching of the cervical spinal cord may lead to dramatic reduction in its perfusion, causing mid-cervical flexion myelopathy and consequent quadriplegia (41,42). Spinal canal stenosis and systemic arterial hypotension are other factors implicated in this dreaded complication, which may be encountered in geriatric patients (43). Since the dorsal spinal columns are perfused by the posterior spinal arteries, monitoring of the somatosensory tract via SSEPs is useful for detecting regional spinal cord ischemia intraoperatively (44).

Postoperative facial nerve palsy is one of the most common postoperative complications seen after surgical resection of posterior fossa tumours (most commonly with acoustic neuromas), which may significantly compromise the patient's quality of life (45). Congress of Neurological Surgeons recommends routine intraoperative facial nerve monitoring during acoustic neuroma surgery to improve long-term facial nerve function. The functional integrity of the facial nerve and its corticobulbar pathway can be evaluated using EMG after direct stimulation of facial nerve (mapping), free running EMG (monitoring), and facial MEP after transcranial stimulation (46).

In contrast to facial nerve monitoring, the role of IONM during acoustic neuroma surgery for hearing preservation is less well defined and less frequently used. However, placement of retractors, tumor dissection and temporal bone drilling during surgery can cause compression of cerebellar tissue which can either involve direct mechanical injury of the cochlea or CN VIII or indirect vascular compromise of the brainstem. According to the recent guidelines by Congress of Neurological Surgeons, intraoperative vestibulocochlear CN monitoring should be used during acoustic neuroma surgery whenever hearing preservation is attempted (47). The most popular techniques for eighth CN monitoring includes BAEP monitoring, electrocochleography, and direct compound nerve action potential monitoring (45). Intraoperative critical BAEP developments, with deterioration or loss, are significant predictors of postoperative hearing function (48).

Analogues to CN VII and VIII, LCN can be monitored by EMG, using needle electrodes within their respective musculature (49). CN X may be monitored with EMG using an endotracheal tube with surface electrodes that stimulate the mucosa of the vocal cords. The afferent and efferent signals are carried along the recurrent laryngeal nerve, a branch of the vagus nerve. Submucosal bipolar electrodes in the soft palate, cricothyroid muscle, trapezius, and tongue, may be used to monitor CN IX, X, XI, and XII, respectively.

Positioning

Neurosurgery for posterior fossa pathology is unique in terms of its challenging patient positioning. Furthermore, the fragile condition of many geriatric patients poses additional challenges as they have an increased risk of spinal stenosis, osteoporosis, arthritic joints, fixed flexion deformities and thin skin which makes them prone to incidental trauma during positioning. Hence, prior to induction, the proposed intraoperative positioning should be simulated and the physiological range of head and neck flexion and rotation should be checked in awake patients. Any symptom, such as paresthesia or numbness of the trunk and/or limbs, should be noted, thus determining the final extent of safe positioning. In the end, the final position should be based not only on lesion characteristics and the patient's preoperative medical condition but also on the experience of the anaesthetic and surgical teams as well.

Head and neck positioning is one of the most important part of patient positioning during neurosurgical procedures to ensure optimal surgical exposure. Extreme care should be taken to allow neck flexion in safe limits in elderly patients with cervical spine stenosis and/or carotid artery stenosis, preferably under electrophysiologic neuromonitoring to minimize cord compression. Furthermore, while fixing head in flexion, a minimum of two-three finger breadths space (3–4 cm) should be kept between the chin and the sternum/ any other bony point in lateral position and neck rotation should be minimized to ensure normal cerebral venous and lymphatic outflow.

During surgery, head elevation or reverse Trendelenburg up to 30° has been recommended to facilitate venous return and decrease ICP. However, it may potentially reduce CPP by causing hypotension. Hence, any intraoperative positioning should be done in a step-wise manner to prevent precipitous fall in mean arterial pressure (MAP), along with controlled fluid loading and judicious use of vasopressors in elderly patients. Proper positioning of upper and lower extremities should be done as per the guidelines stated by the American Society of Anesthesiologists Practice Advisory for the Prevention of Perioperative Peripheral Neuropathies (50). In older patients, prolonged surgical procedures further increase the risk of peripheral nerve injuries and "pressure sores," owing to reduced skin depth, muscle mass and vascularity. Hence, extreme care should be taken during patient positioning in elderly patients, carefully padding all the probable sites of nerve injury with silicone pads and routinely assessing every 30 min throughout the surgery.

Supine position with head and neck rotation to the contralateral side can be used for access to lateral structures in the posterior fossa. Depending on the site of the lesion, maximal lateral rotation may be required by elevating the ipsilateral shoulder using a roll or pillow. However, this technique might not be feasible in elderly patients with restricted neck movement.

The lateral position is utilized for unilateral procedures of the posterior fossa, as it leads to improved surgical access via gravitational retraction of the cerebellum, and drainage of CSF and blood from the surgical field. Spektor et al. reported a slightly lower incidence of VAE (4.4% versus 6.5%, respectively (p = 0.558) and anesthesiological measures of hemodynamic instability in patients, aged 10–83 years, operated in lateral position compared to sitting position, though the differences did not reach statistical significance (51). Park-bench position is a variation of the lateral position and resembles the posture of a person reclining on a park bench. It gives better access to the midline structures when compared with the conventional lateral position. The patient is placed semi-prone with the head rotated and the neck flexed, resulting in the

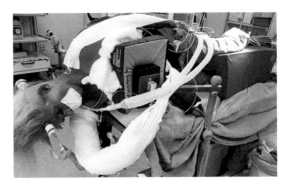

Figure 6.1 Park-bench Positioning in an elderly lady planned for posterior fossa craniotomy via retrosigmoid approach.

forehead facing the floor. (Figure 6.1) The patient is placed so that the dependent arm hangs free of the edge of the operating table, which is slightly flexed and secured with a sling.

Though prone position allows optimal surgical access to the suboccipital region, it may not be feasible in elderly patients with restricted neck mobility. Moreover, prone positioning is logistically difficult, with an increased risk of dislodging the airway, venous catheters and other means of invasive monitoring along with temporary disconnection from ventilator and monitoring equipment, which may be disastrous in elderly patients with severe co-morbidities. Other disadvantages include restricted airway access and the difficulty in providing effective cardiopulmonary resuscitation in the setting of a crisis. The only advantage of this position compared to sitting is a reduced incidence VAE (52,53).

Sitting position provides obvious surgical advantages for posterior fossa lesions including optimal access to the cranio-vertebral junction and the posterior fossa (particularly pineal region and the petroclival junction), gravitational drainage of blood and CSF away from surgical site allowing a cleaner surgical field, less intraoperative venous bleeding, gravity assisted cerebellar retraction allowing better surgical exposure of deep areas and reducing the need for extensive dissection and bipolar coagulation, decreased operating time and better preservation of CN function (20,52,54). The anaesthetic advantages include easy access to the airway and peripheries for monitoring CN's and in the event of any respiratory or cardiac complications, along with favourable changes in ventilatory mechanics (Figure 6.2).

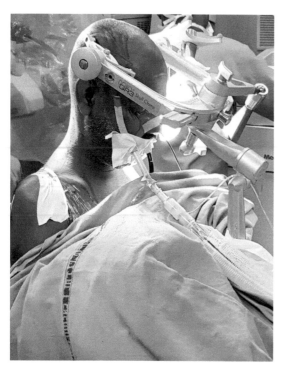

Figure 6.2 Sitting Position in an elderly male patient planned for posterior fossa craniotomy via suboccipital midline approach.

Despite the advantages, its popularity declined steadily due to an increased association with several serious complications, most notably VAE with possible paradoxical air embolism (PAE) and significant haemodynamic instability. Nevertheless, over years, the position has been modified to a semisitting position which includes a Trendelenburg tilt, thus achieving a positive intracranial venous pressure and hence, a reduced incidence of VAE (20,35,36,55).

Recent studies have shown that the semisitting position does not carry any significant additional risk to patients, even in presence of a PFO, as long as the neurosurgical and anesthetic teams performing the surgical procedure follow a strict perioperative protocol with meticulous anesthesia and neurosurgical management and are aware of the risks and remedies associated with the position (20,36,56,57). However, the mean age of the patients in these studies lies somewhere between the 4th to 6th decade of life, with elderly population accounting for a very small proportion. Hence, their result should be carefully extrapolated in elderly patients with significant physiological decline or multiple

comorbidities. Furthermore, sitting position is relatively contraindicated in patients with a restricted cervical spine mobility, cervical canal stenosis and significant carotid artery disease; commonly encountered in elderly patients. Spektor et al. found no obvious advantages in surgical or neurological outcomes for use of either sitting or lateral patient position, in patients undergoing complex posterior fossa surgery (51). Hence, elderly patients may safely undergo surgery for posterior fossa pathologies with acceptable outcomes in an alternative lateral or park-bench position as well. Nevertheless, with an experienced team sitting position may be considered safely in geriatric patients, with minimal or no associated cardiac and respiratory comorbidities, if deemed absolutely necessary by the neurosurgical team.

Intraoperative management

Normal aging decreases the structural, physiologic, and immunologic reserve of the respiratory system (58). Emphysema-like change (called "senile emphysema") occurs in the elderly lungs due to the loss of alveolar architecture leading to reduced lung elasticity and an increase in residual lung volume. Moreover, a loss of supporting elastic tissues contributes to narrowing and closure of the small airways, thus, causing expiratory airflow obstruction and air trapping.

Both expiratory and inspiratory muscles weaken with age. Acute decline in forced expiratory volume measured during the first second (FEV1) is a marker of a weaker cough, which may compound the complications arising from LCN injury in patients undergoing posterior fossa procedures. Decreased functional residual capacity and lung compliance contribute to atelectasis and ventilation/perfusion mismatch (V/Q mismatch), which in turn leads to intrapulmonary shunting, thus reducing baseline oxygen saturation. Alveolar destruction and a reduction in pulmonary capillary density further reduces the surface area available for gas exchange increasing the dead space. Older patients may also have diminished cardiac and ventilatory responsiveness to hypoxemia and hypercapnia.

All these physiological changes associated with aging, combined with gravity induced V/Q mismatch in the sitting and lateral positions and presence of respiratory comorbidity (chronic smoking,

COPD), makes geriatric patient susceptible to hypoxemia and other postoperative respiratory complications. Hence, continuous monitoring of airway pressures and adaptation of inspired fractions of gases and inspiratory pressures according to frequent arterial blood gas values is critical in geriatric patients undergoing posterior fossa craniotomy.

Patients should be mechanically ventilated to maintain either normocapnia or mild hypercapnia (20,28). Lung-protective mechanical ventilation combining low tidal volumes (6–8 mL/kg), positive end-expiratory pressure (PEEP) of 5–8 cm cmH$_2$O, and repeated recruitment maneuvres (application of high airway pressures to open collapsed lung areas) has been shown to result in improvement of intraoperative oxygenation and lung mechanics in elderly patients (59) and also result in improved postoperative outcomes in patients at increased risk for pulmonary complications (60,61).

Use of PEEP is controversial during sitting position craniotomies with some authors avoiding it in view of its adverse effect on haemodynamics and potential for PAE in patients with PFO (62) whereas others recommends its use (at a level from 6 to 10 cm H$_2$O) to lower the incidence of VAE by increasing the intrathoracic pressures (20). Use of PEEP has also been found helpful in elderly patients to prevent the intraoperative deterioration of lung mechanics (63). However, it may cause collapse of alveolar capillaries, causing hypercarbia, which may increase CBF and ICP in the elderly patients. Thus, the decision to use PEEP should be individualized and appears to be safe if euvolemia and normotension is maintained (64).

Analogues to respiratory system, cardiovascular system undergoes profound age-related changes in structure and physiology (23). The autonomic nervous system in the elderly has reduced neuronal mass as compared to younger patients, and this is manifested as a diminished sympathetic response to stress. Decreased responsiveness to β-adrenoceptor agonists and renin–angiotensin–aldosterone system stimulation further limits the ability of aged heart to increase CO and to respond to fluid losses. In addition, an increased aortic outflow resistance, as seen with ageing, and a thickened left ventricle leads to a reduced stroke volume, as well as decreased early diastolic filling due to delayed relaxation. This leads to the tendency for volume intolerance and diastolic dysfunction in the elderly.

Thickening of the aortic valve also results in reduced outflow to tissues such as the brain and coronary arteries. Increased systolic pressure can lead to myocardial hypertrophy and increased myocardial oxygen consumption, while the decreased diastolic pressure leads to decreased coronary perfusion pressure. This mismatch between increased oxygen demand and decreased oxygen supply makes the patient prone to myocardial ischemia and even infarction. Reduced venous compliance further accentuate hypotension by causing a reduced preload in hypovolemic states, as seen with acute blood loss or diuresis.

Arterial wall thickening may lead to chronic hypertension, primarily isolated systolic hypertension, and an increased pulse pressures. Severe hypertension predisposes patients to wide swings in intraoperative blood pressure and consequent cardiac arrhythmias and myocardial ischemia. In patients with chronic hypertension, blood flow to oxygen-sensitive organs such as brain and kidney is reset at higher blood pressure limits, due to a possible rightward shift of the organ autoregulation curves. Hence, elderly hypertensive patients with normotensive blood pressure readings may actually be in a state of hypotension with an increased risk of cerebral and renal ischemia. Sitting and prone positioning also induces significant changes in patients haemodynamics. Changing from the supine to the sitting position leads to a significant decrease of cardiac index, stroke volume index, and MAP along with an increase in pulmonary and systemic vascular resistance. Similarly, in prone position, pressure on the abdomen may occlude the inferior vena cava and decrease pulmonary compliance resulting in higher peak airway pressure and decreased venous return to the heart, thus causing hypotension (especially in elderly patients).

Understanding what constitutes a safe and optimal blood pressure during the perioperative period in elderly patients is thus, a complex decision dependent on several factors, including patient's physiology, preoperative drug compliance, intraoperative patient positioning and surgical need. In the elderly trauma patients (more than 65 years of age), Oyetunji et al. have demonstrated that an systolic blood pressure (SBP) of 117 mmHg is a better diagnostic definition for hypotension and predictor of mortality than the optimal 90 mmHg value for patients younger than 65 years of age (65). A recently conducted Intraoperative Norepinephrine to Control Arterial Pressure (INPRESS) study by Futier and colleagues prospectively compared two intraoperative blood pressure management strategies in a high-risk noncardiac surgical population (66). In this study, 49% of participants were aged 70 years or older and 82% experienced chronic hypertension. Authors found that targeting an individualized SBP within 10% of the reference value (i.e., patient's resting SBP) compared with standard management (treating SBP less than 80 mmHg or lower than 40% from the reference value), reduced the risk of postoperative organ dysfunction. Hence, in elderly patients undergoing posterior fossa surgery, it appears imperative to maintain blood pressures close to pre-induction values to reduce any risk of postoperative cognitive and organ dysfunction. In ideal circumstances, the lower limit of cerebral autoregulation should be continuously assessed using bedside auto-regulation testing tools to identify the minimal acceptable blood pressure in anesthetized seated patients and thus adjusting the intraoperative blood pressure goals accordingly (28).

In a small percentage of patients, use of a vasopressor such as ephedrine or phenylephrine may become necessary to augment MAP so as to maintain CPP. Numerous studies evaluating phenylephrine and ephedrine in neuroanaesthesia have shown that despite an increase in MAP by both agents, brain oxygen saturation remains unaltered by ephedrine administration, but is reduced after phenylephrine administration, possibly explained by their differing effects on the cerebral microcirculation, particularly the capillary transit-time heterogeneity which determines oxygen extraction efficacy (67–69). In upright sitting or beach-chair position, phenylephrine infusion was found to prevent hypotension by maintaining preload and increasing SVR but was associated with a decrease in CO and cerebral oxygen desaturation (69). Currently, a trial is underway evaluating the effect of phenylephrine and ephedrine on brain oxygenation and microcirculation (using magnetic resonance imaging (MRI) and positron emission tomography (PET) scans for measurement of CBF, capillary transit-time heterogeneity, cerebral metabolic rate of oxygen and oxygen extraction fraction; BIS and cerebral oximetry) in patients aged 18–75 years old posted for supratentorial craniotomy in supine position (70). Result of this trial are expected to provide a perfect choice among ephedrine and phenylephrine in anesthetized patients with brain pathology and at risk of cerebral oxygen desaturation.

Considering the current trend of vasopressor preference in elderly patients at high-risk of postoperative adverse outcomes, a recent multicentre observational study has reported ephedrine (43%) to be the most commonly used vasopressor to treat hypotension during general anesthesia, followed by phenylephrine and noradrenaline (61). Even, in the INPRESS study, ephedrine was used as the first-line vasopressor for standard care among high-risk patients undergoing major surgery, rather than phenylephrine or norepinephrine (66). Authors of the trial have recommended active management of hypotension using combined β and α-agonist. Essentially, phenylephrine is a selective α1-adrenergic agonist with a greater risk of negative effects on CO (in contrast to ephedrine or norepinephrine, which have β-adrenergic activity), which may be detrimental in elderly and in patients with significant cardiovascular morbidity.

Intraoperatively, frequent arrhythmias may occur during manipulation of the brain stem, including bradycardia, ST-wave depression and rarely multifocal ventricular bigeminy proceeding to ventricular tachycardia and even cardiac arrest. These arrhythmias represent a warning sign of deleterious surgical stimulation of brainstem CN nuclei and should not be treated pharmacologically (71). Rather, the surgeon should be notified immediately and asked to stop further dissection until resolution of the arrhythmias. During sitting craniotomy, use of intermittent pneumatic compression (IPC) devices on the lower extremities helps prevent venous pooling, thus decreasing intraoperative hypotensive episodes and improving cerebral oxygen saturation (72).

Normoglycemia and normovolemia should be maintained throughout surgery and in the ICU. Studies have shown benefit of goal-directed fluid therapy (GDFT) in improving hemodynamics and limiting infusion volumes during prone position neurosurgeries and sitting craniotomies, especially in patients with decreased brain compliance (55,73). Concerning the cardiac risks associated with fluid challenges and inotropes used during GDFT in high-risk surgical patients with limited cardiopulmonary reserves, no association was observed between the two in a meta-analysis of 22 randomized controlled trials (RCTs) by Arulkumaran and colleagues (74). In subgroup analysis, maximum benefits of GDFT were obtained in patients where oxygen delivery was optimized with fluids and inotropes (supranormal oxygen delivery index achieved), using minimally invasive CO monitors. Elderly patients, however, have a questionable benefit from GDFT in improving outcomes, probably because of their limited ability to increase stroke volume in view of high incidence of diastolic dysfunction (75). Nonetheless, few recent studies have shown a benefit in maintaining stable perioperative hemodynamics and improving microcirculation perfusion in elderly patients, even during prone position surgery (76,77). However, GDFT was found to be associated with a higher infusion of colloidal solutions in elderly patients (76,77) which may limit its applicability in high-risk neurosurgical cases (73). Hence, the prospect of GDFT for intraoperative fluid administration in elderly patients undergoing posterior fossa surgery is still questionable and needs validation through well conducted RCTs. Furthermore, regardless of the technique or monitoring used, fluid therapy should be administered with great care and in divided boluses to allow assessment of response, to avoid overloading or insufficient fluid resuscitation.

In elderly patients, perioperative hypothermia (defined as temperature <36°C) is common and is known to cause decreased drug metabolism, impaired wound healing, increase risk of infection, coagulopathy, perioperative cardiac dysfunction and PD (23). Hence, normothermia should be maintained by utilizing forced air warmers and fluid warmers, taking into account the long surgical duration and difficulty in rewarming elderly patients once hypothermic (2). Deep venous thrombosis prophylaxis is also important in view of prolonged surgical duration during posterior fossa craniotomies and probable longer duration of ICU stay. Perioperative use of elastic stockings, low-molecular-weight heparin and IPC devices along with appropriate fluid therapy and optimal patient positioning plays a vital role in reducing the risk of peri-operative thromboembolism in the elderly (2,78).

Awakening and postoperative care

Emergence after surgeries in the posterior fossa should ideally be smooth, without coughing or straining during endotracheal extubation. The last dose of neuromuscular blocker must be adequately timed as elderly patients require more time to recover from neuromuscular blockade with anti-cholinesterase agents. Early awakening is desired as it allows timely postoperative neurological monitoring. However, patient may require elective mechanical ventilation in the event of preoperative bulbar dysfunction, surgery for large tumors or tumors involving the LCN or their nuclei in the floor of the fourth ventricle (possibly causing postoperative LCN dysfunction), excessive intraoperative manipulation of the brainstem causing impaired consciousness and compromised airway either because of tongue swelling or residual postoperative neuromuscular blockade. Prior to extubation, laryngoscopy should be done to confirm the presence of protective laryngeal reflexes. In the setting of decreased airway reflexes, extubation should be postponed until there is complete return of consciousness. If the decision is made to keep the patient sedated and ventilated postoperatively, ICP monitoring may be considered as an alternative to monitor patients neurological status. Failure to recover from anaesthesia should prompt urgent imaging of the brain to exclude any complications, most importantly pneumocephalus (including tension pneumocephalus), air embolism, and operative site haematoma. Postoperative hypertension should be carefully managed to avoid bleeding complications, particularly in hypertensive elderly patients.

Older patients, in general, report less severe postcraniotomy pain and require a smaller amount of analgesics as compared to younger adults (79,80). However, it is important to realize that frailty, diminished organ reserve, and neurologic diseases (previous stroke) may have a profound effect on how elderly patients perceive and communicate pain. Asking elderly patients to describe pain in their own words is an effective means to assess post-operative pain. Before treating acute postoperative pain, it is important exclude PD and to consider the extent of their frailty and cognitive status. Furthermore, reduction in hepatic, renal, and nervous system reserve mandates cautious drug dosing and avoiding potentially inappropriate drugs (81).

Compared to supratentorial craniotomies, postoperative pain is more common after infratentorial procedures, especially after acoustic neuroma and posterior fossa surgeries, both at movement and at rest (80,82). The difference in the incidence as well as the severity of post craniotomy pain may be explained by a high muscle mass underlying the surgical incision, with extensive resection and consequent spasm of temporalis and posterior cervical muscles after suboccipital and sub-temporal interventions. Hence, elderly patients undergoing posterior fossa interventions may experience substantial amount of pain and considering the pharmacological constraints in elderly patients, require a multi-modal approach for effective pain management (2,83).

Similarly, patients undergoing infratentorial craniotomy are more likely to have postoperative nausea and vomiting (PONV) compared with supratentorial craniotomies, probably because of location of chemoreceptor trigger zone in the infratentorial compartment (84). However, literature shows contradictory association between site of craniotomy and PONV risk and no association between age and PONV risk after craniotomy (84–86).

PD is a common and potentially serious complication seen in approximately 10%–60% of elderly surgical patients, undergoing major surgery (2,34). Though the exact incidence in patients undergoing posterior fossa craniotomy is not known, steps should be taken to prevent its occurrence and to diagnose it immediately (as per recommendations from the American Geriatrics Society) to minimize its serious sequalae including other major postoperative complications, prolonged hospitalization, functional dependence, cognitive decline and death (34). Essentially, PD should be kept in the differential diagnosis of an elderly patient showing acute confusion, agitation or cognitive decline in the immediate postoperative period. At times, other postoperative complications such as myocardial infarction or pulmonary embolism may initially present as delirium in older adults, and hence, need to be properly evaluated.

Complications

Due to the abundance of the neural tracts and vital centres nuclei in the brainstem and their challenging blood supply, even minor damage during posterior fossa surgery can cause devastating complications. These complications are further compounded by the physiological changes associated with non-supine patient positioning and aging

physiology in elderly patients. Hence, a gamut of complications may arise during these surgeries, necessitating constant vigilance and proactive management, both by the neuro-anaesthesiologists and neurosurgical team.

AGE RELATED COMPLICATIONS

Under the stress of anaesthesia and surgery and because of their ageing physiology and multiple comorbidities, elderly patients are potentially at risks of serious or even life-threatening postoperative complications (7). Loss of pulmonary functional reserve and defences makes elderly patients particularly prone for postoperative pulmonary complications (58). These include prolonged mechanical ventilation or unplanned reintubation, atelectasis, COPD exacerbation and pneumonia, which may substantially contribute to prolonged hospitalization and mortality (7,13). Presence of dysphagia in patients with preoperative LCN dysfunction is poorly tolerated in elderly patients compared to young adults, further escalating the risk of postoperative pneumonia (13). Similarly, perioperative cardiac events, are more common in the elderly patients undergoing posterior fossa surgery, ranging from minor ECG changes to arrhythmias, syncopal episode and myocardial infarctions (5,7).

While analysing the NIS for patients undergoing acoustic neuroma surgery, Sylvester et al. found that elderly patients had significantly higher rates of all composite postoperative complications, including surgical, neurological and medical complications, compared to younger adults (7). However, after correcting for patient demographics and presence of individual comorbidities, elderly status was independently associated only with composite medical complications. The most common medical complications included acute cardiac event, urinary tract infections, and mechanical ventilation, all of which had significantly higher rates in the elderly cohort. Acute renal failure, sepsis, infectious pneumonia, and venous thrombosis were also significantly more common in the elderly. On the contrary, Van Abel et al. found no significant difference in length of stay in the ICU and hospital, nor in the frequency of surgical or anesthetic-related complications in between elderly and non-elderly patients undergoing acoustic neuroma surgery, thereby suggesting that tumor size and extent of resection may result in complication more than age alone (5).

The overall reported mortality in elderly patients undergoing acoustic neuroma surgery is reportedly low (5,7,8). Sylvester et al., however, reported significantly higher mortality in elderly patients (less than 10 cases out of 519 patients) than the younger ones (less than 10 cases out of 3616 patients) (7).

POSITIONING RELATED COMPLICATIONS

Older patients are at higher risk of peripheral nerve injuries, especially during prolonged surgeries, including the ulnar nerve and lower back injury when supine; the dependent radial nerve, peroneal nerve and lateral femoral cutaneous nerve injury and the brachial plexus injury (due to axillary artery compression) in the lateral and park-bench positioning; axillary, ulnar and radial neuropathies in prone position, and sciatic nerve or peroneal nerve injury during sitting craniotomies (2). Additionally, if there is excessive traction on the shoulder, the brachial plexus can be stretched and injured.

Sitting position during posterior fossa surgeries is associated with a myriad of significant and potentially life-threatening complications, including VAE and its sequalae (tachyarrythmias, myocardial ischaemia, sudden onset right heart failure, stress-induced Takotsubo cardiomyopathy, pulmonary oedema, cerebral ischaemia, coagulation abnormalities and PAE with consequent stroke or myocardial infarction), haemodynamic instability with hypotension, symptomatic tension pneumocephalus, acute subdural hematoma, peripheral neuropathy, laryngeal edema, macroglossia and quadriplegia (35,54,87–90). Prone position may result in macroglossia, pressure sores, retinal ischemia from orbital compression, VAE and cervical cord compression with quadriplegia (88). Pharyngeal and tracheal edema may also develop during prolonged procedures.

VAE during neurosurgical procedures in head-up position is common because of the negative pressure in the intracranial veins and non-collapsible dural venous sinuses. Historically, sitting position has been implicated as having the highest incidence of VAE because of maximum head elevation compared to other horizontal positions (supine, lateral, park-bench and prone) (52). Nonetheless, recent literature suggests that

with the use of effective preventive strategies (such as hydration, use of IPC devices, correct patient positioning with toes above the level of heart, preoperative endoscopic PFO closure and careful surgical dissection), meticulous monitoring for timely detection of VAE and efficient management by the neurosurgical and neuroanesthetic teams; the incidence of clinically significant VAE and PAE during posterior fossa surgery is low (3,35–37,57). Furthermore, when managed promptly, intraoperative VAE may not result in adverse postoperative outcomes (36,57). Recently, Saladino et al. analyzed data from adult patients (mean age of 47 ± 14 years [range 18–81 years]) undergoing elective cranial surgery in the semi-sitting position. Authors found that even in the presence of intraoperative VAE in 21% of cases (detected by PCD probe), the semisitting position was not related to an increased risk of postoperative neurological deficits (57). Interestingly, younger patients were at higher risk of VAE ($p = 0.03$), while other physiological conditions including patient's sex, ASA Classification, obesity, and pulmonary or cardiac disease, had no effect on its occurrence.

Theoretically, the risk of quadriplegia appears to be high in elderly patients with cervical cord compression or because of hypotensive ischaemia of brainstem or spinal cord (discussed previously). However, no such correlation between age and surgical complications was observed in the study by Saladino and colleagues (57). Nonetheless, more data is required from studies on geriatric patients, including octagenarians to establish the risk-benefit analysis of different patient positioning in elderly patients undergoing posterior fossa surgery.

SURGERY RELATED COMPLICATIONS

Common surgical complications after posterior fossa interventions include CN dysfunction, CSF leak, meningitis, wound infection, hydrocephalus, hematoma in or around the surgical cavity, iatrogenic cerebrovascular infarction/haemorrhage and cerebellar mutism (57,88,91).

Surgeries in which tumor dissection from the brainstem is necessary carry a higher risk than surgeries in which less dissection is required. In extensive approaches, coagulation might add up to decreased venous and/or arterial flow, resulting in cerebral edema and temporary or permanent cerebral ischemia. Compared to younger adults, the incidence of postoperative hematoma (7) and long-term postoperative imbalance (5) has been found to be significantly higher in elderly patients undergoing acoustic neuroma surgery.

CN dysfunction may result from direct operative intervention in and around the CN, particularly in acoustic neuromas when the facial nerve may be functionally or anatomically injured. Studies have found no correlation between facial nerve dysfunction and age of patients, thus dispelling the concern related to poor regenerative capacity of the facial nerve in elderly because of atherosclerosis induced decreased perfusion (5,8). Damage to the motor division of the LCN that run into the jugular foramen leads to hoarseness, dysphagia, stridor and the risk of aspiration pneumonia. Hence, patients with dysphagia should be put on nasogastric tube feeding to minimize aspiration risk while tracheostomy should be considered in patients with persisting deficits.

CONCLUSION

Posterior fossa surgery in elderly patients with age limited physiological reserves, pose significant management challenges because of the small surgical space and the importance of the neural and vascular structures involved and adverse physiological effects of non-horizontal patient positioning. Patients physiologic condition, posterior fossa pathology and location, preoperative functional status, and comorbidities may, however, be more important than chronological age in predicting perioperative complications. Pre-operative assessment of the higher-risk elderly patients with multiple comorbidities involves a structured multifactorial approach, with proactive identification and optimisation of modifiable risk factors. Multidisciplinary perioperative care, strict monitoring as well as meticulous surgical techniques can help minimize the complications and improves outcomes for elderly surgical patients undergoing posterior fossa surgery.

REFERENCES

1. Babu R, Sharma R, Bagley JH, Hatef J, Friedman AH, Adamson C. Vestibular schwannomas in the modern era: Epidemiology, treatment trends, and disparities in management. *J Neurosurg.* 2013;119:121–130.
2. Griffiths R, Beech F, Brown A et al. Association of Anesthetists of Great Britain and Ireland. Peri-operative care of the elderly 2014: Association of Anaesthetists of Great Britain and Ireland. *Anaesthesia.* 2014 Jan;69(Suppl 1):81–98.
3. Sandhu K, Gupta N. Anaesthesia for Posterior Fossa Surgery. In: Prabhakar H (ed.) *Essentials of Neuroanaesthesia,* San Diego: Academic Press, Elsevier 2017. pp. 255–73.
4. Shih RY, Smirniotopoulos JG. Posterior Fossa Tumors in Adult Patients. *Neuroimaging Clin N Am.* 2016 Nov;26(4):493–510.
5. Van Abel KM, Carlson ML, Driscoll CL, Neff BA, Link MJ. Vestibular schwannoma surgery in the elderly: A matched cohort study. *J Neurosurg.* 2013 Jul 19;120(1):207–17.
6. Roehm PC, Gantz BJ. Management of acoustic neuromas in patients 65 years or older. *Otol Neurotol.* 2007;28:708–714.
7. Sylvester MJ, Shastri DN, Patel VM, Raikundalia MD, Eloy JA, Baredes S, Ying YM. Outcomes of Vestibular Schwannoma Surgery among the Elderly. *Otolaryngol Head Neck Surg.* 2017 Jan;156(1):166–172.
8. Nuseir A, Sequino G, De Donato G, Taibah A, Sanna M. Surgical management of vestibular schwannoma in elderly patients. *Eur Arch Otorhinolaryngol* 2012;269:17–23.
9. Kepes JJ, Whittaker KC, Watson K et al. Cerebellar Astrocytomas in Elderly Patients with Very Long Preoperative Histories: Report of Three Cases. *Neurosurgery.* 1989 Aug 1;25(2):258–64.
10. Babu R, Kranz PG, Karikari IO, Friedman AH, Adamson C. Clinical characteristics and treatment of malignant brainstem gliomas in elderly patients. *J Clin Neurosci.* 2013 Oct;20(10):1382–6.
11. Negoto T, Terachi S, Baba Y, Yamashita S, Kuramoto T, Morioka M. Symptomatic brainstem cavernoma of elderly patients: Timing and strategy of surgical treatment: Two case reports and review of the literature. *World Neurosurg.* 2018 Mar;111: 227–234.
12. Chen L, Zhao Y, Zhou L, Zhu W, Pan Z, Mao Y. Surgical strategies in treating brainstem

cavernous malformations. *Neurosurgery.* 2011;68:609–621.

13. Nakamura M, Roser F, Dormiani M, Vorkapic P, Samii M. Surgical treatment of cerebello-pontine angle meningiomas in elderly patients. *Acta Neurochir (Wien).* 2005 Jun; 147(6):603–9; discussion 609–10.

14. Poon MT, Fung LH, Pu JK, Leung GK. Outcome of elderly patients undergoing intracranial meningioma resection – A systematic review and meta-analysis. *Br J Neurosurg.* 2014 Jun;28(3):303–9.

15. Cornu P, Chatellier G, Dagreou F, Clemenceau S, Foncin JF, Rivierez M, Philippon J. Intra-cranial meningiomas in elderly patients. Post-operative morbidity and mortality. Factors predictive of outcome. *Acta Neurochir (Wien).* 1990;102(3–4):98–102.

16. Morgenstern LB, Hemphill JC, 3rd, Anderson C et al. Guidelines for the management of spontaneous intracerebral hemorrhage: A guideline for healthcare professionals from the American Heart Association/American Stroke Association. *Stroke* 2010;41:2108–29.

17. Puffer RC, Graffeo C, Rabinstein A, Van Gompel JJ. Mortality rates after emergent posterior fossa decompression for ischemic or hemorrhagic stroke in older patients. *World Neurosurg.* 2016 Aug;92:166–170.

18. Levine GN, Bates ER, Bittl JA et al. 2016 ACC/AHA Guideline Focused Update on Duration of Dual Antiplatelet Therapy in Patients With Coronary Artery Disease: A Report of the American College of Cardiology/ American Heart Association Task Force on Clinical Practice Guidelines: An Update of the 2011 ACCF/AHA/SCAI Guideline for Percutaneous Coronary Intervention, 2011 ACCF/AHA Guideline for Coronary Artery Bypass Graft Surgery, 2012 ACC/AHA/ACP/AATS/PCNA/SCAI/STS Guideline for the Diagnosis and Management of Patients With Stable Ischemic Heart Disease, 2013 ACCF/AHA Guideline for the Management of ST-Elevation Myocardial Infarction, 2014 AHA/ACC Guideline for the Management of Patients With Non-ST-Elevation Acute Coronary Syndromes, and 2014 ACC/AHA Guideline on Perioperative Cardiovascular Evaluation and Management of Patients Undergoing Noncardiac Surgery. *Circulation.* 2016;134:e123–e155.

19. Duceppe E, Parlow J, MacDonald P et al. Canadian Cardiovascular Society Guidelines on Perioperative Cardiac Risk Assessment and Management for Patients Who Undergo Noncardiac Surgery. *Can J Cardiol.* 2017;33: 17–32.

20. Ammirati M, Lamki TT, Shaw AB, Forde B, Nakano I, Mani M. A streamlined protocol for the use of the semi-sitting position in neurosurgery: A report on 48 consecutive procedures. *J Clin Neurosci.* 2013;20(1): 32–4.

21. Fathi AR, Eshtehardi P, Meier B. Patent fora-men ovale and neurosurgery in sitting posi-tion: A systematic review. *Br J Anaesth.* 2009;102(5):588–96.

22. Akhtar S. Pharmacological considerations in the elderly. *Curr Opin Anaesthesiol.* 2018 Feb;31(1):11–18.

23. Alvis BD, Hughes CG. Physiology consider-ations in geriatric patients. *Anesthesiol Clin.* 2015;33(3):447–56.

24. Pasternak JJ, Lanier WL. Is nitrous oxide use appropriate in neurosurgical and neurologi-cally at-risk patients? *Curr Opin Anaesthesiol.* 2010;23(5):544–50.

25. Pasternak JJ, McGregor DG, Lanier WL, Schroeder DR, Rusy DA, Hindman B, Clarke W, Torner J, Todd MM; IHAST Investigators. Effect of nitrous oxide use on long-term neu-rologic and neuropsychological outcome in patients who received temporary proximal artery occlusion during cerebral aneurysm clipping surgery. *Anesthesiology.* 2009; 110(3):563–73.

26. Myles PS, Leslie K, Chan MT et al. ANZCA Trials Group for the ENIGMA-II investigators. The safety of addition of nitrous oxide to general anaesthesia in at-risk patients having major non-cardiac surgery (ENIGMA-II): A randomised, single-blind trial. *Lancet.* 2014;384(9952):1446–54.

27. Sun R, Jia WQ, Zhang P, Yang K, Tian JH, Ma B, Liu Y, Jia RH, Luo XF, Kuriyama A. Nitrous oxide-based techniques versus nitrous oxide-free techniques for general anaesthesia. *Cochrane Database Syst Rev.* 2015 Nov 6; (11):CD008984.

28. Gracia I, Fabregas N. Craniotomy in sitting position: Anesthesiology management. *Curr Opin Anaesthesiol.* 2014;27(5):474–83.

29. Fayad A, Shillcutt S, Meineri M, Ruddy TD, Ansari MT. Comparative Effectiveness and Harms of Intraoperative Transesophageal Echocardiography in Noncardiac Surgery: A Systematic Review. *Semin Cardiothorac Vasc Anesth.* 2018 Jun;22(2):122–136.

30. Stoddard MF, Longaker RA. The safety of trans-esophageal echocardiography in the elderly. *Am Heart J.* 1993 May;125(5 Pt 1):1358–62.

31. Hilberath JN, Oakes DA, Shernan SK, Bulwer BE, D'Ambra MN, Eltzschig HK. Safety of transesophageal echocardiography. *J Am Soc Echocardiogr.* 2010 Nov;23(11):1115–27.

32. Marik PE, Cavallazzi R. Does the central venous pressure predict fluid responsive-ness? An updated meta-analysis and a plea for some common sense. *Crit Care Med.* 2013 Jul;41(7):1774–81.

33. Mirski MA, Lele AV, Fitzsimmons L, Toung TJ. Diagnosis and treatment of vascular air embo-lism. *Anesthesiology* 2007;106(1):164–77.

34. Postoperative delirium in older adults: Best practice statement from the American Geriatrics Society. American Geriatrics Society Expert Panel on Postoperative Delirium in Older Adults. *J Am Coll Surg.* 2015 Feb; 220(2):136–48.e1.

35. Jadik S, Wissing H, Friedrich K, Beck J, Seifert V, Raabe A. A standardized protocol for the prevention of clinically relevant venous air embolism during neurosurgical interventions in the semisitting position. *Neurosurgery* 2009;64:533–539.

36. Feigl GC, Decker K, Wurms M et al. Neurosurgical procedures in the semisitting position: Evaluation of the risk of paradoxical venous air embolism in patients with a pat-ent foramen ovale. *World Neurosurg* 2014; 81:159–164.

37. Günther F, Frank P, Nakamura M, Hermann EJ, Palmaers T. Venous air embolism in the sitting position in cranial neurosurgery: Incidence and severity according to the used monitoring. *Acta Neurochir (Wien).* 2017 Feb;159(2): 339–346.

38. Buchholz S, Shakil A, Figtree GA, Hansen PS, Bhindi R. Diagnosis and management of pat-ent foramen ovale. *Postgrad Med J.* 2012 Apr;88(1038):217–25.

39. Schubert A, Deogaonkar A, Drummond JC. Precordial Doppler probe placement for optimal detection of venous air embolism during craniotomy. *Anesth Analg.* 2006 May; 102(5):1543–7.

40. Slotty PJ, Abdulazim A, Kodama K, Javadi M, Hänggi D, Seifert V, Szelényi A. Intra-operative neurophysiological monitoring during resection of infratentorial lesions: The surgeon's view. *J Neurosurg.* 2017 Jan; 126(1):281–288.

41. Morandi X, Riffaud L, Amlashi SF, Brassier G. Extensive spinal cord infarction after poste-rior fossa surgery in the sitting position: Case report. *Neurosurgery.* 2004 Jun;54(6):1512–5; discussion 1515–6.

42. Rau CS, Liang CL, Lui CC, Lee TC, Lu K. Quadriplegia in a patient who underwent pos-terior fossa surgery in the prone position. Case report. *J Neurosurg.* 2002 Jan;96(1 Suppl): 101–3.

43. Martínez-Lage JF, Almagro MJ, Izura V, Serrano C, Ruiz-Espejo AM, Sánchez-Del-Rincón I. Cervical spinal cord infarction after posterior fossa surgery: A case-based update. *Childs Nerv Syst.* 2009 Dec;25(12):1541–6.

44. Deinsberger W, Christophis P, Jödicke A, Heesen M, Böker DK. Somatosensory evoked potential monitoring during positioning of the patient for posterior fossa surgery in the semisitting position. *Neurosurgery.* 1998;43(1): 36–40; discussion 40–2.

45. Oh T, Nagasawa DT, Fong BM, Trang A, Gopen Q, Parsa AT, Yang I. Intraoperative neuromonitoring techniques in the surgical management of acoustic neuromas. *Neurosurg Focus.* 2012 Sep;33(3):E6.

46. Acioly MA, Liebsch M, de Aguiar PH, Tatagiba M. Facial nerve monitoring during cerebellopontine angle and skull base tumor surgery: A systematic review from descrip-tion to current success on function predic-tion. *World Neurosurgery* 2013;80(6):e271–300.

47. Vivas EX, Carlson ML, Neff BA, Shepard NT, McCracken DJ, Sweeney AD, Olson JJ. Congress of Neurological Surgeons Systematic Review and Evidence-Based Guidelines on Intraoperative Cranial Nerve Monitoring in Vestibular Schwannoma Surgery. *Neurosurgery.* 2018 Feb 1;82(2):E44–E46.

48. Hummel M, Perez J, Hagen R, Gelbrich G, Ernestus RI, Matthies C. Auditory Monitoring

in Vestibular Schwannoma Surgery: Intraoperative Development and Outcome. *World Neurosurg.* 2016 Dec;96:444–453.

49. Topsakal C, Al-Mefty O, Bulsara KR, Williford VS. Intraoperative monitoring of lower cranial nerves in skull base surgery: Technical report and review of 123 monitored cases. *Neurosurg Rev.* 2008;31(1):45–53.

50. Practice Advisory for the Prevention of Perioperative Peripheral Neuropathies 2018. An Updated Report by the American Society of Anesthesiologists Task Force on Prevention of Perioperative Peripheral Neuropathies. *Anesthesiology.* 2018 Jan;128(1):11–26.

51. Spektor S, Fraifeld S, Margolin E, Saseedharan S, Eimerl D, Umansky F. Comparison of outcomes following complex posterior fossa surgery performed in the sitting versus lateral position. *J Clin Neurosci.* 2015 Apr;22(4): 705–12.

52. Black S, Ockert DB, Oliver WC Jr, Cucchiara RF. Outcome following posterior fossa craniectomy in patients in the sitting or horizontal positions. *Anesthesiology.* 1988 Jul;69(1): 49–56.

53. Orliaguet GA, Hanafi M, Meyer PG, Blanot S, Jarreau MM, Bresson D, Zerah M, Carli PA. Is the sitting or the prone position best for surgery for posterior fossa tumours in children? *Paediatr Anaesth.* 2001;11(5):541–7.

54. Porter JM, Pidgeon C, Cunningham AJ. The sitting position in neurosurgery: A critical appraisal. *Br J Anaesth.* 1999 Jan 1;82(1): 117–28.

55. Lindroos AC, Niiya T, Silvasti-Lundell M, Randell T, Hernesniemi J, Niemi TT. Stroke volume-directed administration of hydroxyethyl starch or Ringer's acetate in sitting position during craniotomy. *Acta Anaesthesiol Scand.* 2013;57(6):729–36.

56. Ganslandt O, Merkel A, Schmitt H, Tzabazis A, Buchfelder M, Eyupoglu I, Muenster T. The sitting position in neurosurgery: indications, complications and results. A single Institution experience of 600 cases. *Acta Neurochirurgica (Wien).* 2013;155(10):1887–93.

57. Saladino A, Lamperti M, Mangraviti A, Legnani FG, Prada FU, Casali C, Caputi L, Borrelli P, DiMeco F. The semisitting position: Analysis of the risks and surgical outcomes in a contemporary series of 425 adult patients

undergoing cranial surgery. *J Neurosurg.* 2017 Oct;127(4):867–876.

58. Tran D, Rajwani K, Berlin DA. Pulmonary effects of aging. *Curr Opin Anaesthesiol.* 2018 Feb;31(1):19–23.

59. Weingarten TN, Whalen FX, Warner DO, Gajic O, Schears GJ, Snyder MR, Schroeder DR, Sprung J. Comparison of two ventilatory strategies in elderly patients undergoing major abdominal surgery. *Br J Anaesth.* 2010 Jan;104(1):16–22.

60. Güldner A, Kiss T, Serpa Neto A, Hemmes SN, Canet J, Spieth PM, Rocco PR, Schultz MJ, Pelosi P, Gama de Abreu M. Intraoperative protective mechanical ventilation for prevention of postoperative pulmonary complications: A comprehensive review of the role of tidal volume, positive end-expiratory pressure, and lung recruitment maneuvers. *Anesthesiology.* 2015 Sep;123(3):692–713.

61. Molliex S, Passot S, Morel J, Futier E, Lefrant JY, Constantin JM, Le Manach Y, Pereira B. Opti-Aged group, Azurea clinical research Network. A multicentre observational study on management of general anaesthesia in elderly patients at high-risk of postoperative adverse outcomes. *Anaesth Crit Care Pain Med.* 2018 Jun 12. (Epub ahead of print)

62. Giebler R, Kollenberg B, Pohlen G, Peters J. Effect of positive end-expiratory pressure on the incidence of venous air embolism and on the cardiovascular response to the sitting position during neurosurgery. *Br J Anaesth.* 1998;80(1):30–5.

63. Marangoni E, Alvisi V, Ragazzi R, Mojoli F, Alvisi R, Caramori G, Astolfi L, Volta CA. Respiratory mechanics at different PEEP level during general anesthesia in the elderly: A pilot study. *Minerva Anestesiol.* 2012 Nov; 78(11):1205–14.

64. Mrozek S, Constantin JM, Geeraerts T. Brain-lung crosstalk: Implications for neurocritical care patients. *World J Crit Care Med.* 2015 Aug 4;4(3):163–78.

65. Oyetunji TA, Chang DC, Crompton JG, Greene WR, Efron DT, Haut ER, Cornwell EE 3rd, Haider AH. Redefining hypotension in the elderly: Normotension is not reassuring. *Arch Surg.* 2011 Jul;146(7):865–9.

66. Futier E, Lefrant JY, Guinot PG et al. INPRESS Study Group. Effect of Individualized vs

Standard blood pressure management strategies on postoperative organ dysfunction among high-risk patients undergoing major surgery: A randomized clinical trial. *JAMA*. 2017 Oct 10;318(14):1346–1357.

67. Meng L, Cannesson M, Alexander BS, Yu Z, Kain ZN, Cerussi AE, Tromberg BJ, Mantulin WW. Effect of phenylephrine and ephedrine bolus treatment on cerebral oxygenation in anaesthetized patients. *Br J Anaesth* 2011; 107(2):209–17.

68. Hahn GH, Hyttel-Sorensen S, Petersen SM et al. Cerebral effects of commonly used vasopressor-inotropes: A study in newborn piglets. *PLOS ONE* 2013;8:e63069.

69. Soeding PF, Hoy S, Hoy G, Evans M, Royse CF. Effect of phenylephrine on the haemodynamic state and cerebral oxygen saturation during anaesthesia in the upright position. *Br J Anaesth* 2013;111(2):229–34.

70. Koch KU, Tietze A, Aanerud J, Öettingen GV, Juul N, Sørensen JCH, Nikolajsen L, Østergaard L, Rasmussen M. Effect of ephedrine and phenylephrine on brain oxygenation and microcirculation in anaesthetised patients with cerebral tumours: Study protocol for a randomised controlled trial. *BMJ Open*. 2017 Nov 17;7(11):e018560.

71. Artru AA, Cucchiara RF, Messick JM. Cardiorespiratory and cranial-nerve sequelae of surgical procedures involving the posterior fossa. *Anesthesiology*. 1980 Jan;52(1): 83–6.

72. Kwak HJ, Lee D, Lee YW, Yu GY, Shinn HK, Kim JY. The intermittent sequential compression device on the lower extremities attenuates the decrease in regional cerebral oxygen saturation during sitting position under sevoflurane anesthesia. *J Neurosurg Anesthesiol* 2011;23(1):1–5.

73. Lindroos AC, Niiya T, Randell T, Niemi TT. Stroke volume-directed administration of hydroxyethyl starch (HES 130/0.4) and Ringer's acetate in prone position during neurosurgery: A randomized controlled trial. *J Anesth*. 2014;28(2):189–97.

74. Arulkumaran N, Corredor C, Hamilton MA, Ball J, Grounds RM, Rhodes A, Cecconi M. Cardiac complications associated with goal-directed therapy in high-risk surgical patients: A meta-analysis. *Br J Anaesth*. 2014 Apr;112(4):648–59.

75. Moppett IK, Rowlands M, Mannings A, Moran CG, Wiles MD. LiDCO-based fluid management in patients undergoing hip fracture surgery under spinal anaesthesia: A randomized trial and systematic review. *Br J Anaesth* 2015;114:444–59.

76. Liu TJ, Zhang JC, Gao XZ, Tan ZB, Wang JJ, Zhang PP, Cheng AB, Zhang SB. Clinical research of goal-directed fluid therapy in elderly patients with radical resection of bladder cancer. *J Cancer Res Ther*. 2018; 14(Supplement):S173–S179.

77. Zhang N, Liang M, Zhang DD et al. Effect of goal-directed fluid therapy on early cognitive function in elderly patients with spinal stenosis: A Case-Control Study. *Int J Surg*. 2018 Jun;54(Pt A):201–205.

78. Chibbaro S, Cebula H, Todeschi J et al. Evolution of Prophylaxis Protocols for Venous Thromboembolism in Neurosurgery: Results from a Prospective Comparative Study on Low-Molecular-Weight Heparin, Elastic Stockings, and Intermittent Pneumatic Compression Devices. *World Neurosurg*. 2018 Jan;109:e510–e516.

79. Ryzenman JM, Pensak ML, Tew JM Jr. Headache: A quality of life analysis in a cohort of 1,657 patients undergoing acoustic neuroma surgery; results from the acoustic neuroma association. *Laryngoscope*. 2005;115(4):703–11.

80. Gottschalk A, Berkow LC, Stevens RD, Mirski M, Thompson RE, White ED, Weingart JD, Long DM, Yaster M. Prospective evaluation of pain and analgesic use following major elective intracranial surgery. *J Neurosurg*. 2007;106(2):210–6.

81. American Geriatrics Society 2015 Updated Beers Criteria for Potentially Inappropriate Medication Use in Older Adults. By the American Geriatrics Society 2015 Beers Criteria Update Expert Panel. *J Am Geriatr Soc*. 2015 Nov;63(11):2227–46.

82. Thibault M, Girard F, Moumdjian R, Chouinard P, Boudreault D, Ruel M. Craniotomy site influences postoperative pain following neurosurgical procedures: A retrospective study. *Can J Anaesth*. 2007 Jul;54(7):544–8.

83. Vacas S, Van de Wiele B. Designing a pain management protocol for craniotomy: A narrative review and consideration of promising practices. *Surg Neurol Int.* 2017 Dec 6;8:291.

84. Hellickson JD, Worden WR, Ryan C, Miers AG, Benike DA, Frank SP, Rhudy LM. Predictors of Postoperative Nausea and Vomiting in Neurosurgical Patients.

85. Irefin SA, Schubert A, Bloomfield EL, DeBoer GE, Mascha EJ, Ebrahim ZY. The effect of craniotomy location on postoperative pain and nausea. *J Anesth* 2003;17:227–231.

86. Latz B, Mordhorst C, Kerz T, Schmidt A, Schneider A, Wisser G, Werner C, Engelhard K. Postoperative nausea and vomiting in patients after craniotomy: Incidence and risk factors. *J Neurosurg.* 2011 Feb;114(2):491–6.

87. Bithal PK, Pandia MP, Dash HH, Chouhan RS, Mohanty B, Padhy N. Comparative incidence of venous air embolism and associated hypotension in adults and children operated for neurosurgery in the sitting position. *Eur J Anaesthesiol* 2004;21:517–522.

88. Rath GP, Bithal PK, Chaturvedi A, Dash HH. Complications related to positioning in posterior fossa craniectomy. *J Clin Neurosci* 2007;14(6):520–5.

89. Raimann F, Senft C, Honold J, Zacharowski K, Seifert V. Mersmann Takotsubo Cardiomyopathy Triggered by Venous Air Embolism During Craniotomy in the Sitting Position. *World Neurosurg.* 2017 Nov;107:1045.e1–1045.e4.

90. Schäfer ST, Sandalcioglu IE, Stegen B, Neumann A, Asgari S, Peters J. Venous air embolism during semi-sitting craniotomy evokes thrombocytopenia. *Anaesthesia* 2011;66(1):25–30.

91. Dubey A, Sung WS, Shaya M, Patwardhan R, Willis B, Smith D, Nanda A. Complications of posterior cranial fossa surgery—an institutional experience of 500 patients. *Surg Neurol* 2009;72(4):369–75.

7

Neurosurgery: Cerebrovascular diseases

PAOLO GRITTI, LUIGI ANDREA LANTERNA, FRANCESCO FERRI,
CARLO BREMBILLA, AND FERDINANDO LUCA LORINI

INTRODUCTION

Cerebrovascular disease (CVD) was defined in 1975 as: "denotes all disorders in which there is an area of brain, transiently or permanently affected by ischemia or bleeding, or in which one or more brain blood vessels are primarily involved in a pathological process, or a combination of the two" (1). "Cerebrovascular" and "cerebral" are used in the original Latin sense, referring to the whole brain and not merely to the hemispheres of the forebrain (1). Since 1975, the definition has not changed. CVD is a term that includes every pathological condition that affects the blood vessels of the brain and the cerebral circulation (2,3). This condition is one of the first in frequency and importance among all the neurologic diseases in adults, including at least 50% of the neurologic disorders in a general hospital (2). Moreover, as population ages and life expectancy increases, the elderly are widely involved in the CVD process (3,4). CVD can encompass a wide variety of medical acute events, such as ischemic or hemorrhagic stroke, to insidious pathological processes, such as atherosclerotic changes and small-vessel diseases (Table 7.1) (2,3).

In the last few decades, new types of imaging technology have been introduced, allowing the physician to make physiologic distinctions between normal, ischemic, and infarcted brain tissue, thus guiding the treatments (2). Because of this great variability in CVD, in this chapter we focus on the management of acute ischemic and hemorrhagic stroke, including subarachnoid hemorrhage (SAH) and venous sinus thrombosis, without considering the specific endovascular approach, since it is treated in detail elsewhere in this book.

CAUSE AND RISK FACTORS

Many individual factors can contribute to CVD and stroke in general. Independent stroke predictors include age, systolic blood pressure (BP), hypertension, diabetes mellitus, current smoking, established cardiovascular disease such as myocardial infarction, angina, or coronary insufficiency, congestive heart failure, intermittent claudication, atrial fibrillation, and left ventricular hypertrophy on ECG (5,6). Other potential risk factors include obesity, BP variability, sleep-disordered breathing, chronic inflammation, chronic kidney

Table 7.1 Causes of cerebral abnormalities from alterations of arteries and veins

1. Atherosclerotic thrombosis
2. Transient ischemic attacks
3. Embolism
4. Hypertensive hemorrhage
5. Ruptured or unruptured saccular aneurysm or AVM
6. Arteritis
   a. Meningovascular syphilis, arteritis secondary to pyogenic and tuberculous meningitis, rare infective types (typhus, schistosomiasis, malaria, mucormycosis, etc.)
   b. Connective tissue diseases (polyarteritis nodosa, lupus erythematosus), necrotizing arteritis, Wegener arteritis, temporal arteritis, Takayasu disease, granulomatous or giant cell arteritis of the aorta, and giant cell granulomatous angiitis of cerebral arteries.
7. Cerebral thrombophlebitis secondary to infection of ear, paranasal sinus, face, etc.; with meningitis and subdural empyema, debilitating states, postpartum, postoperative, cardiac failure, hematologic disease (polycythemia, sickle cell disease), and of undetermined cause.
8. Hematologic disorders: anticoagulants and thrombolytics, clotting factor disorders, polycythemia, sickle cell disease, thrombotic thrombocytopenic purpura, thrombocytosis, intravascular lymphoma, etc.
9. Trauma and dissection of carotid and basilar arteries
10. Amyloid angiopathy
11. Dissecting aortic aneurysm
12. Complications of arteriography
13. Neurologic migraine with persistent deficit
14. With tentorial, foramen magnum, and subfalcial herniations
15. Miscellaneous types: fibromuscular dysplasia, with local dissection of carotid, middle cerebral, or vertebrobasilar artery, x-irradiation, unexplained middle cerebral infarction in closed head injury, pressure of unruptured saccular aneurysm, complication of oral contraceptives
16. Undetermined cause in children

Source: Victor M et al. *Adams & Victor's Principles of Neurology.* 8th ed. New York: McGraw-Hill Medical; 2005. pp. 660–746.
Abbreviation: AVM, arteriovenous malformation.

disease, migraine, hormonal contraception or hormone replacement therapy, psychosocial stress, depression, job strain, and long working hours (7,8). However, among these risk factors, hypertension, smoking, and diabetes are certainly the most important factors leading to CVDs, as they can change the structure of blood vessels and result in atherosclerosis (5,6). These risk factors manifest their effects over time, and as a consequence, CVDs are widespread among the elderly population. In fact, the cumulative effects of aging on the cardiovascular system and the progressive nature of stroke risk factors over a prolonged period substantially increase the risk of ischemic stroke (IS) and intracerebral hemorrhage (ICH) (6). It seems evident that age is the most common and strongest risk factor among cerebrovascular disorders and subclinical cerebral diseases (3–6).

AGING, STROKE, AND SILENT CEREBROVASCULAR DISEASE

Stroke is the most common manifestation of CVD disease among adults. It is typically characterized as a neurological deficit attributed to an acute focal injury of the central nervous system by a vascular cause, including cerebral infarction, ICH, and SAH, and it is a major cause of disability and death worldwide (9). It diverges from transient ischemic attack (TIA) if the symptoms persist longer than 24 h or lead to earlier death, with imaging or autopsy showing focal infarction or hemorrhage relevant to the symptoms (9). The worldwide prevalence of stroke is 25.7 million, with 10.3 million people having a first stroke (5). It is the second leading global cause of death after heart disease, accounting for 11.8% of total deaths worldwide (5). With

795,000 new cases per year, 610,000 as first attacks, and 185,000 recurrent attacks, stroke is a leading cause of serious long-term disability in the United States (5). Narrowed cerebral arteries can lead to IS, but constant elevated BP can also cause tearing of vessels, leading to a hemorrhagic stroke (2). As a consequence, it can be ischemic, due to embolic or thrombotic causes, or hemorrhagic, in the case of hypertensive cerebral or SAHs (2). Prevalence of stroke in the United States increases with age in both men and women, and the elderly are widely involved in stroke and its disability consequences (5). As the population ages, the prevalence of stroke survivors is projected to increase, especially among elderly women (5). Among patients who are ≥65 years old, 6 months after stroke, 26% would be dependent in their daily living activities and 46% would have cognitive deficits (5).

However, not every cerebrovascular illness expresses itself as a clearly delineated stroke. With the introduction of ever more sophisticated imaging technology such as magnetic resonance imaging (MRI) sequences, it is possible to identify subcortical cavities or cortical areas of atrophy and gliosis that may be caused by previous infarction (4). White matter lesions of presumed vascular origin represent areas of demyelination, gliosis, arteriosclerosis, and microinfarction which are assumed to be caused by ischemia (4). They may be visible as areas of white matter hyperintensity on MRI or white matter hypodensity on computed tomography (CT) (4,10). Microbleeds are thought to represent small areas of hemosiderin deposition from previous silent hemorrhages and are visible only by MRI sequences optimized to detect them (Figure 7.1) (10). Some lesions are so clinically silent or cause such insignificant disorders of function that they do not concern the patient at all; however, they are strongly associated with future incidents such as cognitive decline and stroke (11).

The incidence of silent infarcts strongly increases with age, becoming approximately five times higher within the elderly population when compared with the incidence of stroke in the general population (4,10–12). In some studies conducted from 1993 to 2005, the prevalence of silent cerebral infarction was estimated to range from 6% to 28%, with higher prevalence with increasing age (5). Moreover, approximately 25% of people >80 years of age have ≥1 silent brain infarcts (13). The prevalence of silent CVD by far exceeds the prevalence of symptomatic stroke. It has been

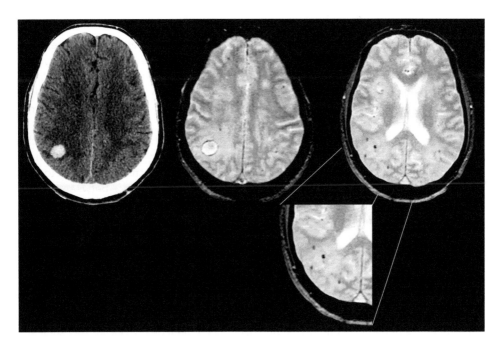

Figure 7.1 Left, hemorrhagic stroke on brain CT scan and (middle) magnetic resonance imaging (MRI) fluid-attenuated inversion recovery (FLAIR) scan. Right, microbleed (enlarged picture) on MRI T2*-weighted gradient-recalled echo sequence.

estimated that for every symptomatic stroke, there are approximately 10 silent brain infarcts (13). Because of this high prevalence, silent CVD is the incidental finding most commonly encountered on brain imaging (10).

STROKE PRESENTATION AND DIAGNOSIS

Stroke presents in a variety of ways and symptoms, and definition of the term *stroke* incorporates a broad range of clinical and tissue criteria (Table 7.2) (9). A rapid and accurate diagnosis is fundamental to increase the chance of a good outcome; however, clinical diagnosis can be complicated because no historical feature distinguishes ischemic from hemorrhagic stroke (2). The diagnosis of stroke can be even more difficult in the initial hours, particularly if the onset is uncertain, the features are atypical, the patient is unwell or agitated, and access to imaging could be delayed or not definitive because during the first hours, CT brain scan seems normal, as in IS (14). Finally, the diagnostic path can be complicated by the lack of pathognomonic signs that distinguish the different causes of stroke and by the context of management of the complications, especially among the elderly, where the lack of collaboration and the presence of comorbidity makes management even more complicated (15,16).

Table 7.2 Updated definition of stroke by the stroke council of the American Heart Association/ American Stroke Association

CNS infarction: Brain, spinal cord, or retinal cell death attributable to ischemia, based on
1. Pathological, imaging, or other objective evidence of cerebral, spinal cord, or retinal focal ischemic injury in a defined vascular distribution; or
2. Clinical evidence of cerebral, spinal cord, or retinal focal ischemic injury based on symptoms persisting ≥24 hours or until death, and other etiologies excluded. (Note: CNS infarction includes hemorrhagic infarctions, types I and II.)

Ischemic stroke: An episode of neurological dysfunction caused by focal cerebral, spinal, or retinal infarction. (Note: Evidence of CNS infarction is defined above.)

Silent CNS infarction: Imaging or neuropathological evidence of CNS infarction, without a history of acute neurological dysfunction attributable to the lesion.

Intracerebral hemorrhage: A focal collection of blood within the brain parenchyma or ventricular system that is not caused by trauma. (Note: Intracerebral hemorrhage includes parenchymal hemorrhages after CNS infarction, types I and II.)

Stroke caused by intracerebral hemorrhage: Rapidly developing clinical signs of neurological dysfunction attributable to a focal collection of blood within the brain parenchyma or ventricular system that is not caused by trauma.

Silent cerebral hemorrhage: A focal collection of chronic blood products within the brain parenchyma, subarachnoid space, or ventricular system on neuroimaging or neuropathological examination that is not caused by trauma and without a history of acute neurological dysfunction attributable to the lesion.

Subarachnoid hemorrhage: Bleeding into the subarachnoid space (the space between the arachnoid membrane and the pia mater of the brain or spinal cord).

Stroke caused by subarachnoid hemorrhage: Rapidly developing signs of neurological dysfunction and/or headache because of bleeding into the subarachnoid space (the space between the arachnoid membrane and the pia mater of the brain or spinal cord), which is not caused by trauma.

Stroke caused by cerebral venous thrombosis: Infarction or hemorrhage in the brain, spinal cord, or retina because of thrombosis of a cerebral venous structure. Symptoms or signs caused by reversible edema without infarction or hemorrhage do not qualify as stroke.

Stroke, not otherwise specified: An episode of acute neurological dysfunction presumed to be caused by ischemia or hemorrhage, persisting ≥24 hours or until death, but without sufficient evidence to be classified as one of the above.

Source: Sacco RL et al. *Stroke.* 2013;44(7):2064–89.
Abbreviation: CNS, central nervous system.

Clinical presentation

Common stroke signs and symptoms may include sudden onset of weakness, hemiparesis, monoparesis, or rarely quadriparesis, hemisensory deficits, visual loss or visual field deficits, diplopia, dysarthria, altered speech, aphasia, facial droop, ataxia, vertigo, nystagmus, and sudden decrease in the level of consciousness (14). Although such symptoms can occur alone, they are more likely to occur in combination. No historical feature distinguishes ischemic from hemorrhagic stroke, although nausea, vomiting, headache, and sudden change in the level of consciousness are the most common in hemorrhagic strokes. In younger patients, a history of recent trauma, coagulopathies, illicit drug use (such as cocaine), migraines, or use of oral contraceptives should be elicited. Associated symptoms vary and usually reflect the cause or the consequence of the stroke. For example, headache occurs in about a quarter of patients with acute IS, half of patients with ICH, and nearly all patients with SAH (14–16). Headache may also reflect the underlying cause of the stroke, such as cervical artery dissection or giant cell arteritis, or be the consequence of cortical ischemia or intracranial hemorrhage (14).

Diagnostically, the Face, Arm, and Speech Test (FAST), a mnemonic to help detect stroke and to facilitate an appropriate response, aids screening for stroke and is as sensitive and specific as the Recognition of Stroke in the Emergency Room (ROSIER) score. The ROSIER score adds to the three items of FAST assessment of the visual field defect, leg weakness, loss of consciousness or syncope, and seizure activity (Table 7.3) (14,15). If these criteria are met, the likelihood of a stroke is higher, in particular among the elderly with a history of prolonged exposure to vascular risk factors (14).

Investigations

It is more difficult to diagnose a stroke in the initial hours, particularly if the onset is uncertain, the features are atypical or changing, the patient is unwell or agitated, and the access to imaging is delayed. One-fifth of the patients (20%–25%) presenting with a stroke syndrome actually have a stroke mimic, which is a non-cerebrovascular cause for their symptoms which confounds the clinical diagnosis of stroke. The five most frequent non-stroke diagnoses are seizure, syncope, sepsis, migraine, and brain tumor (16). Diagnosis of stroke can be confirmed by brain CT or MRI or cerebrospinal fluid examination for subarachnoid blood (14). Noncontrast cranial CT scan has near-perfect sensitivity to detect fresh intracranial hemorrhage, but its sensitivity for diagnosis of IS is even poorer if ischemia is recent, small, or in the posterior fossa (14). The sensitivity

Table 7.3 The Face, Arm, and Speech Test (FAST) and the Recognition of Stroke in the Emergency Room (ROSIER) scores

Face, Arm, and Speech Test (FAST) (14,15)

    Face—Ask the person to smile. Does one side of the face droop?
    Arms—Ask the person to raise both arms. Does one arm drift downward?
    Speech—Ask the person to repeat a simple phrase. Is the speech slurred or strange?
    Time—If you observe any of these signs, call for an ambulance immediately.

Recognition of Stroke in the Emergency Room (ROSIER) Scale to Differentiate Stroke and "Stroke Mimics" (14,15)

    Has there been loss of consciousness or syncope?
    Has there been seizure activity?
    Is there a new onset (or waking from sleep)?
    Asymmetric facial weakness.
    Asymmetric arm weakness.
    Asymmetric leg weakness.
    Speech disturbance.
    Visual field defect.

Note: Stroke is likely if total score >0. Scores of ≤ 0 have low probability of stroke but not excluded
Abbreviation: FAST, Facial drooping, Arm weakness, Speech difficulties, and Time.

of CT is 98% for SAH within 12 hours, 93% at 24 hours, and declines rapidly after 10 days (15).

IS may not be apparent on the initial CT scan, although subtle signs of early ischemia are usually evident. The sensitivity of CT to diagnose acute IS is limited if the focal ischemia is recent, minutes to hours, small, or in the posterior fossa (14).

MRI, in particular diffusion weighted sequences (DWI-MRI), detects acute brain ischemia in about 90% of patients with IS, and about a third of patients with transient symptoms lasting less than 24 hours, while gradient-echo T2-weighted susceptibility MRI is as sensitive as CT for acute hemorrhage and more sensitive for previous hemorrhage (14). CT angiography (CTA) scan of the neck and head may be useful not only in the evaluation of an intracerebral aneurysm, but in the case of acute IS to detect intracranial occlusions, to estimate the extent of the occlusion in the arterial tree, and to provide neurovascular anatomy in the case of endovascular treatment (17). Finally, digital angiography is necessary not only for diagnostic proposes, but in both ischemic and endovascular hemorrhagic treatment (18–20).

ACUTE ISCHEMIC STROKE

Acute ischemic stroke (AIS) is defined as an episode of neurological dysfunction caused by focal cerebral, spinal, or retinal infarction (9). Central nervous system (CNS) infarction is brain, spinal cord, or retinal cell death attributable to ischemia, based on pathological, imaging, or other objective evidence of cerebral ischemic injury in a defined vascular distribution, or to clinical evidence of cerebral, spinal cord, or retinal focal ischemic injury based on symptoms persisting ≥24 hours or until death, and other etiologies excluded (9). The presence of large-vessel occlusion of a major intracranial artery, the most common being the middle cerebral artery or internal carotid artery, is estimated to occur in approximately one-third to one-half of AIS (79). Additional ischemia-modifying factors determine the extent of necrosis. According to the Trial of ORG 10172 in Acute Stroke Treatment (TOAST) classification, IS is caused by large-artery atherosclerosis, cardio-embolism, small-vessel occlusion, stroke of other determined etiology, and stroke of undetermined etiology (21). Another classification is included by the ASCOD (Atherosclerosis, Small-vessel disease,

Cardiac pathology, Other cause, Dissection) phenotyping system (22).

Specific treatment

The goal of early therapy for AIS is to restore perfusion to the ischemic areas of the brain as soon as possible. The speed of occlusion is as important as promptness in the treatment: The earlier the treatment is performed, the better the results are. Outcomes can be improved by a rapid diagnosis and a selection of patients with CT scan, CTA of the brain, and/or magnetic resonance angiography (MRA) to confirm large artery occlusion, and by second-generation devices and techniques that enable higher rates of reperfusion (Figure 7.2) (15,18,19,23). For these reasons, local algorithms and rapid triage and organization are necessary.

The use of intravenous alteplase (rtPA) at the dose of 0.9 mg/kg, administered within 4,5 h of IS, increases the odds of no significant disability at 3–6 months by about a third and does not affect mortality, despite increasing the odds of symptomatic ICH (15,24). Moderate to high quality evidence suggests that compared with medical care alone in a selected group of patients, endovascular thrombectomy as an add-on to intravenous thrombolysis performed within 6–8 hours after large vessel IS in the anterior circulation provides beneficial functional outcomes without increasing detrimental effects (Figure 7.3) (18,23,25,26). The effect is consistent among the elderly (>80 years) and patients ineligible for rtPA (26).

Finally, recent research on patients with acute stroke who had been in good condition 6–24 hours before the stroke and who had a mismatch between clinical deficit and infarct at 90 days, shows better outcomes for disability with thrombectomy plus standard care than with standard care alone (19).

HEMORRHAGIC STROKE

Hemorrhagic stroke is the third most frequent cause of stroke after AIS and TIA (2). Hypertensive hemorrhages (11%–15.5%) compared with hemorrhage due to ruptured aneurysms and vascular malformations (4.5%–7%) have a higher overall incidence in the context of the major CVD (2). Primary hypertensive ICH is the mundane "spontaneous" brain hemorrhage (9). It is predominantly due to chronic hypertension and degenerative changes in

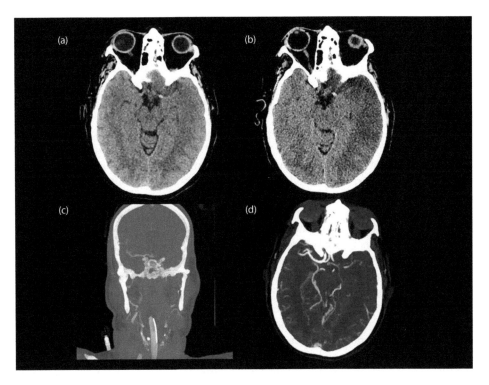

Figure 7.2 Acute obliteration of the left middle carotid artery (MCA) with an hyperdense artery sign suggesting an acute thrombus in the left MCA (a) evolving in ischemia 24 hours later (b). CT angiography shows obliteration of the left MCA (c, d).

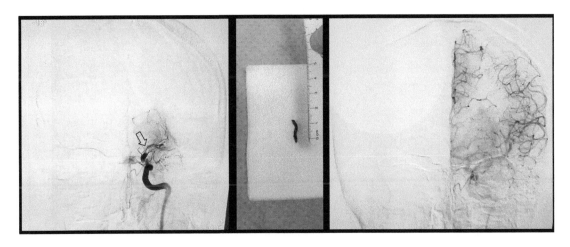

Figure 7.3 A 78-year-old man developed right-sided hemiplegia and aphasia due to left middle carotid artery (MCA) occlusion (left figure). Intravenous actilyse was applied; however, 1 hour later, mechanical thrombectomy of the obliterated left MCA was performed with successful thrombus removal (central and right figure), with almost complete right-sided hemiplegia and aphasia resolved.

cerebral arteries. In recent decades, with increased awareness of the need to control BP, the percentage of hemorrhages caused by factors other than hypertension has greatly increased. In order of frequency, ICH is classified according to its anatomical site or presumed etiology. The most common sites of ICH are supratentorial (85%–95%), including deep (50%–75%) and lobar (25%–40%). The most common causes are hypertension (30%–60%), cerebral amyloid angiopathy (10%–30%), anticoagulation (1%–20%), and vascular structural lesions (3%–8%), while undetermined causes account for about 5%–20% of cases (27).

Specific treatment

BP control is desirable in primary hypertensive ICH. It has been shown that intensive BP reduction within 3–6 h of onset of ICH to a systolic target of 110–139 mmHg does not result in a lower rate of death or disability than a standard reduction to a target of 140–179 mmHg, but the rate of renal adverse events within 7 days after randomization was significantly higher in the intensive-treatment group than in the standard-treatment group (28). Although platelet transfusion after ICH associated with antiplatelet drugs increases death and dependence at 3 months, spontaneous ICH associated with vitamin K antagonist anticoagulation, reversal of the INR to lower than 1.3, and reduction of the systolic BP to lower than 160 mmHg within 4 h is associated with reduced hematoma enlargement (29,30). Normalization of INR with four-factor prothrombin complex concentrate seems superior to fresh frozen plasma, reducing hematoma expansion (31). Idarucizumab can be used for dabigatran-associated ICH, although ICH associated with direct inhibition of thrombin or factor Xa by direct oral anticoagulants can be more complicated, requiring immediate cessation of the direct oral anticoagulants, supportive measures, and consideration of specific reversal agents (32–35).

SURGICAL TREATMENTS FOR ACUTE STROKE COMPLICATIONS

The surgical approach to patients with stroke emergencies in some contexts can greatly reduce the unfavorable outcome and mortality (Figure 7.4a–d). Cerebral edema can be a secondary consequence of a large area of brain infarction as in malignant middle cerebral artery infarctions. Decompressive hemicraniectomy (DHC) versus conventional treatment significantly decreases mortality and

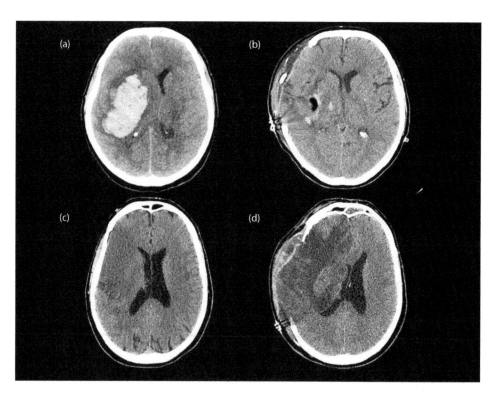

Figure 7.4 Preoperative CT scan showed a large right basal ganglion hemorrhage hematoma (a) followed by clot evacuation and decompressive hemicraniectomy (b). Decompressive hemicraniectomy for malignant right MCA infarction (c, d).

increases the good functional outcome, although it is associated with non-significant difference in severe disability among survivors compared with conservative treatment (36). Although the optimum criteria to perform DHC, such as patient selection, timing of surgery, and acceptable degree of disability in survivors, remains undefined, the operation should be performed before there is a major midline shift causing secondary ischemic brain injury and bleeding in the brainstem (15). The tradeoff between improved survival at the expense of substantial disability is greater for patients older than 60 than for younger ones (36). Also, in cerebellar infarction, suboccipital decompressive craniectomy (SDC) has been taken into account with associated better outcomes compared with decompressive surgery for hemispheric infarctions. Similarly, sensitivity analysis found less mortality in patients with mean age <60 years (37).

Even if there is lively debate and insufficient evidence to justify a general policy of early surgery for patients with spontaneous ICH compared with conservative treatment, surgery could play an important role in patients with ICH, but it is still not clear which patients would benefit most (38). Surgery includes open craniotomy and minimally invasive approaches, such as endoscopic aspiration and stereotactic aspiration, that could reduce the volume of intracerebral hematoma with associated clinical and experimental evidence that clot removal might reduce nervous tissue damage, thereby reducing local ischemia (39). The pathophysiology of ICH is time-dependent, and the removal of blood from the brain should be ideally accomplished as soon as possible with minimal damage to the overlying normal brain parenchyma and without increasing the risk of further growth of hemorrhage (15,38). The STICH trial, one of the largest studies on emergent hematoma evacuation via craniotomy within 72 h of ictus, fails to improve outcome significantly compared to initial medical management, damping the enthusiasm of neurosurgeons to perform surgery (40). The sequel of the study, STICH II, failed to support hypothesis that early surgery compared with initial conservative treatment, with delayed surgery if the patient deteriorates, improves outcome in conscious patients in whom there is a superficial ICH of 10–100 mL and no evidence of intraventricular hemorrhage (41). However, this last study has shown that early open-surgery evacuation of supratentorial

hematomas might be beneficial for patients with a Glasgow Coma Scale (GCS) score of 9–12 who are treated within 8 h of symptom onset (41). In conclusion, although early surgery does not increase the rate of death or disability at 6 months, it could have a small but clinically relevant survival advantage for patients with spontaneous superficial ICH without intraventricular hemorrhage (38,40,41). Finally, minimally invasive drainage by catheter holds promise in the treatment of deep hematomas (42). An external ventricular drain combined with topical fibrinolysis reduces mortality but not functional dependence in intraventricular hemorrhage and hydrocephalus (43). Surgical evacuation of infratentorial ICH is usually indicated if the GCS is lower than 14, the hematoma diameter is higher than 30–40 mm, its volume higher than 7 cm^3, or if there is obliteration of the fourth ventricle. Finally, an external ventricular drain is usually inserted if there is associated hydrocephalus (15,38).

SUBARACHNOID HEMORRHAGE

Subarachnoid hemorrhage (SAH) is a severe subtype of stroke with a third of patients involved who do not survive, and at least one of five of those who survive are unable to regain functional independence (44). Rupture of arterial aneurysms is the major cause of SAH and the fourth most frequent and devastating cerebrovascular disorder, with an estimated incidence of approximately 7–9 cases per 100,000 inhabitants per year (5,45). Saccular aneurysm takes the form of small, thin-walled blisters protruding from arteries of the circle of Willis or its major branches, and its rupture releases blood directly into the cerebrospinal fluid under arterial pressure (Figure 7.5) (2,45). The bleeding usually lasts only for a few seconds, but it can cause an increase of intracranial pressure (ICP), which can be followed by severe headache, seizure, nausea, vomiting, focal neurologic deficit, or stiff neck. If the bleeding is violent and continuous, the increase of ICP and the dropping of the cerebral perfusion pressure explains the transient or persisting decreased consciousness, deep coma, or death (2,45). Etiology and risk factors of SAH aneurysm rupture could also include familial predisposition and heritable connective tissue diseases as polycystic kidney disease, Ehlers–Danlos syndrome type IV, neurofibromatosis type 1, and Marfan syndrome, but cigarette smoking may also predispose

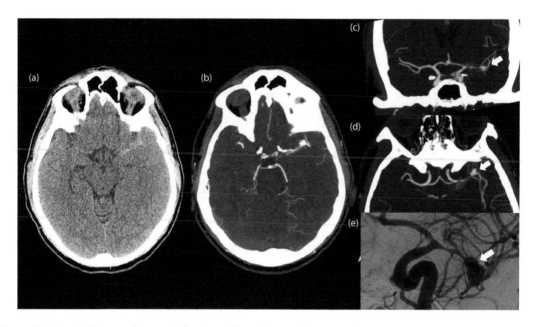

Figure 7.5 Brain CT scan shows a left subarachnoid hemorrhage (a) due to bilobar saccular aneurysms at the left middle cerebral artery bifurcation (b). The sequence (c), (d), and (e) shows the aneurysm and an initial vasospasm of the proximal M1 artery at the angiograms.

to aneurysmal SAH, whereas moderate- to high-level alcohol consumption is an independent risk factor (2,46).

AGE and subarachnoid hemorrhage

Autopsy studies show that cerebral aneurysms are common in adults, with a prevalence ranging between 1% and 5% (47), and recent data suggest that with the aging in general populations, there is an increasing admission rate of elderly patients suffering from SAH (48). Although the age-specific incidence of SAH increases with advanced age, a recent study suggests that elderly patients may run less risks of rupture compared with younger ones (49). Females show decreasing relative aneurysmal SAH incidence after around 65, while the age is around 53 years old for males (49). Age still remains, according to World Federation of Neurological Surgeons (WFNS) grade on admission, the strongest prognostic independent predictive factor of bad outcome in patients with SAH due to aneurysm rupture (50). The risk of poor outcome is significantly higher after the age of 60 years (50,51), when there is a linear association between advancing age and worse outcome with an odds ratio of 1.32 for each decade increase in age, and 60 days mortality (52). Several factors

may be involved, including increased rates of diabetes, myocardial disease, arterial hypertension, and cerebrovascular and pulmonary disease (52). Moreover, the incidence of severe complications during the treatment that increases with advancing age and the fact that the aging brain has a less optimal response to the initial bleeding could explain the increased worse outcome in the elderly (52).

Clinical investigations

Brain CT with or without lumbar puncture allows the diagnosis of SAH, as it can identify signs of bleeding in the cerebrospinal fluid (CSF) or hyperdense signals provided by the extravasated blood in the basal cisterns at the brain scan CT (53). The location and spreading of the bleeding can often suggest the location of the ruptured aneurysm. The highest sensitivity of head CT is in the first 6–12 hours after SAH, decreasing in the subsequent days. A subsequent CTA or MRA, which are noninvasive tests, can be useful for screening and presurgical planning. Both CTA and MRA can identify aneurysms from 3 to 5 mm or larger with a high degree of sensitivity, but they do not achieve the resolution of conventional angiography (54). Digital subtraction angiography (DSA) can be performed in cases of uncertainty; it has increased sensitivity in diagnosing and allows better characterization of the morphology, orientation, neck size, adjacent vessels, and detects any additional aneurysm or vascular malformations (53,54).

Grading SAH, the risk of vasospasm, and prognosis

There are several grading systems used in practice to standardize and classify patients with SAH based upon the initial neurologic examination and finding on CT scan imaging. The most widely used are the Hunt and Hess, and the WFNS, which combine GCS and neurological evaluation of patients with the presence of a motor deficit (Table 7.4, right side) (55,56). The Fisher and Claassen grading score is an index of vasospasm risk based upon a CT-defined hemorrhage pattern (Table 7.4, left side) (57,58).

Two other scales used in classification of the SAH patients are the Vasograde, a three-category scale based on the WFNS, and modified Fisher that predicts the risk of delayed cerebral ischemia, and the Ogilvy and Carter scale, which incorporates a number of features that may impact on outcome, including age, Hunt and Hess grade, Fisher grade, and aneurysm size (59,60). More recently, several prediction models and risk scores have been developed for patients with SAH. FRESH is the first SAH prognostication tool to combine functional outcome with cognitive and quality of life outcomes (61). The last one is the Subarachnoid Hemorrhage International Trialists (SAHIT) score, a clinical prediction model developed with individual patient data coming from 10.936 patients derivate by the SAHIT data repository, available on line (http://sahitscore.com). It is constituted by seven items divided into a core model, a neuroimaging

Table 7.4 Grading systems used in practice to standardize and classify patients with SAH based upon the initial neurologic examination and finding on CT scan imaging

Fisher grade of cerebral vasospasm risk in SAH	Classen grade of cerebral vasospasm risk in SAH	Grade	Hunt and Hess grading system neurologic status	WFNS	
				GCS	Motor deficit
No blood detected	No SAH or IVH	1	Asymptomatic or mild headache and slight nuchal rigidity	15	Absent
Diffuse deposition or thin layer with all vertical layers less than 1 mm thick	Minimal SAH and no IVH	2	Severe headache, stiff neck, no neurologic deficit except cranial nerve palsy	13–14	Absent
Localized clot and/or vertical layers 1 mm or more in thickness	Minimal SAH with bilateral IVH	3	Drowsy or confused, mild focal neurologic deficit	13–14	Present
Intracerebral or intraventricular clot with diffuse or no subarachnoid blood	Thick SAH (completely filling one or more cistern or fissure) without bilateral IVH	4	Stuporous, moderate or severe hemiparesis	7–12	Present or absent
	Thick SAH (completely filling one or more cistern or fissure) with bilateral IVH	5	Coma, decerebrate posturing	3–6	Present or absent

Source: Hunt WE, Hess RM. J Neurosurg. 1968;28(1):14–20 (55); J Neurosurg. 1988;68(6):985–6 (56); Fisher CM et al. Neurosurgery. 1980;6(1):1–9 (57); Claassen J et al. Stroke. 2001;32(9):2012–20.

Abbreviations: GCS, Glasgow Coma Scale; WFNS, World Federation of Neurological Surgeons.

model, and a treatment modality on admission to predict risk of functional outcome with a good discrimination and an area under the receiver operator characteristics curve (AUC) of 0.81 (IC 0.79–0.83) (50).

Specific treatment

After aneurysmal SAH, the risk of early aneurysm rebleeding is higher, particularly in the first hours, with reported rates of occurrence between 4% and 13.6% within the first 24 hours (62). Aneurysmal rebleeding occurs frequently within the first 6 hours and could be associated with high systolic pressure, the presence of an intracerebral or intraventricular hematoma, poor Hunt-Hess grade (III−IV), aneurysms in the posterior circulation, and aneurysm size (10 mm) (63). Rebleeding often results in very poor outcomes and with an estimated mortality of 70% (62,63). Therefore, urgent evaluation and treatment of patients with suspected SAH is recommended, since aneurysm repair is the only effective treatment to prevent this occurrence and should be performed within 24–72 hours with

an antifibrinolytic therapy to prevent bleeding (62). Microsurgical clip obliteration of intracranial aneurysms both with endovascular approach and with electrolytically detachable coils are the two pivotal ways of treating aneurysm (Figures 7.6 and 7.7) (62). However, in the last few decades the treatment of aneurysms has changed, especially from clipping to coiling, and treatment of aneurysms takes place more often as soon as it is possible (64). Algorithms to determine the proper patient population and aneurysmal characteristics for each treatment are continually undergoing refinement (62). To current knowledge, middle cerebral artery aneurysms can be difficult to treat with coil embolization, and surgical treatment is preferable (62). Moreover, an elderly age may confer a reduced risk of aneurysmal recurrence after endovascular coiling (65), providing further evidence that coiling should be considered as first-line therapy in elderly patients with a ruptured aneurysm and in patients presenting it during the vasospasm period (62,65). On the other hand, patients with intraparenchymal hematoma should preferentially undergo clipping treatment with a rapid hematoma evacuation (62).

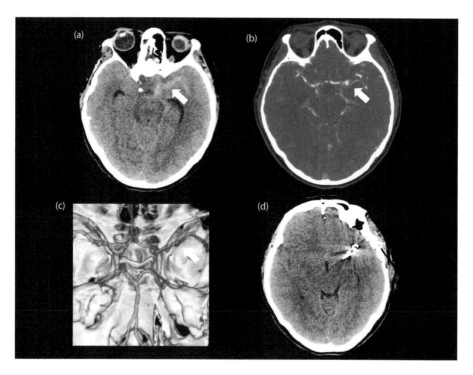

Figure 7.6 Comparison of section images from brain CT (a), CT angiography (b), to 3D representation (c) in a patient with severe subarachnoid hemorrhage and aneurysm of left MCA bifurcation before and after clipping (d).

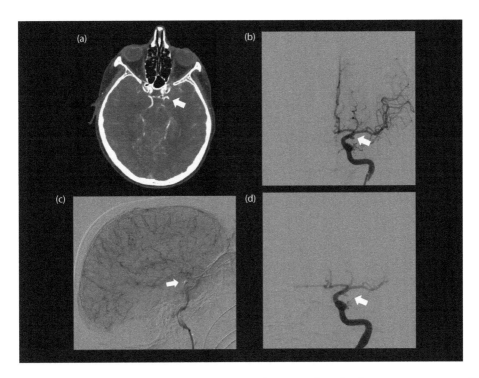

Figure 7.7 A section of images from brain CT angiography **(a)** to digital subtraction angiogram **(b, c)** in a patient with a left internal carotid aneurysm (white arrows) before and after embolization **(d)**.

CEREBRAL VENOUS SINUS THROMBOSIS

Thrombosis of the cerebral venous sinuses (CVT), although infrequent, varying from 0.5%–1% of all form of strokes, causes approximately 5 deaths per million annually (66,67). Due to the increasing availability of neuroimaging of the last few decades, CVT has become a more easily recognized disease and appears to be more common than previously believed (66). It may develop in relation to infections of the adjacent ear and paranasal sinuses or to bacterial meningitis, or non-infectious venous occlusion resulting from one of the many hypercoagulable states such as pregnancy and puerperium, cancer, cyanotic congenital heart disease, cachexia in infants, sickle cell disease, antiphospholipid antibody syndrome, Behcet disease, factor V Leiden mutation, protein S or C deficiency, antithrombin III deficiency, resistance to activated protein C, primary or secondary polycythemia and thrombocythemia, and paroxysmal nocturnal hemoglobinuria (2,68). However, the two most common risk factors are an underlying thrombophilia (34%) or exposure to oral contraceptives

(54%); at least one risk factor was identified in 85% of cases, and two or more in 44% of patients (68). The clinical features of CVT are nonspecific, varying from mild headache and focal neurologic signs to catastrophic progressive rise in ICP leading to neurological deterioration and death. It may also lead to a number of important neurologic syndromes (2,67). Focal or generalized seizures are frequent, occurring in 40% of patients; moreover, bilateral brain involvement is not infrequent (67). This is particularly notable in cases that involve the deep venous drainage system, when bilateral thalamic involvement may occur, causing alterations at level of consciousness without focal neurological findings. Bilateral motor signs, including paraparesis, may also be present due to sagittal sinus thrombosis and bihemispheric injury. Finally, patients with CVT often present with slowly progressive symptoms. However, within the elderly population these symptoms may be different, with rare case presentation as isolated intracranial hypertension, whereas mental status and alertness disturbances are common, and CVT often resulting in a worse prognosis (69). Clinical and laboratory findings may demonstrate suggestive abnormalities of an underlying hypercoagulable state, an infectious process, or an inflammatory state, all of which may contribute to the development of CVT (67). CT without contrast is often normal but may demonstrate findings that suggest CVT. The primary sign of acute CVT on a noncontrast CT is hyperdensity of a cortical vein or dural sinus. Thrombosis of the posterior portion of the superior sagittal sinus may appear as a dense triangle, the dense or filled delta sign. An ischemic lesion that crosses usual arterial boundaries or in close proximity to a venous sinus is suggestive of CVT (67). Contrast-enhanced CT may show enhancement of the dural lining of the sinus with a filling defect within the vein or sinus. Brain parenchymal lesions of CVT are better visualized and depicted on MRI than on CT (Figure 7.8). Focal edema without hemorrhage is visualized on CT in 8% of cases and on MRI in 25% of cases, while CVT is diagnosed on MRI with the detection of thrombus in a venous sinus. Cerebral angiography and direct cerebral venography are reserved for situations in which the MRA or CTA results are inconclusive, or if an endovascular procedure is being considered and the venous phase of cerebral angiography shows a filling defect in the thrombosed cerebral vein/sinus (Figure 7.8) (67). Normally, the early veins begin became opaque about 4–5 seconds after injection of contrast material into the carotid artery, and the complete cerebral venous system becomes opaque in 7–8 seconds. If cerebral veins or dural sinuses are not visualized in the normal sequences of cerebral angiography, the possibility of acute thrombosis is suspected (67).

Specific treatment

On the basis of the available data, anticoagulation appears safe and effective in the management of patients with CVT. If anticoagulation is given, there are no data supporting differences in outcome with the use of unfractionated heparin (UFH) in adjusted doses or low molecular weight heparins (LMWH) in CVT patients (70). However, in the setting of deep vein thrombosis and pulmonary embolism, in a recent systematic review and meta-analysis of 29 studies, major hemorrhage and recurrent venous thromboembolism occurred less frequently in participants treated with LMWH than in those treated with UFH (OR 0.69, 95% CI 0.50–0.95; P = 0.02 and OR 0.71, 95% CI 0.56–0.90; P = 0.005, respectively) (70). Although patients with CVT may recover with an anticoagulation therapy, 9%–13% have poor outcomes despite anticoagulation (68). Many invasive therapeutic procedures have been reported to treat CVT. These include direct catheter chemical thrombolysis and direct mechanical thrombectomy with or without thrombolysis (67,71). Decompressive craniotomy may be needed as a life-saving measure if a large venous infarction leads to a significant increase in ICP (71). However, there are no randomized controlled trials to support these interventions compared with anticoagulation or with each other,

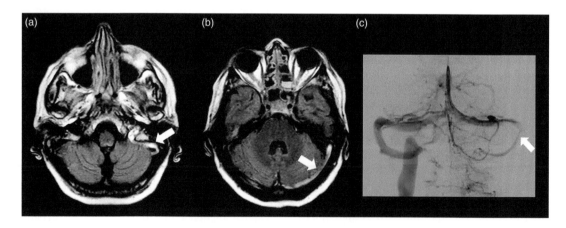

Figure 7.8 A series of images that show an axial plane FLAIR MRI sequence with hyperintensity in the left transverse sinus path (white arrows) that corresponds to thrombosis (a, b). Digital subtraction angiography and venous phase of direct carotid angiogram (c) shows left transverse sinus thrombosis (white arrows).

but most evidence is based on small case series or anecdotal reports (67,71).

MAIN TREATMENT PRINCIPLES

General considerations

Patients with CVD are at risk of hemodynamic instability and neurologic deterioration. Airway support and ventilator assistance are recommended for the treatment of patients with acute stroke who have decreased consciousness or who have bulbar dysfunction that causes failures of the airway (72). Moreover, they benefit from the close neurologic and hemodynamic monitoring provided in the ICU or stroke unit to minimize the risk of secondary injury due to development of malignant edema, or due to the hemorrhagic transformation of ischemia (73–75). In hemorrhagic stroke or SAH due to aneurysm rupture, coagulopathy and low platelet count below 50,000 should be urgently treated with some combination of intravenous vitamin K, fresh frozen plasma, platelet transfusions, and prothrombin complex concentrates (62,75). Finally, patients with SAH are at risk of hemodynamic instability and neurologic deterioration that often occurs in one-third of patients, complicated by pulmonary edema and cardiac arrhythmias in 23% and 35% of patients, respectively (75).

Decline in neurological status

The patient's cognitive status may be a useful guide because if the patient is alert, then cerebral perfusion pressure is adequate. It is important to consider the broad range of causes of neurological deterioration, since appropriate treatments will vary. Physical examination may show further evidence of herniation or a new seizure requiring treatment. Diagnosing the cause of CVD as soon as possible can be lifesaving and prevent or minimize permanent neurologic damage. The history may provide clues to these diagnoses, but early triage of the patient to CT scan or MRI is critical (73–76). However, it is important to assess and optimize vital physiologic function before sending the patient for an imaging study. Therefore, after subsequent early intensive treatment, it may be advisable to repeat a CT scan, as it may show herniation, edema, ultra-early rebleeding, development of hydrocephalus, or development of an intraparenchymal or subdural hematoma (75,76). Moreover, it is important to stabilize respiratory and hemodynamic status of the patient because hypotension will decrease cerebral perfusion pressure, while hypoxia may result from neurogenic pulmonary edema. Arrhythmias may also lead to hypotension. Cardiovascular collapse could be the result of increasing hydrocephalus or brain herniation, neurocardiogenic shock from Takotsubo cardiomyopathy, or respiratory failure from neurogenic pulmonary edema (75,76).

Blood pressure

The arterial BP is often elevated in patients with CVD, and this is due to chronic hypertension, which is a major risk factor for IS, but also to an appropriate response to maintain brain perfusion in cerebral edema or ICP due to SAH. Regular BP monitoring should be undertaken after a CVD event, and it is preferable to have a continuous BP monitoring via arterial line in those with unstable hemodynamic and those who are intubated and ventilated, where it has the advantage of facilitating arterial blood gas analysis (75). There are currently no data to suggest significant risks with the use of arterial lines in those undergoing thrombolysis (76). The decision to treat BP requires a balance between the potential danger of severe increases in BP and a possible decline in neurologic functioning when BP is lowered. There is a U-shaped relationship between BP and outcome after AIS, with both high and low BP having adverse effects on outcome (76). Although high BP is independently associated with poor outcome after AIS, the effect of acute BP lowering is not clear. Some patients may benefit from BP augmentation, for example, those with severe carotid stenosis; conversely, severe hypotension will compromise cerebral perfusion and potentially increase infarct volume. However, further data are required to assess long-term outcomes (76).

In conclusion, there are controversies surrounding optimal BP targets and the reluctance to lower BP in the acute setting, except in relation to thrombolysis where guidelines recommend that BP should be less than 185/110 mmHg before commencing and for 24 h after treatment (72). In the SAH guidelines, the lack of quality data about BP control suggests that BP should be monitored and controlled to "balance the risk of stroke, hypertension-associated rebleeding, and maintenance of the cerebral perfusion pressure" (62). Therefore, it is preferable to use antihypertensive medications that are short acting, easily titratable, and can be administered as a continuous infusion to reduce the systolic pressure to below 160 mmHg, or the MAP < 110 mmHg (62).

Endotracheal intubation and tracheostomy

The decision to perform an endotracheal intubation is based on the ability of the patient to control his or her airway, the presence of hyperventilation or hypoventilation, hypoxia resistant to supplemental oxygen, or an anticipated clinical decompensation, especially if transfer to another facility is planned (75,76). Patients with CVD can present with a decreased respiratory drive or muscular airway obstruction. Hypoventilation, with a resulting increase in the partial pressure of carbon dioxide, may lead to cerebral vasodilation, which further elevates ICP. Intubation may be necessary to restore adequate ventilation and to protect the airway, in particular by vomiting, which occurs commonly with increased ICP, and oral secretions. Clinicians should be prepared to intubate at any time, given that the neurological examination can decline, particularly in the setting of acute cerebral edema, aneurysm re-rupture, acute hydrocephalus, or herniation (75). Dysphagia is common after both hemispheric and brainstem stroke and increases the risk of aspiration pneumonia (77). Between 15% and 35% of AIS patients managed in the ICU setting require tracheostomy, usually those with severe dysphagia and bulbar palsies resulting from brainstem and large hemispheric infarcts, the elderly, or those patients who require prolonged periods of mechanical ventilation (78).

Specific considerations in AIS

The recent guidelines for the management of patients with AIS clearly impose an intensive treatment to support the vital function of these patients (72). Supplemental oxygen should be provided to maintain oxygen saturation >94%; hypotension and hypovolemia should be corrected to maintain systemic perfusion levels necessary to support organ function. Although the benefit of induced hypothermia to treat patients with IS is not well established, sources of hyperthermia (temperature >38°C) should be identified and treated with antipyretic medications (72). Moreover, it is reasonable to treat hyperglycemia to achieve blood glucose levels in a range of 140–180 mg/dL and to closely monitor to prevent hypoglycemia (72,76).

In patients undergoing fibrinolytic therapy, physicians should be prepared to treat potential emergent adverse effects, including bleeding complications and angioedema that may cause partial airway obstruction, and maintaining BP <180/105 mmHg for at least the first 24 hours after IV alteplase treatment (72). Also, elderly patients (>80 years old) presenting in the 3–4.5 h window could undergo fibrinolytic therapy (0.9 mg/kg, maximum dose 90 mg over 60 min with initial 10% of dose given as bolus over 1 min) (72). Outcomes after AIS are improved if patients are managed by multidisciplinary teams in an acute stroke unit, and all patients administered with alteplase should be admitted to an intensive care or stroke unit for monitoring (72,75,76).

Specific considerations in SAH

In the period following diagnosis and before definitive aneurysm treatment, when definitive treatment of the aneurysm is unavoidably delayed and there are no other contraindications to treatment, short-term therapy (<72 h) with tranexamic acid or aminocaproic acid is reasonable (62). Patients with SAH often develop increased ICP that is usually due to acute hydrocephalus and reactive hyperemia after hemorrhage. Ventriculostomy allows treatment of ICP by drainage of CSF in appropriate patients, and consent to direct measurement of ICP (62,75,80). When it is not possible to place a catheter in the ventricles, then the use of osmotic therapy with mannitol or hypertonic saline solutions could be utilized, lowering ICP and improving cerebral perfusion (74,75). Finally, when it is not possible to place a ventriculostomy and osmotic therapy is insufficient to reduce ICP, decompressive craniectomy (DC) may be needed as extreme treatment, although in poor-grade aneurysmal SAH it is associated with high rates of unfavorable outcome and death (77,80). Physiologic derangements occur frequently in the acute phase of SAH and might worsen the diffuse brain injury, so stabilization of the patient aims to avoid hypoxemia, metabolic acidosis, hyperglycemia, and BP instability. Moreover, intravenous fluid administration should target euvolemia and normal electrolyte balance (62). Anemia, fever, infections, and endocrine dysfunction in SAH patients are common and should be recognized, and treated. The management of seizures in CVD and in particular associated with SAH are controversial (80). The recent AHA guidelines suggest that use of prophylactic anticonvulsants may be considered in the immediate post hemorrhagic period; however, the routine long-term use of anticonvulsants is not recommended but may be considered for patients with known risk factors to delay seizure disorder, such as prior seizure, intracerebral hematoma, intractable hypertension, infarction, or aneurysm at the middle cerebral artery (62). Therefore, a very short course of prophylactic anticonvulsants may be recommended in the period following diagnosis and before definitive aneurysm treatment. As phenytoin may lead to worse long-term cognitive outcomes, the use of a different agent, such as levetiracetam, could be considered (62,75).

CONCLUSION

Elderly patients are at increased risk to develop CVD; however, the care of these diseases, such as IS or hemorrhage stroke has dramatically transformed over the past few decades due to diagnostic, medical, endovascular, and surgical advances. This progress has certainly helped to not exclude the elderly from the principal treatments of CVD because of their advanced age. Time remains the main limiting factor for the outcome of these patients together with the necessity of a dedicated center in which to treat, follow, and guide these patients until an early rehabilitation phase.

REFERENCES

1. National Institutes of Health. A classification and outline of cerebrovascular diseases. II. *Stroke*. 1975;6:564–616.
2. Victor M, Ropper AH, Adams RD et al. *Adams & Victor's Principles of Neurology*. 8th ed. New York: McGraw-Hill Medical; 2005. pp. 660–746.
3. Seidel GA, Giovannetti T, Libon DJ. Cerebrovascular disease and cognition in older adults. *Curr Top Behav Neurosci*. 2012;10:213–41.
4. Vermeer SE, Longstreth WT Jr, Koudstaal PJ. Silent brain infarcts: A systematic review. *Lancet Neurol*. 2007;6(7):611–9.
5. Benjamin EJ, Blaha MJ, Chiuve SE et al. Heart disease and stroke statistics—2017 update: A report from the American Heart Association. *Circulation*. 2017;135(10):e146–603.
6. Meschia JF, Bushnell C, Boden-Albala B et al. Guidelines for the primary prevention of stroke: A statement for healthcare professionals from the American Heart Association/American Stroke Association. *Stroke*. 2014;45(12):3754–832.
7. O'Donnell MJ, Chin SL, Rangarajan S et al. Global and regional effects of potentially modifiable risk factors associated with acute stroke in 32 countries (INTERSTROKE): A case-control study. *Lancet*. 2016;388(10046): 761–75.
8. Feigin VL, Roth GA, Naghavi M et al. Global burden of stroke and risk factors in 188 countries, during 1990–2013: A systematic analysis for the Global Burden of Disease Study 2013. *Lancet Neurol*. 2016;15(9):913–24.
9. Sacco RL, Kasner SE, Broderick JP et al. An updated definition of stroke for the 21st century: A statement for healthcare professionals from the American Heart Association/ American Stroke Association. *Stroke*. 2013; 44(7):2064–89.
10. Vernooij MW, Ikram MA, Tanghe HL et al. Incidental findings on brain MRI in the general population. *N Engl J Med*. 2007; 357(18):1821–8.
11. Smith EE, Saposnik G, Biessels GJ et al. Prevention of stroke in patients with silent cerebrovascular disease: A scientific statement for healthcare professionals from the American Heart Association/American Stroke Association. *Stroke*. 2017;48(2):e44–71.
12. Fanning JP, Wong AA, Fraser JF. The epidemiology of silent brain infarction: A systematic review of population-based cohorts. *BMC Med*. 2014;12:119.
13. Leary MC, Saver JL. Annual incidence of first silent stroke in the United States: A preliminary estimate. *Cerebrovasc Dis*. 2003;16:280–5.
14. Hankey GJ, Blacker DJ. Is it a stroke? *BMJ*. 2015;350:h56.
15. Hankey GJ. Stroke. *Lancet*. 2017;389(10069): 641–54.
16. Gibson LM, Whiteley W. The differential diagnosis of suspected stroke: A systematic review. *J R Coll Physicians Edinb*. 2013;43(2):114–48.
17. Menon B, Demchuk AM. Computed tomography angiography in the assessment of patients with stroke/TIA. *Neurohospitalist*. 2011;1(4): 187–99.

18. Goyal M, Demchuk AM, Menon BK et al. Randomized assessment of rapid endovascular treatment of ischemic stroke. *N Engl J Med.* 2015;372(11):1019–30.

19. Nogueira RG, Jadhav AP, Haussen DC et al. Thrombectomy 6 to 24 hours after stroke with a mismatch between deficit and infarct. *N Engl J Med.* 2018;378(1):11–21.

20. Molyneux A, Kerr R, Stratton I et al. International Subarachnoid Aneurysm Trial (ISAT) of neurosurgical clipping versus endovascular coiling in 2143 patients with ruptured intracranial aneurysms: A randomised trial. *Lancet.* 2002;360(9342):1267–74.

21. Adams HP Jr, Bendixen BH, Kappelle LJ et al. Classification of subtype of acute ischemic stroke. Definitions for use in a multicenter clinical trial. TOAST. Trial of Org 10172 in Acute Stroke Treatment. *Stroke.* 1993;24(1):35–41.

22. Amarenco P, Bogousslavsky J, Caplan LR et al. The ASCOD phenotyping of ischemic stroke (Updated ASCO Phenotyping). *Cerebrovasc Dis.* 2013;36(1):1–5.

23. Rodrigues FB, Neves JB, Caldeira D, Ferro JM, Ferreira JJ, Costa J. Endovascular treatment versus medical care alone for ischaemic stroke: Systematic review and meta-analysis. *BMJ.* 2016;353:i1754.

24. Emberson J, Lees KR, Lyden P et al. Effect of treatment delay, age, and stroke severity on the effects of intravenous thrombolysis with alteplase for acute ischaemic stroke: A meta-analysis of individual patient data from randomised trials. *Lancet.* 2014;384:1929–35.

25. Badhiwala JH, Nassiri F, Alhazzani W et al. Endovascular thrombectomy for acute ischemic stroke: A meta-analysis. *JAMA.* 2015; 314(17):1832–43.

26. Goyal M, Menon BK, van Zwam WH et al. Endovascular thrombectomy after large-vessel ischaemic stroke: A meta-analysis of individual patient data from five randomised trials. *Lancet.* 2016;387(10029):1723–31.

27. Rannikmae L, Woodfield R, Anderson CS et al. Reliability of intracerebral haemorrhage classification systems: A systematic review. *Int J Stroke.* 2016;11(6):626–36.

28. Qureshi AI, Palesch YY, Barsan WG et al. Trial investigators and the neurological emergency treatment trials network. Intensive blood-pressure lowering in patients with acute cerebral hemorrhage. *N Engl J Med.* 2016;375(11):1033–43.

29. Baharoglu MI, Cordonnier C, Salman RA et al. Platelet transfusion versus standard care after acute stroke due to spontaneous cerebral haemorrhage associated with antiplatelet therapy (PATCH): A randomised, open-label, phase 3 trial. *Lancet.* 2016;387(10038): 2605–13.

30. Kuramatsu JB, Gerner ST, Schellinger PD et al. Anticoagulant reversal, blood pressure levels, and anticoagulant resumption in patients with anticoagulation-related intracerebral hemorrhage. *JAMA.* 2015;313(8):824–36.

31. Steiner T, Poli S, Griebe M et al. Fresh frozen plasma versus prothrombin complex concentrate in patients with intracranial haemorrhage related to vitamin K antagonists (INCH): A randomised trial. *Lancet Neurol.* 2016; 15(16):566–73.

32. Pollack CV Jr, Reilly PA, Eikelboom J et al. Idarucizumab for dabigatran reversal. *N Engl J Med.* 2015;373(6):511–20.

33. Siegal DM, Curnutte JT, Connolly SJ et al. Andexanet alfa for the reversal of factor Xa inhibitor activity. *N Engl J Med.* 2015;373(25): 2413–24.

34. Ansell JE, Bakhru SH, Laulicht BE et al. Use of PER977 to reverse the anticoagulant effect of edoxaban. *N Engl J Med.* 2014;371(22): 2141–42.

35. Aronis KN, Hylek EM. Who, when, and how to reverse non-vitamin K oral anticoagulants. *J Thromb Thrombolysis.* 2016;41(2):253–72.

36. Li YP, Hou MZ, Lu GY et al. Neurologic functional outcomes of decompressive hemicraniectomy versus conventional treatment for malignant middle cerebral artery infarction: A systematic review and meta-analysis. *World Neurosurg.* 2017;99:709–25.

37. Ayling OGS, Alotaibi NM, Wang JZ et al. Suboccipital decompressive craniectomy for cerebellar infarction: A systematic review and meta-analysis. *World Neurosurg.* 2018;110: 450–9.

38. Akhigbe T, Zolnourian A. Role of surgery in the management of patients with supratentorial spontaneous intracerebral hematoma: Critical appraisal of evidence. *J Clin Neurosci.* 2017;39:35–8.

39. Nehls DG, Mendelow DA, Graham DI, Teasdale GM. Experimental intracerebral haemorrhage: Early removal of a spontaneous mass lesion improves late outcome. *Neurosurgery*. 1990;27:674–82.

40. Mendelow AD, Gregson B, Fernanades HM et al. Early surgery versus initial conservative treatment in patients with spontaneous supratentorial intracerebral haematoma in the International Surgical Trial in Intracerebral Haemorrhage (STICH): A randomised clinical trial. *Lancet*. 2005;365(9457):387–97.

41. Mendelow AD, Gregson BA, Rowan EN et al. Early surgery versus initial conservative treatment in patients with spontaneous supratentorial lobar intracerebral haematomas (STICH II): A randomised trial. *Lancet*. 2013; 382(9890):397–408.

42. Mould WA, Carhuapoma JR, Muschelli J et al. Minimally invasive surgery plus recombinant tissue-type plasminogen activator for intracerebral hemorrhage evacuation decreases perihematomal edema. *Stroke*. 2013;44(3): 627–34.

43. Ziai WC, Tuhrim S, Lane K et al. A multicenter, randomized, double-blinded, placebo-controlled phase III study of Clot Lysis Evaluation of Accelerated Resolution of Intraventricular Hemorrhage (CLEAR III). *Int J Stroke*. 2014;9(4):536–42.

44. Al-Khindi T, Macdonald RL, Schweizer TA. Cognitive and functional outcome after aneurysmal subarachnoid hemorrhage. *Stroke*. 2010;41(8):e519–36.

45. Feigin VL, Lawes CM, Bennett DA, Barker-Collo SL, Parag V. Worldwide stroke incidence and early case fatality reported in 56 population-based studies: A systematic review. *Lancet Neurol*. 2009;8(4):355–69.

46. Grasso G, Alafaci C, Macdonald RL. Management of aneurysmal subarachnoid hemorrhage: State of the art and future perspectives. *Surg Neurol Int*. 2017;8:11.

47. Wiebers DO, Whisnant JP, Huston J 3rd et al. Unruptured intracranial aneurysms: Natural history, clinical outcome, and risks of surgical and endovascular treatment. *Lancet*. 2003;362(9378):103–10.

48. Brawanski N, Kunze F, Bruder M et al. Subarachnoid hemorrhage in advanced age: Comparison of patients aged 70–79 years and 80 years and older. *World Neurosurg*. 2017;106:139–44.

49. Wáng YXJ, Zhang L, Zhao L et al. Elderly population have a decreased aneurysmal subarachnoid hemorrhage incidence rate than Middle aged population: A descriptive analysis of 8144 cases in mainland China. *Br J Neurosurg*. 2018;17:1–7.

50. Jaja BNR, Saposnik G, Lingsma HF et al. Development and validation of outcome prediction models for aneurysmal subarachnoid haemorrhage: The SAHIT multinational cohort study. *BMJ*. 2018;360:j5745.

51. Lanzino G, Kassell NF, Germanson TP et al. Age and outcome after aneurysmal subarachnoid hemorrhage: Why do older patients fare worse? *J Neurosurg*. 1996;85(3):410–8.

52. Risselada R, Lingsma HF, Bauer-Mehren A et al. Prediction of 60 day case-fatality after aneurysmal subarachnoid haemorrhage: Results from the International Subarachnoid Aneurysm Trial (ISAT). *Eur J Epidemiol*. 2010;25(4):261–6.

53. Perry JJ, Spacek A, Forbes M, Wells GA, Mortensen M, Symington C, Fortin N, Stiell IG. Is the combination of negative computed tomography result and negative lumbar puncture result sufficient to rule out subarachnoid hemorrhage? *Ann Emerg Med*. 2008;51(6):707–13.

54. Li MH, Cheng YS, Li YD et al. Large-cohort comparison between three-dimensional time-of-flight magnetic resonance and rotational digital subtraction angiographies in intracranial aneurysm detection. *Stroke*. 2009;40(9):3127–9.

55. Hunt WE, Hess RM. Surgical risk as related to time of intervention in the repair of intracranial aneurysms. *J Neurosurg*. 1968;28(1):14–20.

56. Report of World Federation of Neurological Surgeons Committee on a Universal Subarachnoid Hemorrhage Grading Scale. *J Neurosurg*. 1988;68(6):985–6.

57. Fisher CM, Kistler JP, Davis JM. Relation of cerebral vasospasm to subarachnoid hemorrhage visualized by computerized tomographic scanning. *Neurosurgery*. 1980;6(1):1–9.

58. Claassen J, Bernardini GL, Kreiter K et al. Effect of cisternal and ventricular blood on risk of delayed cerebral ischemia after subarachnoid hemorrhage: The Fisher scale revisited. *Stroke*. 2001;32(9):2012–20.

59. De Oliveira Manoel AL, Jaja BN, Germans MR et al. The VASOGRADE: A simple grading scale for prediction of delayed cerebral ischemia after subarachnoid hemorrhage. *Stroke.* 2015;46(7):1826–31.

60. Ogilvy CS, Carter BS. A proposed comprehensive grading system to predict outcome for surgical management of intracranial aneurysms. *Neurosurgery.* 1998;42(5):959–68.

61. Witsch J, Frey HP, Patel S et al. Prognostication of long-term outcomes after subarachnoid hemorrhage: The FRESH score. *Ann Neurol.* 2016;80(1):46–58.

62. Connolly ES Jr, Rabinstein AA, Carhuapoma JR et al. Guidelines for the management of aneurysmal subarachnoid hemorrhage: A guideline for healthcare professionals from the American Heart Association/american Stroke Association. *Stroke.* 2012;43(6):1711–37.

63. Tang C, Zhang TS, Zhou LF. Risk factors for rebleeding of aneurysmal subarachnoid hemorrhage: A meta-analysis. *PLOS ONE.* 2014;9(6):e99536.

64. Gritti P, Akeju O, Lorini FL, Lanterna LA, Brembilla C, Bilotta F. A narrative review of adherence to subarachnoid hemorrhage guidelines. *J Neurosurg Anesthesiol.* 2017; 30(3):203–16.

65. Rinaldo L, Lanzino G. Increased age associated with reduced likelihood of recurrence after coiling of ruptured aneurysms. *World Neurosurg.* 2017;100:381–7.

66. Kernan WN, Ovbiagele B, Black HR et al. Guidelines for the prevention of stroke in patients with stroke and transient ischemic attack: A guideline for healthcare professionals from the American Heart Association/American Stroke Association. *Stroke.* 2014; 45(7):2160–236.

67. Saposnik G, Barinagarrementeria F Jr, Brown RD et al. Diagnosis and management of cerebral venous thrombosis: A statement for healthcare professionals from the American Heart Association/American Stroke Association. *Stroke.* 2011;42(4):1158–92.

68. Ferro JM, Canhão P, Stam J et al. Prognosis of cerebral vein and dural sinus thrombosis: Results of the International Study on Cerebral Vein and Dural Sinus Thrombosis (ISCVT). *Stroke.* 2004 r;35(3):664–70.

69. Ferro JM, Canhão P, Bousser MG, Stam J, Barinagarrementeria F, ISCVT Investigators.

Cerebral vein and dural sinus thrombosis in elderly patients. *Stroke.* 2005;36(9):1927–32.

70. Robertson L, Jones LE. Fixed dose subcutaneous low molecular weight heparins versus adjusted dose unfractionated heparin for the initial treatment of venous thromboembolism. *Cochrane Database Syst Rev.* 2017; 2:CD001100.

71. Lanterna LA, Gritti P, Manara O, Grimod G, Bortolotti G, Biroli F. Decompressive surgery in malignant dural sinus thrombosis: Report of 3 cases and review of the literature. *Neurosurg Focus.* 2009;26(6):E5.

72. Powers WJ, Rabinstein AA, Ackerson T et al. 2018 Guidelines for the early management of patients with acute ischemic stroke: A guideline for healthcare professionals from the American Heart Association/American Stroke Association. *Stroke.* 2018;49(3):e46–110.

73. Bevers MB, Kimberly WT. Critical care management of acute ischemic stroke. *Curr Treat Options Cardiovasc Med.* 2017;19(6):41.

74. Solenski NJ, Haley EC Jr, Kassell NF et al. Medical complications of aneurysmal subarachnoid hemorrhage: A report of the multicenter, cooperative aneurysm study. Participants of the Multicenter Cooperative Aneurysm Study. *Crit Care Med.* 1995;23(6): 1007–17.

75. Edlow BL, Samuels O. Emergency neurological life support: Subarachnoid hemorrhage. *Neurocrit Care.* 2017;27(Suppl. 1):116–23.

76. Kirkman MA, Citerio G, Smith M. The intensive care management of acute ischemic stroke: An overview. *Intensive Care Med.* 2014;40(5):640–53.

77. Alotaibi NM, Elkarim GA, Samuel N et al. Effects of decompressive craniectomy on functional outcomes and death in poor-grade aneurysmal subarachnoid hemorrhage: A systematic review and meta-analysis. *J Neurosurg.* 2017;127(6):1315–1325.

78. Bösel J. Tracheostomy in stroke patients. *Curr Treat Options Neurol.* 2014;16(1):274.

79. Smith WS, Lev MH, English JD et al. Significance of large vessel intracranial occlusion causing acute ischemic stroke and TIA. *Stroke.* 2009;40(12):3834–40.

80. Gritti P, Lorini FL, Lanterna LA et al. Periprocedural management of patients with subarachnoid hemorrhage. *Curr Opin Anaesthesiol.* 2018;31(5):511–519.

8

Neurosurgery: Neuroendocrine lesions

KIRAN JANGRA

INTRODUCTION

The proportion of elderly subjects is expanding throughout the world, and similarly the frequency of various diseases, including pituitary tumors, is also increasing in this population subset (1,2). The possible explanations for this rising trend include increasing proportion of elderly subjects and more frequent use of neuroimaging techniques for medical conditions, such as cerebrovascular disease and dementia (3). In elderly patients, the frequency of nonfunctioning pituitary tumors (NFPTs) is more common than the functional tumors, which are usually underrepresented, especially prolactinomas (4,5). The signs and symptoms of pituitary tumors in elderly patients are usually concealed by various comorbidities and physiological effects of aging that might delay the diagnosis. As a result of this, these patients commonly present with the symptoms of mass effect. The surgical resection of these tumors is associated with more complications due to the presence of associated comorbidities. This chapter focuses on the characteristics of pituitary adenomas in elderly patients and anesthetic concerns of surgical resection of pituitary.

CLINICAL ANATOMY AND RELATIONSHIPS OF THE PITUITARY GLAND

The pituitary gland is situated in a saddle-shaped depression (sella turcica) in the sphenoid bone, also known as hypophyseal fossa (6). Boundaries of the hypophyseal fossa are formed by tuberculum sellae (elevation in the sphenoid bone) anteriorly, dorsum sellae posteriorly, the sphenoid sinus inferiorly, and folds of dura joining the anterior and posterior clinoid processes (diaphragmatic sella) superiorly. Dural reflections enclosing cavernous sinuses form the lateral wall of hypophyseal fossa. The carotid arteries and cranial nerves (III, IV, VI, V1, and V2) traverse through these sinuses (Figure 8.1).

Superiorly, the pituitary gland is connected to the hypothalamus via the pituitary stalk, passing through an opening in the diaphragmatic sella. In addition to this, the optic chiasm lies in the subarachnoid space just superior to the diaphragmatic sella. Vigorous removal of the pituitary tumor may cause cerebrospinal fluid (CSF) leak.

The pituitary gland is separated both structurally and functionally as the anterior pituitary

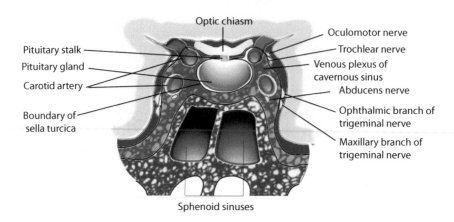

Figure 8.1 Coronal section of the sella turcica demonstrating the anatomic relationship between the pituitary gland and cranial nerves, carotid arteries, and the cavernous and sphenoid sinuses.

gland (adenohypophysis) and posterior pituitary gland (neurohypophysis). The adenohypophysis contains both secretory (hormone secreting) and non-secretory cells (null cells, supportive cells). Various hormones secreted by anterior pituitary include growth hormone (GH), prolactin (PRL), adrenocorticotropic hormone (ACTH), thyroid-stimulating hormone (TSH), follicle-stimulating hormone (FSH), and luteinizing hormone (LH). Aging causes interstitial fibrosis in adenohypophysis but a substantial number of hormone-secreting cells remain intact. These morphological changes of aging in the pituitary gland may not cause its functional derangement. Capillaries of the posterior pituitary receive the hormones (oxytocin and vasopressin) directly released by the

axons of the supraoptic and paraventricular nuclei of the hypothalamus. Anterior pituitary hormones are controlled by the hypothalamus, which secretes releasing hormone to stimulate pituitary hormones, which in return inhibit the hypothalamic hormones. This feedback control is known as the hypothalamo–pituitary axis. Prolactin, which is usually inhibited by dopamine released by the hypothalamus, is one exception to this. Compression on the pituitary stalk by any space-occupying lesion causes a decrease in production of most of the anterior pituitary hormones except prolactin, which is increased. This phenomenon is known as the stalk syndrome (Figure 8.2). Deficiency of posterior pituitary hormones is not commonly found preoperatively. If the patient

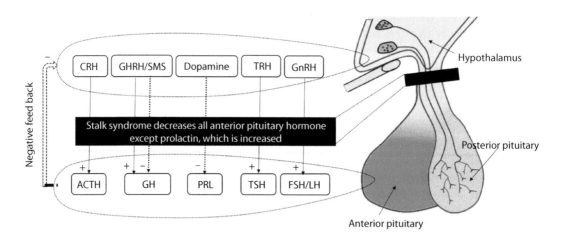

Figure 8.2 Diagram showing hypothalamo–pituitary axis and stalk syndrome.

presents with vasopressin deficiency, known as diabetes insipidus (DI), preoperatively, then the diagnosis for other suprasellar lesions, such as craniopharyngiomas, is made.

PATHOLOGY

Most of the pituitary adenomas in the elderly age group are nonfunctioning (80%), while functional adenomas are approximately 20% of all pituitary tumors. In a series of 39 elderly patients, NFPTs represented 80%, acromegaly 13%, and prolactinomas 7% of the cases (7). Similarly, other studies also reported the dominancy of NFPTs and preponderance of growth hormone—secreting tumors among the functional tumors (1,4,5,8,9). A few studies also suggest that gonadotroph adenomas and prolactinomas tend to increase with age, especially in men, and are usually included erroneously in the NFPT category (10,11). With aging, the rate of cellular proliferation decreases, which accounts for the slow growth of pituitary tumors in elderly patients (11,12). Functional tumors tend to remain intrasellar, except for prolactinomas (1,4,7,8). Cushing disease is rare in the elderly and presents by rule as microadenomas (1,8). The microprolactinomas are generally diagnosed only on autopsy (13). The presence of comorbidities such as hypertension or anticoagulation might favor spontaneous apoplexy (1).

CLINICAL PRESENTATION OF PITUITARY TUMORS WITH AGING

The diagnosis of pituitary adenomas in elderly patient may be disguised by associated comorbid conditions and polypharmacy, and is usually missed more often than in younger adults (4). Despite the advancement of diagnostic tools, diagnosis of pituitary adenomas is delayed by several years after the onset of specific symptoms. There are various factors that contribute to such delay in elderly patients (3). Hypogonadism, which is the earliest and most common symptom in nonfunctioning adenomas, is usually clinically silent in postmenopausal women, and is often ascribed to the normal physiological decline in sexual function due to aging in men. Other symptoms due to pituitary hypofunction, such as hypothyroidism and hypoadrenalism, are also not so prominent in elderly patients. In addition, interpretation of the endocrinological and biochemical profile may be altered as compared to the younger population (14). Visual disturbances are the most common presenting symptom of pituitary tumor enlargement in younger patients. In elderly patients, this symptom is usually misinterpreted initially as having other age-related ocular pathologies, such as cataract and macular or retinal degeneration (3).

The diagnosis of hypersecreting tumors such as acromegaly and Cushing disease is also delayed due to the presence of age-related comorbidities such as hypertension, diabetes, cardiovascular disease, asthenia, depression, joint pains, and fractures with trivial trauma. The common presentations of these tumors in geriatric patients are enumerated in Table 8.1.

INDICATIONS FOR SURGERY IN ELDERLY PATIENTS

The decision to operate on these patients should be based on the risk and benefit between surgical management and the patient's associated comorbidities. In addition, decreased physiological reserve predisposing this population to increased surgical and anesthesia-related complications, must be considered (15–17). Pituitary tumors can be approached either by craniotomy or transsphenoidal (endoscopic or microscopic) routes. The endonasal approach has several advantages over the microscopic approach, including panoramic view of the surgical site and fewer complications. The current use of intraoperative neuronavigation and imaging studies has drastically enhanced the safety and improved the outcome during surgery.

Transsphenoidal surgery (TSS) can be performed safely in patients over the age of 70, particularly when perioperative risk is low. As the most common presenting feature in these patients is mass effect, surgery becomes the best option (18).

ANESTHETIC MANAGEMENT

Preoperative evaluation

Elderly patients tend to have decreased physiological reserve and systemic illnesses (Table 8.2). Various physiological changes with aging are described elsewhere in this book. A detailed

Table 8.1 Clinical presentations of pituitary tumors

Local mass effect

Headache

Superior extension

- Visual symptoms (most common)
- Bitemporal hemianopia
- Monocular or homonymous field defects
- Complete blindness
- Hypothalamic dysfunction
- Obstructive hydrocephalus (rare)
- Lateral extension in cavernous sinus—cranial nerve palsy
  - Dysfunction of extraocular muscles and diplopia
  - Sensory disturbances of the face
- Extension in temporal lobe seizures (rare)
- Inferior extension causing expansion of sella headache (most common)

Generalized mass effect—Features of elevated ICP

Hypersecretory pituitary adenomas (1,4,8,9)

- Prolactin prolactinomas (4.5%–10%)
- ACTH-secreting Cushing disease (0%–6%)
- GH acromegaly (9%–17%)
- Thyrotropin-secreting hormone adenoma—hyperthyroidism (rare)

Pituitary apoplexy

- Sudden onset of severe headaches
- Compromise of vision
- Ocular paresis
- Vomiting
- Acute adrenal insufficiency

Stalk effect

- Hyperprolactinemia
- Suppression of function of the pituitary stalk

Abbreviations: ICP, intracranial pressure; ACTH, adrenocorticotropic hormone; GH, growth hormone.

history, examination, and investigations should focus on physiological reserve and polypharmacy. In addition to this, the elderly patient with pituitary tumor should be evaluated for neurologic findings (visual field defects/extraocular muscle weakness), signs and symptoms of raised intracranial pressure (ICP), and neuroimaging for size, location, and extension of tumor (Figure 8.3). Endocrine workup must be done in all patients with pituitary adenoma and should be optimized prior to elective surgery. The common endocrinological abnormalities

requiring replacement therapy include hypothyroidism, hypocortisolism, and adrenal insufficiency. Endocrinology experts should be consulted for the need of perioperative steroid cover. NFPTs usually do not affect the various body systems directly, so the decision for advanced testing, such as echocardiography, is based on associated systemic diseases and functional capacity.

In patients with Cushing disease and acromegaly, echocardiography is mandatory to rule out disease-associated effects on the myocardium. These patients should also be screened for obstructive sleep apnea and difficult airway. Patients with Cushing disease may suffer from gastroesophageal reflux disease.

Intraoperative management

NFPTs may not pose a risk to the airway but aging and acromegaly do have significant effects on airway management. Elderly edentulous patients along with features of acromegaly may pose a difficulty in both mask-holding as well as intubation (19). Patients with acromegaly have 13% higher incidence of difficult airway as compared to those with non-acromegalic features (20,21). Even a clinically apparent normal airway might turn out to be difficult in acromegaly. This difficulty increases with aging, as cervical joints become fixed and teeth are often absent (19). Therefore, one has to be prepared for the management of difficult airway in these patients. An endotracheal tube (ETT) should be fixed in the corner of the mouth opposite the surgeon's dominant operating hand. A right-handed surgeon will operate from the right side of the patient, so the tube should be fixed on the left corner of mouth. A throat pack should be inserted to prevent blood and debris from entering into the stomach which can increase the risk of postoperative nausea and vomiting.

Monitoring

In addition to routine monitoring, direct arterial pressure monitoring is also indicated during pituitary resection surgery due to various factors, including pre-existing cardiovascular disease, need of controlled hypotension, and potential vascular complications due to close proximity of the internal carotid artery (ICA) to the surgical site. The arterial cannulation site should be chosen carefully, as patients with acromegaly can have ulnar

Table 8.2 Preoperative evaluation of patients with pituitary tumors

Screening for	Systems assessed	Investigations/assessments
	Comorbidity/severity	
	• Cardiovascular	• Vital signs, electrocardiography, echocardiography
	• Respiratory	• Chest x-ray, S_pO_2 (pulmonary function tests and arterial blood gases, if indicated)
	• Hematological	• Full blood count including platelet count
	• Renal	• Urea and electrolytes, estimated glomerular filtration rate
	• Endocrinological	• Blood sugar
	• Nutritional	• Weight, body mass index, albumin (liver function tests)
	Previous anesthesia	Inquire about problems during previous exposure (difficult airway, cardiovascular liability, emergence delirium, delayed awakening)
	Medication review Anticoagulant therapy Relevant allergies	Coagulation screen
	Use of functional aids	
	Visual, hearing, dentures	Glasses, hearing aids
Pituitary tumor–specific	Neurologic findings	Glasgow Coma Scale, visual field defects/extraocular muscle weakness, signs and symptoms of raised intracranial pressure
	Neuroimaging	Size, location, and extension/invasion of tumor Relation to the carotid arteries
	Endocrine workup	Serum tests include • Adrenocorticotrophic hormone • Growth hormone • Insulin-like growth factor • Prolactin • Follicular stimulating hormone • Luteinizing hormone • Testosterone (may be physiologically declined) • Thyroid-stimulating hormone
	Ophthalmological examination	Visual acuity Visual field testing
	Acromegaly	Evaluate the history of obstructive sleep apnea (OSA) and hoarseness of voice (if present, get indirect laryngoscopy) X-ray of the soft tissues of the neck Echocardiography is mandatory Screen and optimize diabetes mellitus
	Cushing disease	Echocardiography is mandatory Screen and optimize diabetes mellitus Evaluate for difficult airway

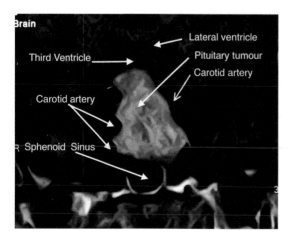

Figure 8.3 Magnetic resonance imaging of coronal section depicting pituitary tumor and its extension.

insufficiency. In patients with ulnar insufficiency, alternate sites such as the dorsalis pedis artery should be selected for cannulation (22). Even if there is a potential for venous air embolism (VAE), central venous catheterization (CVC) is not performed routinely, as the risk of VAE is very low. CVC may be inserted if indicated due to systemic illnesses. Urine output should also be monitored, especially in postoperative period, as there is a likelihood of DI postoperatively. End-tidal carbon dioxide (EtCO$_2$) monitoring should be closely watched. EtCO$_2$ is usually kept in the high-normal range to push the suprasellar extension down toward the sella during transsphenoidal surgeries. Previously, a lumbar drain was also inserted to push the suprasellar pituitary in the sella by injecting air or saline through the lumbar drain, but currently this practice is not popular (23). The use of neurophysiological monitoring during these surgeries is debatable. Even though reported to be associated with improved postoperative visual fields, there is a lack of strong evidence, and it is also associated with a high incidence of false-positive rates with the use of visual evoked potentials (VEPs) (24). VEPs are exquisitely sensitive to anesthetic agents and are technically difficult to monitor intraoperatively, and hence not advocated to be routinely used during TSS.

Anesthesia technique

The major goals of anesthetic management for TSS are airway management, good hemodynamic control, providing a good surgical field, and rapid emergence to facilitate early neurological evaluation. Perioperative steroids should be supplemented, if indicated. The head is placed on horseshoe head rest or head ring if microscopic and endoscopic TSS is planned, and on head pins during neuronavigation-guided surgery. The ETT tube should be secured properly, using water-resistant material, on the site opposite the dominant hand of the chief surgeon. Long extensions are required for breathing circuits, and arterial and venous lines. During endoscopic TSS, the nasal mucosa is prepared using adrenaline, which can incite severe hypertension, various malignant arrhythmias, and even myocardial infarction (25,26). These episodes are managed by deepening the anesthesia, using additional opioids, and use of appropriate antihypertensive medications. During microscopic TSS, insertion of a nasal speculum causes an intense sympathetic surge that should also be managed in a similar way. In addition to these techniques, bilateral maxillary nerve block has also shown to decrease these hemodynamic responses (27). Similarly, bilateral sphenopalatine and infraorbital nerve blocks are known to decrease the anesthetic agent requirement, blood loss, emergence time, time to achieve Aldrete score of 9, and also to provide more stable intraoperative hemodynamics (28).

Another important intraoperative complication is trigeminocardiac reflex (TCR) (29). Stimulation of the trigeminal nerve can precipitate severe bradycardia, hypotension, and even asystole (30). During TSS, cavernous sinus manipulation can stimulate TCR. It is usually recovered spontaneously on stopping the surgical stimulus. If still persists, then anticholinergics may be used, particularly atropine. Recurrent TCR is managed by a temporary pacemaker.

Various techniques are employed to facilitate the resection of the suprasellar pituitary including the Valsalva maneuver, high normocapnia (PaCO$_2$ = 40–45 mmHg), and intrathecal administration of air or normal saline (31,32). Controlled hypercapnia up to a limit of 60 mmHg is described in the literature for successfully lowering the suprasellar portion of the tumor, but it has deleterious effects (33). The lumbar drain may be inserted prophylactically preoperatively in anticipation of a CSF leak, or in the postoperative period if a definite leak occurs.

Blood loss is usually minimal during TSS, but there is a potential for major vascular injuries, including trauma to the internal carotid artery. Anesthesiologists should remain vigilant and be prepared for these complications. If such complication occurs, the surgical field is obscured completely, and it becomes difficult to control the bleeding. Anesthesiologists can assist the surgeons by decreasing systolic blood pressure and providing transient bilateral carotid compression so that the site of the bleed can be visualized. The surgical site is then packed, and once the patient is hemodynamically stable, he should be transferred immediately to the neuro-intervention suite for exact localization and sealing the defect. As geriatric patients have poor physiological reserve, euvolemia should be maintained and the threshold for blood transfusion should be kept on the lower side. A few surgeons may ask to provide a Valsalva maneuver (30–40 sec pressure) before closure to assess the quality of hemostasis and CSF leak.

EMERGENCE FROM ANESTHESIA

The pharyngeal pack should be removed under vision after ensuring that no fresh blood is trickling in the throat. A rapid and smooth emergence is desirable after TSS so that neurological status can be rapidly assessed. Coughing and bucking on tube can result in hematoma formation in the tumor bed and may dislodge the fat graft, leading to CSF leak postoperatively. Tumor bed hematoma may manifest as delayed awakening, so an urgent computed tomography scan (CT) is warranted if unexplained delayed awakening is encountered. A retrospective study reported the incidence of tumor bed hematoma to be approximately 8.97% (34).

POSTOPERATIVE MANAGEMENT

Patients should be nursed in the head-up position, which helps in surgical hemostasis. Immediate postoperative complications include upper airway obstruction, bleeding, loss of consciousness, and neurological deterioration.

Upper airway obstruction may occur due to forgotten pharyngeal pack, blood clot obstructing the larynx, laryngospasm due to blood trickling in the larynx, or obstruction of both nostrils with the nasal pack, especially in acromegaly. These complications should be managed as per the cause, and counseling should be done preoperatively regarding retention of nasal packing in the postoperative period.

The cause of bleeding should be explored. If bleeding is through the nasal mucosa, external compression and cauterization of the bleeding site should be done, while bleeding through the tumor bed should be re-explored in the operating theater under general anesthesia. If the patient develops neurological deterioration, first take care of the airway (cleared of obstruction), breathing (supplement oxygen/definite airway insertion), and circulation (hemodynamic support), followed by urgent CT scan to find out the cause. Bag-and-mask ventilation should be avoided in the immediate postoperative period and in patients with CSF leak, as it may dislodge the hemostatic clot or graft from the surgical site and may increase the risk of meningitis by forcing the nasal flora into the surgical bed.

As soon as the patient regains consciousness, visual function should be assessed immediately in the postoperative period. Acute tumor bed hematoma may cause sudden onset of blindness and ophthalmoplegia associated with altered consciousness, warranting urgent CT scan.

Other postoperative complications include CSF leak and endocrinological abnormalities (17.9%) (34). CSF leak is managed by anterior cranial fossa floor repair using fat/muscle graft and lumbar drain. Common endocrine abnormalities include DI, syndrome of inappropriate antidiuretic hormone secretion (SIADH), hypocortisolism (in Cushing disease), while other endocrinopathies occurring due to mass effect of tumor usually improve after surgery.

POSTOPERATIVE ANALGESIA

A large series by Flynn and Nemergut reported that the requirement for postoperative analgesics is minimal in patients after transsphenoidal surgery (35). The authors hypothesized that the pituitary gland contains the highest concentration of endogenous opioids, which are released during surgical manipulation. Most patients present with headache, which can be managed by nonopioid analgesics like paracetamol. In addition to this, bilateral maxillary nerve block, infraorbital nerve, and sphenopalatine blocks are reported to be effective in controlling postoperative pain after TSS (27,28).

Opioid use should be judicious, as it might aggravate airway obstruction, especially in patients with OSA, and also geriatric patients are more sensitive to opioids.

CONCLUSION

Perioperative management of neuroendocrine tumors is quite challenging in elderly patients. Endonasal transsphenoidal surgery, being minimally invasive, is usually well tolerated. Perioperative complications are more severe and are influenced by age-related decline in physiological reserve. A multidisciplinary team approach including surgeon, anesthesiologist, and endocrinologist is must in perioperative period for preoperative optimization and postoperative care.

REFERENCES

1. Turner HE, Adams CBT, Wass JAH. Pituitary tumours in the elderly: A 20 year experience. *Eur J Endocrinol.* 1999;140:383–9.
2. Radhakrishnan K, Mokri B, Parisi JE, O'Fallon WM, Sunku J, Kurland LT. The trends in incidence of primary brain tumors in the population of Rochester, Minnesota. *Ann Neurol.* 1995;37:67–73.
3. Losa M. Pituitary tumors in the elderly. *Eur J Endocrinol.* 1999;140:378–80.
4. Cohen DL, Bevan JS, Adams CBT. The presentation and management of pituitary tumours in the elderly. *Age Ageing.* 1989;18:247–52.
5. Benbow SJ, Foy P, Jones B, Shaw D, MacFarlane IA. Pituitary tumours presenting in the elderly: Management and outcome. *Clin Endocrinol.* 1997;46:657–60.
6. Mancall EL, Brock DG (eds). Cranial fossae. In: *Gray's Clinical Anatomy.* Elsevier Health Sciences; 2011. p. 154.
7. Ferrante L, Trillo G, Ramundo E, Celli P, Jaffrain-Rea ML, Salvati M, Esposito V, Roperto R, Osti MF, Minniti G. Surgical treatment of pituitary tumors in the elderly: Clinical outcome and long-term follow-up. *J Neurooncol.* 2002;60:185–91.
8. Fraioli B, Pastore FS, Signoretti S, De Caro GMF, Giuffre R. The surgical treatment of pituitary adenomas in the eighth decade. *SurgNeurol.* 1999;51:261–7.
9. Pospiech J, Stolke D, Pospiech FR. Surgical treatment of pituitary adenomas in the elderly. *Acta Neurochir Suppl (Wien).* 1996;65:35–6.
10. Ho MD, Hsu CY, Ting LT, Chiang H. The clinicopathological characteristics of gonadotroph cell adenoma: A study of 118 cases. *Hum Pathol.* 1997;28:905–11.
11. Jaffrain-Rea ML, Di Stefano D, Minniti G, Esposito V, Bultrini A, Ferretti E, Santoro A, Faticanti Scucchi L, Gulino A, Cantore G. A critical reappraisal of MIB-1 labelling index significance in a large series of pituitary tumours: Secreting versus non-secreting adenomas. *Endocr Relat Cancer.* 2002;9:103–13.
12. Losa M, Franzin A, Mangili F, Terreni MR, Barzaghi R, Veglia F, Mortini P, Giovanelli M. Proliferation index in non-functioning pituitary adenomas: Clinical characteristics and long-term follow up. *Neurosurgery.* 2000;47:1313–8.
13. Kovacs K, Ryan N, Horvath E, Singer W, Ezrin C. Pituitary adenomas in old age. *J Gerontol.* 1980;35:16–22.
14. Tayal SC, Bansal SK, Chadha DK. Hypopituitarism: A difficult diagnosis in elderly people but worth a search. *Age Aging.* 1994;23:320–2.
15. Black P, Kathiresan S, Chung W. Meningioma surgery in the elderly: A case-control study assessing morbidity and mortality. *Acta Neurochir (Wien).* 1998;140:1013–6.
16. Brandes A, Fiorentino MV. Treatment of high-grade gliomas in the elderly. *Oncology.* 1998;55:1–6.
17. Pietila TA, Stendel R, Hassler WE, Heimberger C, Ramsbacker J, Brock M. Brain tumour surgery in geriatric patients: A critical analysis in 44 patients over 80 years. *Surg Neurol.* 1999;52:259–63.
18. Sheehan JM, Douds GL, Hill K, Farace E. Transsphenoidal surgery for pituitary adenoma in elderly patients. *Acta Neurochir (Wien).* 2008;150(6):571–4.
19. Moon HY, Baek CW, Kim JS, Koo GH, Kim JY, Woo YC, Jung YH, Kang H, Shin HY, Yang SY. The causes of difficult tracheal intubation and preoperative assessments in different age groups. *Korean J Anesthesiol.* 2013;64(4):308–14.

20. Messick JM Jr, Cucchiara RF, Faust RJ. Airway management in patients with acromegaly. *Anesthesiology.* 1982;56:157.

21. Schmitt H, Buchfelder M, Radespiel-Tr.ger M, Fahlbusch R. Difficult intubation in acromegalic patients: Incidence and predictability. *Anesthesiology.* 2000;93:110–4.

22. Tagliafico A, Resmini E, Nizzo R, Derchi LE, Minuto F, Giusti M, Martinoli C, Ferone D. The pathology of the ulnar nerve in acromegaly. *Eur J Endocrinol.* 2008;159(4):369–73.

23. Aghamohamadi D, Ahmadvand A, Salehpour F, Jafari R, Panahi F, Sharifi G, Meshkini A, Safaeian A. Effectiveness of lumbar drain versus hyperventilation to facilitate transsphenoidal pituitary (Suprasellar) adenoma resection. *Anesth Pain Med.* 2013;2(4):159–63.

24. Chacko AG, Babu KS, Chandy MJ. Value of visual evoked potential monitoring during trans-sphenoidal pituitary surgery. *Br J Neurosurg.* 1996;10(3):275–8.

25. Pasternak JJ, Atkinson JL, Kasperbauer JL, Lanier WL. Hemodynamic responses to epinephrine-containing local anesthetic injection and to emergence from general anesthesia in transsphenoidal hypophysectomy patients. *J Neurosurg Anesthesiol.* 2004;16:189–95.

26. Chelliah YR, Manninen PH. Hazards of epinephrine in transsphenoidal pituitary surgery. *J Neurosurg Anesthesiol.* 2002;14:43–6.

27. Chadha R, Padmanabhan V, Rout A, Waikar HD, Mohandas K. Prevention of hypertension during trans-sphenoidal surgery—The effect of bilateral maxillary nerve block with local anaesthetics. *Acta Anaesthesiol Scand.* 1997;41:35–40.

28. Ali AR, Sakr SA, Rahman MA. Bilateral sphenopalatine ganglion block as adjuvant to general anaesthesia during endoscopic trans-nasal resection of pituitary adenoma. *Egypt J Anaesth.* 2010;26:273–80.

29. Schaller B. Trigemino-cardiac reflex during transsphenoidal surgery for pituitary adenomas. *Clin Neurol Neurosurg.* 2005 t;107(6): 468–74.

30. Cho JM, Min KT, Kim EH, Oh MC, Kim SH. Sudden asystole due to trigeminocardiac reflex during transsphenoidal surgery for pituitary tumor. *World Neurosurg.* 2011;76(5): 477.e11–5.

31. Lim M, Williams D, Maartens N. Anaesthesia for pituitary surgery. *J Clin Neurosci.* 2006;13: 413–8.

32. Nath G, Korula G, Chandy MJ. Effect of intrathecal saline injection and Valsalva maneuver on cerebral perfusion pressure during transsphenoidal surgery for pituitary macroadenoma. *J Neurosurg Anesthesiol.* 1995;7:1–6.

33. Korula G, George SP, Rajshekhar V, Haran RP, Jeyaseelan L. Effect of controlled hypercapnia on cerebrospinal fluid pressure and operating conditions during transsphenoidal operations for pituitary macroadenoma. *J Neurosurg Anesthesiol.* 2001;13:255–9.

34. Gondim JA, Almeida JP, Albuquerque LA et al. Endoscopic endonasal approach for pituitary adenoma: Surgical complications in 301 patients. *Pituitary.* 2011;14:174–83.

35. Flynn BC, Nemergut EC. Postoperative nausea and vomiting and pain after transsphenoidal surgery: A review of 877 patients. *Anesth Analg.* 2006;103:162–7.

9

Neurosurgery: Spine surgery

M.V.S. SATYA PRAKASH AND M. SENTHILNATHAN

Introduction	135	Premedication	138
Common problems for which spine surgeries		Type of anesthesia	139
are performed in geriatric population	135	Regional anesthesia in spine surgery	143
Preoperative assessment	136	Postoperative care	144
Antiplatelet drugs	136	References	145
Preoperative investigations	138		

INTRODUCTION

As advances in modern medicine are reaching every corner of the world, the average expected life span of individuals is increasing as a whole, which leads to an increase in the amount of geriatric population worldwide. With the increase in the amount of geriatric population in combination with improvements in modern medicine, the number of geriatric patients undergoing surgery is also increasing. It is common for those in the geriatric population to have problems in the skeletal system because of aging-related complications. Geriatric patients have increased risk for falls because of disturbances in the autonomic system due to polypharmacy, peripheral neuropathy, and autonomic dysregulation (1). As the age increases, there is increased bone resorption leading to osteoporosis and osteopenia, especially in postmenopausal women. These factors lead to increased risk for fractures. At the same time, the elderly are more prone to malignancies, which may also occur in skeletal system or may metastasize to the spine. As modern medicine is advancing, so, too is the number of surgeries on geriatric patients, including

spine surgery. Spine surgery is one of the five most common surgeries for older adults (2).

COMMON PROBLEMS FOR WHICH SPINE SURGERIES ARE PERFORMED IN GERIATRIC POPULATION

1. Degenerative diseases of spine can be divided in to four types:
   a. *Degenerative disc disease*: Occurs due to reduced water content, decrease in disc space, and alteration of the collagen content in the disc.
   b. *Spondylolisthesis*: Slipping or displacement of the one vertebra over another. It is common at L4/L5 (3).
   c. *Prolapse of the disc*: Leads to radicular pain of the nerve roots. This occurs due to the irritation and inflammation of the nerve root by the biologically active tissue within the disc, such as nucleus pulposus.
   d. *Spinal stenosis*: Due to narrowing of the spinal canal.
2. Scoliosis: Idiopathic and degenerative scoliosis (4).

3. Autoimmune diseases such as rheumatoid arthritis.
4. Neuromuscular diseases leading to spine problems.
5. Benign and malignant tumors. Secondary, arising from metastatic malignant diseases.
6. Trauma to the spine requiring surgery (Spinal Trauma).

In traumatic spine cases, the patient may be in the state of spinal shock. Spinal shock starts immediately after injury and lasts for up to 3 weeks (5). Physiological sympathectomy occurs below the lesion. If the lesion is at or above T6, the patient will have hypotension, and if the lesion is higher than the cardiac sympathetic outflow then patient will also have bradycardia. This hypotension responds poorly to intravenous (IV) fluids, and vasopressors are the treatment of choice. Hypoxia or manipulation of larynx or trachea may cause severe hypotension in these cases. Intermittent positive pressure ventilation (IPPV) causes hypotension due to inability to raise systemic vascular resistance (SVR). Even though C4–C8 spine injuries spare the diaphragm, intercostal and abdominal muscles become paralyzed, leading to inadequate cough and paradoxical rib movements on spontaneous ventilation. This in turn leads to reduction in vital capacity (by 50%), functional residual capacity (by 85% of predicted), and loss of dynamic expiration. Spinal trauma causes increased risk of venous thromboembolism because of impaired rheology, increased gastric emptying time, and hyperkalemia (on administration of succinylcholine). Autonomic dysreflexia occurs within 3–6 weeks of spinal trauma, causing extreme hemodynamic responses such as hypertension and tachycardia if stimulated below the lesion.

PREOPERATIVE ASSESSMENT

Geriatric patients are frequently suffering from multiple diseases and might be on polypharmacy. Medication errors are common in these patients (in 8% of population) (6). All these patients should be carefully interviewed regarding past medical history, details of medications, and comorbid conditions. These patients might be on analgesics preoperatively for the present condition. During the preoperative visit, the dependency of the patient on any analgesics should be assessed with regard to the patient's daily routine activities, so that their postoperative requirement for dependency can be predicted and explained to the relatives.

Changes in the structure of collagen in geriatric patients can lead to stiffness of the joints, which necessitates thorough assessment of the airway for ease of intubation. If the clinical airway examination warrants further imaging studies, lateral x-ray or CT scan of the neck can be done to assess the ease of intubation. Stability of the cervical spine is dependent on the ligaments and vertebrae. If damage has occurred to any of these structures, there will be instability of the cervical spine. Instability of the cervical spine can be suspected when one of the following conditions is found:

1. All the anterior or posterior elements are destroyed
2. There is more than 3.5 mm displacement of one vertebra with other vertebra in the lateral x-ray
3. There is more than 11° rotation of one vertebra over other vertebra

Jefferson fractures, disruption of the tectorial and alar ligaments, and occipital condylar fractures cause atlantooccipital instability (7).

A medication review must be done and the drugs that are necessary should be continued on the night before the surgery and the morning of surgery; the drugs that need to be skipped should be advised accordingly during the preoperative visit. Perioperative management of patient medications is depicted in Table 9.1.

ANTIPLATELET DRUGS

Aspirin

If the surgery is of low risk for bleeding, short duration, and the patient does not have any indwelling stents or materials, it is better to continue the drug (1). If the surgery has risk for bleeding, prolonged duration, and the patient has coronary arterial stents or materials in the body which necessitate the antiplatelet therapy, it is better to discuss continuation of the drugs with the surgeon, and a combined decision will be made depending on the risk for increased bleeding and the care for the materials in the body on case-by-case basis.

Table 9.1 Management of medications taken by the patient during perioperative period

Drugs	Night before surgery	Morning of surgery	Drug reactions
Tricyclic antidepressants	Should be continued	Should be continued	Anticholinergic symptoms such as dry mouth, prolonged gastric emptying, urinary retention, postoperative delirium Cardiac symptoms such as PR prolongation, exaggerated responses to the vasopressors, hypotension due to interaction with the anesthetic induction drugs, and hemodynamic instability
Selective serotonin reuptake inhibitors	Should be continued	Should be continued	Increased risk of serotonin syndrome, headache, and agitation
Monoamine oxidase inhibitors	Should be continued	Should be continued	Hypertensive crisis with tyramine-containing drugs and foods
Non-opioid analgesics	To be discussed with surgeon for the need to continue, depending on the type of surgery planned on individual basis	To be discussed with surgeon for the need to continue, depending on the type of surgery planned on individual basis	Increased risk of bleeding intraoperatively, increased chance of epidural hematoma
Opioid analgesics	Should be continued	Should be continued	Opioid dependency leads to increased perioperative opioid requirement
Oral hypoglycemic agents	Should be continued	Should be skipped	Care should be taken that the patient should be maintained in euglycemic state during perioperative period
Insulin	Long-acting insulins which act for more than 24h should be replaced proportionately by short-acting insulins	Should be skipped	Care should be taken that the patient should be maintained in euglycemic state during perioperative period
Antihypertensive drugs	Should be continued	Should be continued except ACE inhibitors and angiotensin receptor–blocking drugs	May cause unresponsive hypotension due to hypovolemic state
Gabapentin	Should be continued	Should be continued	
Thyroid supplements	Should be continued	Should be continued	

Thenopyridines

These medicines cause increased risk of bleeding during surgery and increased incidence of formation of epidural hematoma and postoperative bleeding complications. Depending on their half-life, they should be discontinued preoperatively, but it should be seen that stents, if present, thrombosis of stents should be prevented by prescribing bridging therapy peri-operatively.

PREOPERATIVE INVESTIGATIONS

Geriatric patients might have diabetes mellitus and/or hypertension. The status of these conditions should be investigated. As spine surgeries are done in the prone position and under general anesthesia, the respiratory system should be thoroughly evaluated. Depending on the degree of impairment of the functional integrity of the respiratory system and functional reserve, the need of postoperative elective ventilation should be assessed and should

be explained to the patient. If the preoperative vital capacity is less than 30%–35% of predicted, it is better to plan for postoperative elective ventilation. As the cardiac reserve of the geriatric patient is decreased, a proper evaluation of the cardiovascular system should be done. Common investigations in geriatric patients posted for spine surgery are described in Table 9.2.

PREMEDICATION

Elderly patients are more prone to the adverse effects of drugs. As the age increases, there is increased sensitivity to drugs due to loss of neuronal tissue and other systems in the body which warrant reduction in anesthetic drug dosage (8). Anticholinergics such as glycopyrrolate can be considered to prevent soiling of adhesive tapes of the endotracheal tube. Patients with spine disease will be on chronic use of opioids, which needs to be continued perioperatively. Therefore an increased amount of opioid drugs needs to be prescribed to

Table 9.2 Evaluation of geriatric patient posted for spine surgery

System	Investigations to be done	Reason
Hematology	Hemoglobin, total blood count, platelet count	As baseline investigations
Biochemical tests	Blood sugar, renal function tests including electrolytes, liver function tests	As baseline investigations
Respiratory system	Bedside pulmonary function tests to be done; if abnormal, then further testing should include spirometry and ABG	To assess the pulmonary reserve
Cardiovascular system	ECG should be done; if abnormal ECG or if patient has comorbidities affecting cardiovascular system, further testing should include echocardiogram and stress testing such as tread mill test (TMT) or dobutamine stress test	To assess the functional status of cardiovascular system
Central nervous system	Cognitive function, motor, and sensory functions of the patient should be assessed and documented	For medicolegal problems and to assess whether the patient has developed new onset delirium postoperatively
Airway	If structural abnormality is suspected, then x-ray neck AP and lateral view, and if necessary, a CT scan may be ordered	To assess the difficulty of intubation

get the same effect, but at the same time the anesthesiologist needs to keep in mind the sedative and respiratory depression effects of these drugs.

Geriatric patients are more prone to develop postoperative venous thromboembolism. Studies had shown that the incidence of thromboembolism following spine surgery decreases from around 15% to 0.39% if proper thromboprophylaxis is provided (9). It is necessary to provide thromboprophylaxis against venous thromboembolism. Nonpharmacological forms of prophylaxis such as compression stockings or intermittent pneumatic compression boots may be preferred over pharmacological agents.

Preoperative fasting orders should be modified according to the patient's existing comorbid conditions. Antibiotic prophylaxis should be given according to the individual hospital protocol.

TYPE OF ANESTHESIA

Spine surgeries can be done either under regional block or general anesthesia.

General anesthesia

Advantages

1. All spine surgeries can be done under general anesthesia.
2. There is no time restriction for the surgeon.
3. As the majority of spine surgeries are done in the prone position, the patient will be more comfortable under general anesthesia.
4. The anesthesiologist has full control over the airway.
5. In cases of massive bleeding, there is no need to change the type of anesthesia.
6. There are decreased medicolegal problems due to the development of new-onset neurological complications, questioning the type of anesthesia administered.

Disadvantages

1. Polypharmacy
2. More chances of development of postoperative delirium
3. Greater consumption of analgesics

PREOXYGENATION

Geriatric patients should be preoxygenated properly, as these patients have reduced pulmonary reserve.

INDUCTION

Depending on the condition of the patient, either inhalational induction or IV induction can be done. The hemodynamics of the patient should be maintained to the preoperative values. If the patient is in spinal shock, the anesthesiologist must be extremely vigilant during induction to maintain hemodynamics.

INTUBATION

Denervation of the spinal cord may respond with exaggerated hyperkalemia if succinylcholine is given. This response commonly starts 48 hours after injury and lasts for 9 months, which necessitates avoidance of succinylcholine in patients with spinal cord injury (10).

In patients with cervical spine injury and patients with cervical collar or cervical spine stabilization devices, it is better to proceed with awake fiberoptic intubation, as these cases are difficult to intubate without atlantooccipital extension. In anterior cervical spine surgeries, it is better to use flexometallic endotracheal tubes to prevent kinking of the tube, as the workspace for the surgeon is near the airway. If the thoracic or lumbar spine surgery is being done by the anterior approach, the surgeon may ask for lung collapse for approaching the spine. Depending on the pulmonary functional reserve of the geriatric patient, a decision has to be made regarding the use of double-lumen tube or other lung isolation techniques.

INTRAOPERATIVE PERIOD

Once the patient is intubated, the remaining monitors (such as central venous pressure and/or invasive blood pressure) should be secured. Spine surgeries are commonly done in the prone position. Supine (especially for anterior cervical procedures), lateral (especially for anterior lumbar or thoracic vertebral procedures), jackknife, frog-leg, or knee–chest positions (for lumbar spinal procedures) are the other positions, which are rarely used for spine surgeries. As the prone position is commonly used, care should be taken not to compress the abdomen so that the epidural veins do not engorge, causing more bleeding during surgery. One method to assess whether the abdomen is compressed is to pass the hand below the abdomen after attaining the prone position. If the hand can be placed below the abdomen freely, it is confirmed that the abdomen is free. At the same time, compression on the chest should be avoided, which can be confirmed by checking the peak airway pressure (P_{aw}) before and after prone positioning. If the P_{aw} is increased less than 10% of the pre-position value, then the chest is said to be free. Compression on the chest leads to suboptimal delivery of tidal volume, which results in hypercarbia and leads to exaggerated bleeding due to venous engorgement. Geriatric patients have reduced fat pad in the body and on the subcutaneous tissue of the body, which leads to increased risk of pressure-related neurological damage in the prone position, so the susceptible areas should be padded appropriately.

Some spine surgeries are known to cause major blood loss, so strategies to reduce blood loss should be considered. Blood conservation strategies such as autologous blood transfusion are contraindicated in geriatric patients, as their functional reserve is less. However, other strategies for reduced blood loss can be applied. These strategies include use of antifibrinolytic agents such as ε-aminocaproic acid (5 g of loading dose over 30 min followed by 15 mg/kg/h), tranexamic acid (10 mg/kg over 10–20 min as a loading dose and 10 mg/kg/h), and aprotinin (one million KIU load over 30 min followed by 0.25 million KIU/h) (7,11). It has been found that use of one of these drugs starting before skin incision and ending at the time of skin closure will reduce the blood loss. The anesthesiologist should be careful in using these agents in geriatric patients, as they may have multiple comorbidities and increased sensitivity to the drugs, which may increase the likelihood of hypercoagulable state.

Hypotensive anesthesia can be given so that blood loss will be minimal. Problems in geriatric patients in conducting hypotensive anesthesia are their age, multiple comorbid conditions including coronary artery disease, reduced functional reserve. Hypotensive anesthesia can be considered only if the patient does not have any comorbid conditions and has good functional reserve, and if surgery warrants hypotension to minimize the blood loss. However, mean arterial pressure should be maintained at least above 60 mmHg.

Monitoring

ECG, SpO_2, noninvasive blood pressure, urine output, temperature, end tidal gases, and P_{aw} should be monitored. Depending on the duration of surgery,

site of surgery (such as cervical surgery where handling of carotid artery/carotid sinus is done), and the expected amount of blood loss, a decision should be made on arterial blood pressure and central venous pressure monitoring. The other monitors that are used are neurological monitoring such as somatosensory-evoked potentials (SSEP), motor-evoked potentials (MEP), somato-cortical-evoked potentials, electromyogram (EMG), and electroencephalography (EEG). Central venous pressure is not reliable during prone position, as there is increased intrathoracic pressure leading to reduced ventricular compliance and compression of the inferior vena cava (IVC) (12).

Neuro-monitoring

During spinal cord surgeries, many corrective forces are applied, leading to compromise in the blood supply to parts of the spinal cord. To prevent iatrogenic spinal cord injury, to identify the impending damage, and to take corrective measures, it is advisable to do spinal cord monitoring during spine surgeries. It has been found that electrophysiological monitoring of the spinal cord detects the onset of irreversible damage to the spinal cord by 5–6 minutes earlier in animal studies (13). The common neuromonitors used during spine surgery are SSEP, MEP, Stagnara wakeup test, and ankle clonus test. Among these, SSEP and MEP are the most commonly used. Wakeup test and ankle clonus test are reserved to those centers where SSEP and MEP are not available. The main problem of monitoring evoked potentials in the elderly is that they require quiet deeper planes of anesthesia to prevent patient movement intraoperatively and to prevent injuries. Deeper planes of anesthesia are commonly maintained by using total intravenous anesthesia (TIVA), and these drugs may have their effect for a prolonged period of time due to altered physiology in geriatric persons. This may lead to increased chances of postoperative delirium, and long-term effects of these drugs in elderly patients has not been clear until now (14,15). Hypotension during surgery and the presence of comorbidities such as diabetes mellitus and hypertension may cause alteration in the signals and their quality, leading to difficulty in interpreting the signals. Hence it is preferable to record a baseline signal and analyze its characteristics before skin incision for comparison with the intraoperative signals.

ANKLE CLONUS TEST

This was the first test that was designed to detect over distraction of the spine during spine surgery.

Timing of the test: It should be done only during the emergence from anesthesia when the muscular paralysis is completely antagonized but the patient is still under the effect of anesthetic drugs.

Physiology of the test: In a neurologically intact or awake patient, the higher cortical centers discharge descending inhibitory influence on the spinal reflex, and clonus is not observed after ankle stretch. During anesthesia, the cortical centers are inhibited, and the discharge of descending inhibitory influence is absent, which causes elicitation of clonus upon stretching of the ankle.

How to perform the test: When the muscular paralysis is completely antagonized and the patient is still under anesthesia, the foot is sharply dorsiflexed at the ankle joint.

Interpretation of the result: If the clonus is present during the test, either the patient is completely awake, or if the patient is under anesthesia the spinal cord is intact without damage caused by distraction forces applied during surgery. If the clonus is absent, either the patient had spinal cord damage due to distraction forces applied due to the surgery or inadequate or too-deep planes of anesthesia.

Disadvantages

1. The test can be done only once, at a particular point of time.
2. The test does not provide full proof that the spinal cord is damaged or not damaged if the operator performs the test at the incorrect time or ineffectively.
3. This test does not give the surgeon sufficient time to rectify over-distraction.
4. The test can only detect intactness of the descending pathway. If any other part of the spinal cord is damaged, this test cannot detect it.

STAGNARA WAKEUP TEST

Preoperatively, patient needs to be educated about this test so that the test can be performed properly.

Timing of the test: Once the surgeon applies all the distraction or corrective forces, this test can be done.

Physiology of the test: If the patient is awake and follows and performs all the orders including the motor functions, then the spinal cord is intact.

How to perform the test: Muscular paralysis is antagonized, and the patient is awakened by stopping all the anesthetic drugs after the application of all the corrective forces in the surgical position before the surgery is completed. Once the patient is awake, he/she is asked to perform a motor activity related to a part of the spinal cord above the level of surgery where the spinal cord is expected to be intact and not being operated upon. Commonly, the patient will be asked to perform a movement in the upper limb. If the patient is able to perform this movement, then the patient has achieved status to perform the wakeup test necessary to determine the spinal cord damage. Now the patient is asked to perform a motor movement in the lower limb (commonly to move toes of the both the lower limbs).

Interpretation of the result: If the patient correctly performs the motor movement of the lower limb, then the spinal cord is intact.

Disadvantages

1. The test requires full cooperation of the patient. Therefore it cannot be performed on all patients.
2. The patient needs to be awakened during the test in the middle of the procedure, which may cause violent movement of the patient leading to untoward incidents such as fall from the surgical table or injury.
3. The patient may feel the pain of surgical incision.
4. The motor or sensory deficit of the spinal cord damage may appear after 20 minutes of application of the damaging corrective forces (13). Therefore, the wakeup test can be normal, but the patient may still have spinal cord damage.
5. The result of the test varies depending on the operator who performs the test.
6. The test gives the measure of the motor functions only; other functions are not measured.
7. The test shows intactness of motor functions during a particular time but cannot monitor the spinal cord functions continuously.

8. False negative results are high, as the geriatric patient more commonly has delirium if the anesthesiologist rapidly awakens the patient from anesthesia.

Advantages

1. The test does not require any extra equipment to perform.
2. It gives a reliable insight to intactness of the spinal cord if performed correctly at a particular point in time.

Somatosensory evoked potentials

Here an electrically mixed nerve such as posterior tibial, peroneal, or sural nerve is stimulated by electrodes, and the electrical impulses are recorded at a different level of the spinal cord at which surgery is performed and interpreted. A square wave stimulus of 0.1–0.3 ms at a rate of 3–7 Hz and an intensity of 25–40 mA will be given. Recording electrodes are placed at the scalp or spinous process of the cervical spine, or at the epidural space during the surgery. A baseline response is recorded before the skin incision and this will be compared with the responses recorded during surgery. If there is a decrease in amplitude by 50% and an increase in latency by 10%, this suggests to the surgeon that the spinal cord is supposedly getting stress, and impending damage is expected to occur if corrective steps are not taken immediately. SSEP has a sensitivity of 92% and specificity of 98.9% in detecting spinal cord functional integrity (16).

There are two assumptions in the design of the test:

1. It tests only dorsomedial tracts of the spinal cord but not the motor pathways or anterolateral sensory tracts of the spinal cord. Damage to the aforementioned tracts may be missed by SSEPs.
2. Perfusion to different spinal tracts is by different arteries. Hypo-perfusion can occur in one territory and not in other. If hypo-perfusion occurs in only the tracts that are not measured by SSEPs, the recordings may not reflect damage. Hence SSEPs recording may be normal but the patient may still develop spinal cord damage (17).

Factors that affect SSEP recordings:

1. Inhalational anesthetics and nitrous oxide (N_2O) cause a dose-dependent reduction in SSEP amplitude and increase in latency (18,19).

It is recommended that 60% N_2O with 0.5 minimum alveolar concentration (MAC) inhalational agents may cause the least effect on SSEP recordings (20).

2. IV anesthetic agents such as propofol, midazolam, etc. may also interfere in SSEP recordings. However, it has been found that there is less interference caused by IV agents than inhalational agents (19). Opioids, either intrathecal or IV, cause little effect on SSEPs. Neuromuscular-blocking drugs cause no effect on SSEPs.
3. Deliberate or induced or controlled hypotension causes reduction in SSEP signals. SSEP signals are lost at mean arterial pressure less than 60 mmHg.
4. 1°C reduction in temperature decreases 7% amplitude and 1% increase in latency of SSEP recordings.

Motor-evoked potentials

Principle: Stimulation of the spinal cord cranial to the site of spinal cord surgery causes stimulation of motor tracts in the spinal cord and spread of the impulses caudal to the surgery. If the motor tracts get damaged, then there is reduction in amplitude and increase in latency.

Techniques

- Depending on the site of stimulation: Motor cortex or spinal cord
- Depending on the method of stimulation: Electrical potential or magnetic field
- Depending on the site of recording: Spinal cord, peripheral mixed nerve or muscle

Effect of anesthesia on MEPs

1. Myogenic responses are not recordable in the deeper plane of neuromuscular blockade. Thus, neuromuscular block should be maintained continuously at 10%–20% of first twitch of train of four responses by continuous infusion of neuromuscular blocking agents. Neurogenic responses are not altered by the block of neuromuscular agents.
2. IV induction agents such as propofol cause dose-dependent reduction in the MEP amplitude and increase in latency. Midazolam and etomidate are known to cause a significant but smaller alteration in MEP. Inhalational induction agents at a MAC of 0.87 can abolish MEP.

Ketamine-based techniques are also found to cause interference in MEP. Hence, it is advocated that an IV infusion of propofol with fentanyl or remifentanil can be used to maintain anesthesia so that there is an optimum level of anesthesia where an anesthesiologist can record MEPs which are sufficient to detect damages in the spinal cord (21).

Disadvantages

1. MEP is less reliable in patients with pre-existing neurological deficits.
2. It cannot detect or cannot reliably detect damage in the dorsomedial tracts of the spinal cord.

Maintenance of general anesthesia

Maintenance can be by either inhalational or IV agents, depending on the monitors used for spinal cord monitoring. Intraoperative analgesia can be maintained by opioids. Geriatric patients are commonly on opioids preoperatively to reduce the pain, so they may have developed some tolerance, leading to increased dosing. It has been found that the development of dependence for opioids by geriatric patients is tenfold lower when compared to young adults. Using ketamine infusion intraoperatively can reduce the dose of opioids postoperatively, with reduction in complications associated with opioids (22). Non-opioid analgesics such as paracetamol and gabapentin can also be used intraoperatively to reduce opioid dosages postoperatively. Depending on the organ function of the geriatric patient, neuromuscular blocking agent can be chosen. Generally, atracurium is preferable because of its shorter duration of action and its non-dependency on the organ function of the body.

If the patient is not planned for elective ventilation, has a shorter duration of surgery, blood loss is minimal, and normothermia is maintained, the patient can be reversed and extubated on the table.

REGIONAL ANESTHESIA IN SPINE SURGERY

Subarachnoid block, epidural block, and combined subarachnoid and epidural block have been tried in certain spine surgeries (23–25). Procedures that can be performed under regional anesthesia include decompression of spinal stenosis, discectomy, fusion for degenerative instability, and laminectomy. Regional anesthesia techniques can be used as a sole technique of anesthesia for lumbar spine and lower thoracic spine surgeries only in view of anatomical and technical limitations. When the anesthesiologist decides to use a subarachnoid block, it should be given at least one level above or below the level of the operating site. When the anesthesiologist decides to use an epidural block, the epidural catheter should be fixed such a way that it will not interfere in the surgical field.

Criteria to be followed for spine surgery under regional anesthesia:

1. The patient should be educated about the procedure preoperatively, and should be cooperative.
2. Surgery should be of a short duration (preferably less than 3 h).
3. Expected blood loss should be minimal.
4. The surgeon should be ready to flood the operative area with local anesthetic drug if the surgery exceeds the duration of action of the regional block.

Advantages

1. There is decreased blood loss and less chance of thromboembolism compared to general anesthesia.
2. The patient is awake during the entire procedure so there is no or less chance of delirium postoperatively.
3. Advantages of the prone position in respiratory mechanics can be used in an awake patient for better recovery of the patient.
4. There is decreased need of analgesics postoperatively (25).
5. There is good cardiovascular stability perioperatively compared to general anesthesia.
6. There is less chance of perioperative complications such as nausea, vomiting, and urinary retention.
7. There is less chance of pulmonary complications compared to general anesthesia (26).
8. The patient can do self-positioning for the surgery so that pressure-related complications such as brachial plexus injury, abdominal compression, and chest compression can be minimized.
9. Spontaneous ventilation during surgery results in less distension of epidural veins, leading to a good surgical field.

Disadvantages

1. As the patient is in the prone or lateral position, the airway is not under the control of anesthesiologist. If the patient loses their airway, it is difficult to get the control.
2. There are medico-legal issues associated with it.
3. There is time restriction for duration of the surgery.
4. There is a chance of developing post-dural puncture headache (PDPH), but it has been found that the development of PDPH is less than a patient undergoing non-spine surgery under subarachnoid block. It has been scientifically explained that the spine surgery causes the effect of an epidural blood patch, leading to less chance of PDPH (27).

POSTOPERATIVE CARE

The surgical colleague expects the patient to be wide awake, conscious, and able to respond to commands in the immediate postoperative period for early neurological assessment. It is also important for the anesthesiologist, as the awake patient can expectorate and cough well, and the respiratory functions are better when compared to a drowsy patient.

Postoperative elective ventilation

Indications

1. If the preoperative vital capacity is less than 35% of predicted.
2. Comorbidities such as preoperative coronary cardiac diseases leading to cardiac instability.
3. Obesity.
4. Prolonged duration of surgery.
5. Major blood loss.
6. Hypothermia.
7. Metabolic derangements.
8. Debilitated elderly patient whose functional reserve is low.

Postoperative analgesia

Geriatric patients are sensitive to drugs because of the physiological changes of aging. They may be on opioid drugs preoperatively and have developed opioid tolerance. Parenteral opioids can cause complications such as respiratory depression, nausea, vomiting, sedation, and ileus. NSAIDs may cause epidural hematoma. Therefore, it is a fine line for the anesthesiologist to prescribe analgesic treatment. It is always better to have a multimodal approach.

Epidural analgesia, either with local anesthetics alone in combination with opioids, can be given. In this type of technique, the surgeon leaves the epidural catheter in the epidural space at the completion of surgery. Patient-controlled epidural analgesia can also be given. The main complication that hinders the surgeon's agreeing to this technique is increased chance of infection and formation of epidural abscess. The signs of epidural hematoma or abscess are masked by postoperative pain and pre-existing abnormal neurological symptoms.

Intrathecal analgesia is another method in which surgeon injects the opioid alone or opioid along with the local anesthetic drug into the intrathecal space at the end of surgery. A dose of 2–5 µg/kg of intrathecal morphine provides analgesia for 24 h with lesser incidence of side effects (28).

Disadvantages of this technique are need for use of an alternative technique after 24 h and increased risk of infection.

Advantage of this technique is that the analgesic requirement will be less compared to without this technique even after the completion of effect of intrathecal opioids.

Intrapleural infusion of local anesthetics alone or in combination of opioids is also used as a method for postoperative analgesia for thoracic spine surgery patients. It has been found that the intrapleural technique is inferior to the epidural technique (29).

Recently bilateral erector spinae plane block (ESP) with or without catheter has emerged as a newer technique for providing post-operative analgesia for spine surgeries.

Parenteral analgesics can be opioids, NSAIDs, acetaminophen, or COX-2 inhibitors. Parenteral opioid analgesics may cause more complications in geriatric patients due to increased sensitivity to the drugs. Patient-controlled analgesia (PCA) can be tried. PCA may not be possible in geriatric patients, as delirium is a common postoperative side effect after general anesthesia. Hence, it is preferable to combine parenteral analgesic with any regional technique to prevent complications while providing adequate analgesia. A combination of two techniques along with a combination of groups of two to three drugs is a successful formula for providing adequate and complete pain relief with minimal complications postoperatively in elderly patients.

Airway complications

Surgeries on the cervical spine can cause airway compromise because of hematoma formation or supra-glottic edema due to venous and lymphatic obstruction (30). Incidence of airway compromise is reported up to 1.9% (31). Risk factors for airway compromise are major blood loss, longer duration of surgery, combined anterior and posterior approach, previous spine surgery, and spine surgery at multiple levels. This complication can develop up to 36 hours postoperatively. It can present as neck swelling, change in voice quality, agitation, and respiratory distress. Reopening of the wound can be helpful in this condition.

Thromboembolism

Prophylaxis should be started preoperatively in the form of non-pharmacological methods as mentioned previously. Postoperative use of pharmacological methods to prevent thromboembolism can increase the chances of epidural hematoma and increased blood loss. If deep venous thrombosis occurs, insertion of IVC filter might be considered.

Respiratory complications

Respiratory complications can include respiratory depression due to higher dose of opioids, pneumonitis, infection, atelectasis, and adult respiratory distress syndrome.

Problems with prone position

Can include corneal abrasion, optic neuropathy, retinal artery occlusion, and damage to major vessels due to mechanical compression or hypotension.

Postoperative delirium

This is a common problem in geriatric patients in the postoperative period. The reported incidence for this complication is 0.49%–21% after spine surgeries (32). Risk factors include cervical spine surgery, major blood loss, cerebrovascular disease, hypertension, gender, preoperative alcohol or drug abuse, preoperative treatment of psychiatric drugs, and neurological disorders. Delirium results in increased hospital stay, increase in morbidity and mortality, and increase in cost to the patient postoperatively. It is always better to prevent rather than treat any complication, especially postoperative delirium in elderly. Prevention methods include identifying risk factors and controlling them or treating them permanently. If the patient develops postoperative delirium, the anesthesiologist should first identify the cause and try to remove or treat it. If delirium persists, then it should be treated with nonpharmacological methods such as daily physical activity, cognitive reorientation, allowing bedside presence of a family member, sleep enhancement by frequent change in environment, early mobility and/or physical rehabilitation, adaptations for visual and hearing impairment, pain management, providing good nutrition, adequate oxygenation, prevention of constipation, and minimization of catheters. If delirium persists, then pharmacological treatment with haloperidol, risperidone or olanzapine, or dexmedetomidine can be initiated (33).

Other complications include persistent hypotension, hemorrhage, nerve root damage, cauda equina syndrome, and urinary retention.

REFERENCES

1. Brallier JW, Deiner S. The elderly spine surgery patient: Pre- and intraoperative management of drug therapy. *Drugs Aging.* 2015 Aug;32(8):601–9.
2. Deiner S, Westlake B, Dutton RP. Patterns of surgical care and complications in elderly adults. *J Am Geriatr Soc.* 2014 May;62(5):829–35.
3. Sharma A, Lawmin J-C, Irwin MG. Anaesthesia for spinal surgery. *Anaesth Intensive Care Med.* 2015 Mar;16(3):108–10.
4. Drazin D, Al-Khouja L, Lagman C et al. Scoliosis surgery in the elderly: Complications, readmissions, reoperations and mortality. *J Clin Neurosci.* 2016 Dec;34:158–61.
5. Hambly PR, Martin B. Anaesthesia for chronic spinal cord lesions. *Anaesthesia.* 1998 Mar;53(3):273–89.
6. Picone DM, Titler MG, Dochterman J et al. Predictors of medication errors among elderly

hospitalized patients. *Am J Med Qual.* 2008 Apr;23(2):115–27.

7. Raw DA, Beattie JK, Hunter JM. Anaesthesia for spinal surgery in adults. *Br J Anaesth.* 2003 Dec;91(6):886–904.

8. Prabhakar H, Mahajan C, Kapoor I. *Manual of Neuroanesthesia: The Essentials.* [Internet]. CRC Press; 2017. Available from: https:// books.google.co.in/books?id=MAsqDwA AQBAJ

9. Oda T, Fuji T, Kato Y, Fujita S, Kanemitsu N. Deep venous thrombosis after posterior spinal surgery. *Spine.* 2000 Nov 15;25(22):2962–7.

10. John DA, Tobey RE, Homer LD, Rice CL. Onset of succinylcholine-induced hyperkalemia following denervation. *Anesthesiology.* 1976 Sep;45(3):294–9.

11. Willner D, Spennati V, Stohl S, Tosti G, Aloisio S, Bilotta F. Spine surgery and blood loss: Systematic review of clinical evidence. *Anesth Analg.* 2016;123(5):1307–15.

12. Toyota S, Amaki Y. Hemodynamic evaluation of the prone position by transesophageal echocardiography. *J Clin Anesth.* 1998 Feb; 10(1):32–5.

13. Owen JH, Naito M, Bridwell KH, Oakley DM. Relationship between duration of spinal cord ischemia and postoperative neurologic deficits in animals. *Spine.* 1990 Sep;15(9):846–51.

14. Sieber FE, Zakriya KJ, Gottschalk A et al. Sedation depth during spinal anesthesia and the development of postoperative delirium in elderly patients undergoing hip fracture repair. *Mayo Clin Proc.* 2010 Jan;85(1):18–26.

15. Radtke FM, Franck M, Lendner J, Krüger S, Wernecke KD, Spies CD. Monitoring depth of anaesthesia in a randomized trial decreases the rate of postoperative delirium but not postoperative cognitive dysfunction. *Br J Anaesth.* 2013 Jun;110 Suppl 1:i98–105.

16. Nuwer MR, Dawson EG, Carlson LG, Kanim LE, Sherman JE. Somatosensory evoked potential spinal cord monitoring reduces neurologic deficits after scoliosis surgery: Results of a large multicenter survey. *Electroencephalogr Clin Neurophysiol.* 1995 Jan;96(1):6–11.

17. Pelosi L, Jardine A, Webb JK. Neurological complications of anterior spinal surgery for kyphosis with normal somatosensory evoked potentials (SEPs). *J Neurol Neurosurg Psychiatry.* 1999 May;66(5):662–4.

18. Lam AM, Sharar SR, Mayberg TS, Eng CC. Isoflurane compared with nitrous oxide anaesthesia for intraoperative monitoring of somatosensory-evoked potentials. *Can J Anaesth.* 1994 Apr;41(4):295–300.

19. Clapcich AJ, Emerson RG, Roye DP et al. The effects of propofol, small-dose isoflurane, and nitrous oxide on cortical somatosensory evoked potential and bispectral index monitoring in adolescents undergoing spinal fusion. *Anesth Analg.* 2004 Nov;99(5):1334–40; table of contents.

20. Peterson DO, Drummond JC, Todd MM. Effects of halothane, enflurane, isoflurane, and nitrous oxide on somatosensory evoked potentials in humans. *Anesthesiology.* 1986 Jul;65(1):35–40.

21. Pelosi L, Stevenson M, Hobbs GJ, Jardine A, Webb JK. Intraoperative motor evoked potentials to transcranial electrical stimulation during two anaesthetic regimens. *Clin Neurophysiol.* 2001 Jun;112(6):1076–87.

22. Nielsen RV, Fomsgaard JS, Siegel H et al. Intraoperative ketamine reduces immediate postoperative opioid consumption after spinal fusion surgery in chronic pain patients with opioid dependency: A randomized, blinded trial. *Pain.* 2017 Mar;158(3):463–70.

23. Tu PY, Tung HC, Chao CC, Lin HJ, Cheng HC, Lin SY. Epidural anesthesia for spine surgery. *Ma Zui Xue Za Zhi Anaesthesiol Sin.* 1990 Jun;28(2):203–7.

24. Khajavi MR, Asadian MA, Imani F, Etezadi F, Moharari RS, Amirjamshidi A. General anesthesia versus combined epidural/general anesthesia for elective lumbar spine disc surgery: A randomized clinical trial comparing the impact of the two methods upon the outcome variables. *Surg Neurol Int.* 2013;4:105.

25. Lessing NL, Edwards CC, Brown CH et al. Spinal anesthesia in elderly patients undergoing lumbar spine surgery. *Orthopedics.* 2017 Mar 1;40(2):e317–22.

26. Erbas YC, Pusat S, Yilmaz E, Bengisun ZK, Erdogan E. Posterior lumbar stabilization surgery under spinal anesthesia for high-risk patients with degenerative spondylolisthesis, spinal stenosis and lumbar

compression fracture. *Turk Neurosurg.* 2015;25(5):771–5.

27. Tetzlaff JE, Dilger JA, Kodsy M, al-Bataineh J, Yoon HJ, Bell GR. Spinal anesthesia for elective lumbar spine surgery. *J Clin Anesth.* 1998 Dec;10(8):666–9.

28. Boezaart AP, Eksteen JA, Spuy GV, Rossouw P, Knipe M. Intrathecal morphine. Double-blind evaluation of optimal dosage for analgesia after major lumbar spinal surgery. *Spine.* 1999 Jun 1;24(11):1131–7.

29. Gaeta RR, Macario A, Brodsky JB, Brock-Utne JG, Mark JB. Pain outcomes after thoracotomy: Lumbar epidural hydromorphone versus intrapleural bupivacaine. *J Cardiothorac Vasc Anesth.* 1995 Oct;9(5):534–7.

30. Nowicki RW. Anaesthesia for major spinal surgery. *Contin Educ Anaesth Crit Care Pain.* 2014 Aug;14(4):147–52.

31. Sagi HC, Beutler W, Carroll E, Connolly PJ. Airway complications associated with surgery on the anterior cervical spine. *Spine.* 2002 May 1;27(9):949–53.

32. Kobayashi K, Imagama S, Ando K et al. Risk factors for delirium after spine surgery in extremely elderly patients aged 80 years or older and review of the literature: Japan Association of Spine Surgeons with Ambition Multicenter Study. *Global Spine J.* 2017 Sep;7(6):560–6.

33. Mohanty S, Rosenthal RA, Russell MM, Neuman MD, Ko CY, Esnaola NF. Optimal perioperative management of the geriatric patient: A best practices guideline from the American College of Surgeons NSQIP and the American Geriatrics Society. *J Am Coll Surg.* 2016 May;222(5):930–47.

10

Neurosurgery: Minimally invasive neurosurgery

CHARU MAHAJAN, INDU KAPOOR, AND HEMANSHU PRABHAKAR

INTRODUCTION

The specialty of neuroanesthesia has greatly increased in terms of advancement over the past two decades, keeping pace with ever-growing technological developments in neurosurgery. The new surgical approaches and procedures bring new perioperative concerns—a few already known and others still emerging as incorporation of newer techniques in practice steadily increases. As life expectancy has increased, more and more geriatric patients present for operative procedures. The functional impact of surgery and associated comorbidities has a negative effect on the complication profile and may increase morbidity and mortality. These patients may have other coexisting systemic diseases which have important anesthetic concerns (Table 10.1). Minimally invasive surgical practice has flourished secondarily to the advancement in computer-assisted technology, imaging, optics, and surgical instruments. Neuroimaging modalities such as computed tomography (CT) and magnetic resonance imaging (MRI) have been

integrated with various advanced computerized software, which enable the surgeon to obtain a three-dimensional (3-D) view of an area of interest while operating. Stereotactic systems use co-registration of the patient with a preoperative imaging study and enable the surgeon to relate the location of instruments in the surgical field with preoperative imaging data. For the geriatric population, this translates into less invasive approach with minimal/no tissue retraction, resulting in less neural tissue damage, a more precise job, less pain, early recovery, and better outcomes. Fiberoptics have revolutionized visualization of the surgical area. Special endoscopes are inserted through a small incision, allowing visualization of even hidden areas, resulting in minimal dissection, less pain, minimal scarring, short surgical time, and earlier recovery. Lack of depth perception is a limitation that may be overcome by newer, more expensive 3-D endoscopy. Once the steep learning curve associated with use of endoscopes is surpassed, it is certainly advantageous overall. Robots in neurosurgical practice aid in carrying out minimally

Table 10.1 Common coexisting diseases in geriatric patients

Cardiovascular system	Atherosclerosis
	Hypertension
	Coronary artery disease (CAD)
	Myocardial ischemia
	Congestive cardiac failure
	Arrhythmias
	Valvular heart disease
Respiratory system	Blunted response to hypercarbia and hypoxia
	Emphysema
	Chronic bronchitis
	Pneumonia
	Lung cancer
Endocrine	Diabetes mellitus
Renal system	Compromised renal function
	Decreased ability to handle salt/water load
Hepatobiliary	Decreased ability to metabolize drugs
Neurological	Depression
	Dementia
	Cognitive decline
	Parkinson's disease
	Alzheimer's disease
Musculoskeletal system	Reduced muscle mass
	Degenerative changes of spine
	Osteoporosis
	Rheumatoid arthritis
	Ankylosing spondylitis
Adipose tissue	Decreased total body water and increased adipose tissue affect

invasive surgeries. These integrate navigation and surgical planning with a robotic arm resulting in smaller incisions, more precision, and better access to the surgical area. Table 10.2 enumerates the various minimally invasive neurosurgical procedures.

The preoperative workup of these patients is same as for any open surgery. Presence of coexisting systemic diseases needs further focused specialist examination and special investigations. The anesthesia goals remain the same as for all neurosurgical procedures (Table 10.3). The minimally invasive procedures are individually discussed in detail here.

CRANIAL PROCEDURES

Endoscopic transnasal transsphenoidal hypophysectomy

The endoscopic approach has taken over the earlier microscopic approach for resection of pituitary tumors. Computer-assisted navigation uses co-registration of the patient points on preoperative MRI images, which helps in directing the trajectory toward the focus. A small flexible endoscope is inserted through a nasal cavity toward the tumor base, followed by lateralization of turbinates and sphenoidotomy to reach the sella. An extended approach may be required for removal of parasellar or suprasellar tumors. Intraoperative MRI provides information about the tumor remnants, enabling its more thorough removal and also helps in detection of any hematomas. The main advantages of an endoscopic approach are broader, clearer field visualization and ability to see hidden areas which usually remain inaccessible when using a microscope. Other advantages are less pain, shorter operative times, better airflow, earlier recovery, shorter hospital stay, and better short-term sinonasal quality of life and endocrinological outcome (1–4). Although the evidence varies

Table 10.2 Minimally invasive neurosurgical procedures in the geriatric population

Endoscopic cranial	• Endoscopic transnasal hypophysectomy
	• Endoscopic third ventriculostomy
	• Endoscopic ventriculoperitoneal shunts
	• Endoscopic removal of tumors, colloid cysts, fenestration of cysts, drainage of hematomas
	• Brain biopsy
	• Endoscope assisted aneurysm clipping
	• Stereotactic deep brain surgery
Endoscopic spinal	• Microdiscectomy
	• Laminectomy
	• Microforaminectomy
	• Video-assisted thoracoscopic surgery
	• Tumor resection
	• Spinal fusion
	• Percutaneous kyphoplasty/vertebroplasty
Robotic	• Robotic stereotactic assisted (ROSA) ETV
	• Brain tumor resection
	• Endoscopic procedures
	• Epilepsy surgery
	• Deep brain stimulation
	• Spinal instrumentation

Table 10.3 General anesthetic goals for minimally invasive neurosurgery

1. Adequate depth of anesthesia to keep the patient perfectly immobile
2. Maintenance of hemodynamics and cerebral perfusion pressure
3. Management of intracranial pressure
4. Facilitation of intraoperative neurophysiologic monitoring techniques
5. Rapid emergence for neurologic assessment

regarding long-term sinonasal quality, the recent trend is more toward the endoscopic approach.

The main anesthesia goals are the same as microscopic image-guided resection—to ensure complete patient immobility, be vigilant for sudden increase in intracranial pressure (ICP), and plan for an early emergence for prompt neurologic examination. Geriatric patients may have history of hypertension, diabetes, CAD, compromised renal function, etc. Drug history should be taken, and all organ systems should be properly evaluated. Loss of dentition may make mask ventilation difficult, and arthritic changes in the spine may cause difficulty during laryngoscopy. Cotton pads soaked in an adrenaline and local anesthetic mixture are packed deep in nasal cavity to decongest and widen the space for negotiation of the endoscope. In microscopic procedures, the nasal cavity dilatation with a speculum induces a pressor response and leads to hypertension. On the other hand, in endoscopic procedures, a binasal approach is used, omitting the need to retract the nasal cavity; thus the pressor response may be less intense. Strict control of blood pressure is essential to avoid any bleeding, which may obscure the operating field. Propofol or dexmedetomidine infusion may be used as aids to regulate the blood pressure and prevent any sudden upsurge (5,6). Also, it has been found to decrease total blood loss (6). The different nerve blocks such as maxillary, infraorbital, sphenopalatine, and pterygopalatine have been used as adjuvants to general anesthesia (GA) during resection of these tumors to control the hemodynamic surge and provide analgesia

(7–10). Sevoflurane–remifentanil has been found to provide a faster recovery than a propofol–remifentanil infusion (11). In a recent US health claims database, the incidence of postoperative complications such as diabetes insipidus, syndrome of inappropriate ADH secretion, cerebrospinal fluid (CSF) rhinorrhea, CSF leak, and fever were found to be higher in endoscopic techniques than microscopic procedures (12). This can have an important implication, as it may imply that the burden of perioperative complications may increase. This may be clearer in the future, with more contradictory data coming up (13).

ENDOSCOPIC THIRD VENTRICULOSTOMY

This is a minimally invasive technique in which an endoscope is placed through a burr hole, inside the ventricular system of brain. It is directed toward the third ventricle, where an opening is made in the floor of the third ventricle using the endoscope. This allows CSF movement directly into the basal cisterns, bypassing any obstruction beyond the third ventricle. The preoperative management and optimization are the same as for any patient having elevated intracranial pressure. Fluid and electrolyte abnormalities should be corrected. Sedatives are usually avoided in premedication. The standard anesthetic induction is followed by endotracheal intubation and maintenance of anesthesia with air/inhalational agent or total intravenous anesthesia. Nitrous oxide is avoided due to concern of expansion of air bubbles in the ventricular system. Standard American Society of Anesthesiologists (ASA) monitoring includes ECG, blood pressure, pulse oximetry, capnography, and urine output monitoring. Arterial line monitoring allows beat-to-beat blood pressure monitoring, helping in the hemodynamic management. Intraoperative rate arrhythmias because of elevated ICP or stimulation of adjacent structures such as the hypothalamus and brainstem may occur. The basilar artery lies beneath the floor of the third ventricle, and may be injured rarely. This may lead to massive hemorrhage and blood loss. During neuroendoscopy of ventricles, a continuous fluid irrigation is performed. This is associated with increase in ICP and decrease in cerebral perfusion pressure (CPP) (14). The volume of fluid infused through the ventriculoscope should also be allowed to exit to prevent any sudden increase in ICP. This can be easily monitored by pressure inside the neuroendoscope by a fluid-filled catheter transmitting pressure from the inlet channel to a pressure transducer (15). In an in vitro study, pressure at the inlet was found to overestimate and pressure at the rinsing outlet to underestimate the pressures. The authors found that pressure measured from an electronic tip sensor placed at the distal end of the lumen of the rinsing channel of the endoscope were equal to ventricular pressure (16). Warm Ringer lactate is most commonly used as an irrigation fluid. Irrigation with a large amount of cold fluid can affect the hypothalamus (forming the lateral wall of the third ventricle) resulting in temperature dysregulation and hypothermia. Other perioperative complications are delayed awakening, pneumocephalus, infection, and convulsions. Blood transfusion is generally not required intraoperatively until or unless massive hemorrhage occurs, which is rare. The trachea is extubated postoperatively in uneventful cases; however, delayed awakening may occur in some cases.

ENDOSCOPIC VENTRICULOPERITONEAL SHUNTS

Intraoperative use of ultrasound or frameless stereotaxy for placement of ventricular end of shunt increases the chance of accurate catheter placement and reduces proximal shunt failures (17,18). Minimally invasive laparoscopic approach for insertion of distal catheter as compared to conventional laparotomy results in reduction in operating times and reduced shunt failures and abdominal malposition (19). There is no major difference in anesthetic implications for this minimally invasive approach compared to a conventional freehand technique.

ANEURYSM CLIPPING

The classic pterional craniotomy is associated with retraction of the temporalis muscle, which may cause delayed atrophy/scarring, subsequent facial asymmetry, possibility of temporomandibular joint dysfunction, pain on mastication, and injury to frontal branch of facial nerve (20). It is also associated with exposure of a large area of cerebral cortex. Shorter operative times, less pain, better cosmesis, reduced cost, and improved patient acceptability has turned the trend toward minimal invasive microsurgery such as keyhole or mini-craniotomies and endoscope-assisted aneurysm surgery (21,22). The endoscope is used for either (a) inspection before clipping to visualize the hidden areas, (b) clipping under endoscopic view, or (c) post-clipping evaluation to ensure the aneurysm is completely clipped and the perforators are intact. Purely endoscopic aneurysm surgery still is not very popular.

STEREOTACTIC PROCEDURES

Stereotaxy helps in assessment of depth and direction so that this guided instrumentation causes minimal trauma with improved precision. However, in frame-based stereotactic procedures, the frame is a hindrance for access to the airway. The newer frameless stereotaxy uses scalp markers as fiducial points which help in relating the computer-generated 3-D image to surgical instruments. Stereotaxy may be used for biopsy or excision of brain tumors, drainage of abscess/hematoma, and deep brain stimulation (DBS) for patients having Parkinson's disease.

Patients presenting for DBS are usually elderly, having disease-specific and age-related issues and may also have respiratory, cardiovascular, and autonomic dysfunction along with drug therapy side effects. The goals of anesthetic management are provision of good operating conditions, patient comfort, management of intraoperative complications, and facilitation of intraoperative neuromonitoring. This is usually carried out as a frame-based stereotactic surgery in which the head is placed in a fixed rigid metallic ring frame having fixed fiducials and an instrument holder attached to frame. This is followed by brain imaging and computerized superimposition to obtain a 3-D image. The first stage of surgery is placement of electrodes at the target nuclei of basal ganglia and is usually undertaken as awake surgery under monitored anesthesia care. Anesthetics affect the microelectrode readings by potentiating inhibitory action of gamma amino butyric acid (GABA), so these are generally avoided. Patients should be fully awake and able to cooperate during microelectrode recordings (MER). All options for securing the airway should be kept ready in the operating room, including a wrench to open the frame if the need arises. The patient is positioned in a comfortable manner on soft padding. In addition to standard ASA monitors, invasive blood pressure monitoring and measurement of urinary output is also carried out. Anesthetics such as benzodiazepines, barbiturates, propofol, and volatile agents potentiate the inhibitory action of GABA. Dexmedetomidine does not affect GABA action and can be considered for sedation (23). All sedatives are stopped so that the patient can be awake and cooperative at the time of brain stimulation. Alteration in motor symptoms during brain stimulation helps with proper stimulator lead placement.

In those patients who are unable to undergo awake procedure, are uncooperative, or have severe movement disorder, GA is administered. GA makes clinical testing impossible and masks detection of any adverse effect during stimulation testing, so the correct placement of electrodes is done under MRI guidance. The various intraoperative complications are airway obstruction, respiratory dysfunction, hypertension, orthostatic hypotension, venous air embolism, seizures, and loss of cooperation. The second stage of surgery is battery placement, performed under GA using a laryngeal mask airway or an endotracheal tube. Postoperative concerns are nausea, vomiting, exacerbation of off-drug state, and rarely, intracerebral hemorrhage or pneumocephalus.

Stereotactic radiosurgery is a noninvasive technique in which a beam of radiation is focused on a particular pathological area with an aim to destroy it. The patient is awake and is instructed to remain immobile for the duration of the procedure. Patients who are uncooperative, have movement disorders, or who cannot lie still for a long duration are administered GA. This is a modality of treatment for conditions such as arteriovenous malformations, acoustic neuroma, and trigeminal neuralgia.

SPINAL PROCEDURES

Geriatric patients having multiple comorbidities frequently present for spine surgeries, for prolapsed disc, canal stenosis, spondylolisthesis, spinal tumors, or spinal trauma requiring instrumentation. A minimally invasive approach may provide these patients with a better chance to recuperate, especially those who are considered at high-risk to conventional open surgery.

Endoscopy is increasingly being used as a less invasive approach to the spine, causing minimal muscle dissection, less injury to epidural blood supply, decreased blood loss, less operative time, decreased postoperative pain, earlier mobilization, shorter recovery time, shorter hospital stay, and better cosmesis. This allows early functional recovery and return to daily work. However, this approach has a steep learning curve and requires careful patient selection and complete understanding of the anatomy. The reduced anatomical and visual exposure of the nerve roots as compared to the open techniques makes them vulnerable to injury. This makes intraoperative neurophysiological monitoring especially important. Spine surgery in the elderly is associated with occurrence of postoperative delirium; the incidence varies between 5%–13%. The probable risk factors are older age, greater blood loss, longer operative times, and cerebral vascular disease (24). The minimally invasive technique reduces overall blood loss and operative time, which may be beneficial in this aspect. However, no definite evidence regarding delirium after minimally invasive spinal surgery is present, and this needs to be further studied. The steep learning curve and technical difficulty are its shortcomings.

MINIMALLY INVASIVE SURGERY FOR INTERVERTEBRAL DISC HERNIATION

This is one of the most commonly performed procedures. The three techniques for this condition are micro-discectomy using a tubular retractor system, percutaneous laser disc decompression, or selective endoscopic discectomy. Initially, endoscopic technique was used for lumbar discectomy, but now its use has extended to cervical and thoracic levels as well. In a retrospective cohort study, patients who underwent microendoscopic laminectomy had less incidence of major postoperative complications, surgical site infection, and postoperative delirium (25). GA is the most commonly used anesthesia for these procedures but may be associated with an increased probability of neurological complications. This requires intraoperative neurophysiological monitoring. The main advantage for procedures carried out under local anesthesia is that the patient

can warn the surgeon in the case of any nerve root impingement. Maintaining prone position is a challenge for patients who are not anesthetized. For percutaneous endoscopic discectomy, spinal/epidural anesthesia or local anesthesia along with conscious sedation is an option. Intravenous sedative agents such as propofol and midazolam have been taken over by dexmedetomidine in view of its safer respiratory profile (26). In cases of respiratory depression, conversion to GA may require repositioning the patient and securing of the airway. Data from a retrospective study comparing GA and epidural anesthesia (EA) in patients undergoing lumbar microdiscectomy shows that EA is a cost-effective technique associated with less nerve root manipulation and greater comfort, efficacy, and reliability (27). In another retrospective study, EA was compared to local anesthesia for lumbar transforaminal endoscopic surgery. The authors found that EA is safe, feasible, and is associated with a higher patient satisfaction rate (28).

ENDOSCOPIC MICROFORAMINOTOMY

This is another minimally invasive decompression surgery that helps to relieve the pressure on the spinal cord or nerve roots. Compared to open cervical foraminotomy, it is associated with lower blood loss, less pain, and shorter duration of hospital stay. These procedures are usually carried out under general endotracheal anesthesia. The intraoperative evoked potential monitoring requires total intravenous-based anesthesia with omission of muscle relaxants. The anterior cervical foraminotomy helps to treat ventral radiculopathy without the need for discectomy, obviating the need for any arthrodesis or neck collar. Injury may occur to nerve root, blood vessels, or to sympathetic chain, resulting in Horner syndrome. Posterior cervical microforaminotomy is used to treat foraminal stenosis due to degenerative changes such as osteophytes or lateral disc herniation (29). It may be carried out in the prone or sitting position. Injury to dura, nerve root, or blood vessels may occur. Vertebral artery injury is a dreaded complication and requires control with gelfoam packing. In an uneventful case, patients are woken and trachea extubated at the end of surgery.

VIDEO-ASSISTED THORACOSCOPIC SPINE SURGERY

Video-assisted thoracoscopic spine surgery (VATS) is becoming a more popular approach to anterior thoracic and thoracolumbar junction spine for scoliosis/kyphosis correction and spine trauma patients. Fiberoptic technique is used for visualization of T1–T12 spine through percutaneous keyholes. This technique obviates the need for open thoracotomy, resulting in reduced chest wall morbidity such as incisional pain and intercostal neuralgia (30). There is decreased shoulder and pulmonary dysfunction and better cosmesis. These patients should be evaluated preoperatively, especially for cardiac system and pulmonary reserve. The special anesthesia requirement is single-lung ventilation by means of double-lumen endotracheal tube, which allows complete collapse of the lung ensuring full view through the videoscope. The patient is placed in the lateral decubitus position and all relevant concerns of positioning should be dealt with. Cervical spine involvement is common in the elderly and should be taken care of. Nitrous oxide is usually avoided. Evoked potential monitoring such as somatosensory-evoked potentials (SSEPs) and motor-evoked potentials (MEPs) requires omission of high doses of volatile agents and muscle relaxants. Total intravenous anesthesia with propofol and opioid is the preferred technique. An arterial line is inserted for continuous beat–beat monitoring and repeated gas analysis during long surgeries. Multilevel spine surgery and corpectomy may be associated with significant blood loss. Any inadvertent large vessel injury may obscure the visual field and may require immediate conversion to open thoracotomy. Chest tubes are inserted at end of the procedure. Atelectasis may be a problem in the postoperative period and requires deep breathing exercises and good chest physiotherapy. Adequate pain relief aids in early recovery.

PERCUTANEOUS KYPHOPLASTY AND VERTEBROPLASTY

Patients presenting with fractured vertebrae are usually elderly and may have significant medical comorbidities. The fractured vertebrae are cemented with polymethylmethacrylate through the percutaneous approach. Positioning should be done very carefully, as osteoporosis is common. These procedures are usually performed under GA or local anesthesia with sedation. Intravenous midazolam along with fentanyl boluses are sufficient for vertebroplasty. Kyphoplasty is comparatively more painful and requires additional opioid boluses at the time of balloon tamp insertion for re-expanding the vertebrae. Lee et al. found that dexmedetomidine when compared to remifentanil for monitored anesthesia care during these procedures produced less respiratory depression, lower blood pressure and heart rate, but had less analgesic effect. However, there were no significant between-group differences in terms of recovery time, investigators' satisfaction scores, or patients' overall pain experiences (31). In addition to the conventional local anesthesia, additional extrapedicular infiltration during these percutaneous procedures provides good local anesthesia without any adverse nerve root effects (32). If multiple levels need to be treated, GA is preferable, as the patient may not tolerate lying in the prone position for a very long time. Intraoperative extravasation of bone cement to veins and epidural space may result in pulmonary embolization or spinal cord or nerve root compression. These are usually done as day care procedures, but the stay may be prolonged depending on the general physical condition of the patient and comorbidities.

MINIMALLY INVASIVE LUMBAR SPINE FUSION

Lumbar spine stabilization is often required in geriatric patients having trauma, degenerative changes, infection, or malignancy. Minimally invasive techniques for spinal fusion are anterior lumbar interbody fusion (ALIF), posterior lumbar interbody fusion, transforaminal lumbar interbody fusion, intertransverse fusion, and pedicle screw/rod placement. Decreased muscle and soft tissue injury, decreased operative time, less blood loss, less pain, earlier mobilization, and faster return to work are important advantages of minimally invasive surgery. ALIF can be done through either the laparoscopic transperitoneal or retroperitoneal route. The transperitoneal route provides the best access to the L5–S1 level, as the bifurcation of great vessels lies above this level.

However, injury to the bowel, superior hypogastric plexus, and blood vessels are potential concerns. Retroperitoneal lumbar fusion is performed either in the supine or lateral decubitus position using carbon dioxide (CO_2) insufflation, balloon insufflation, or a combination of both to create and maintain the retroperitoneal working cavity. The related concerns of laparoscopic surgery such as trendelenburg position hypercapnia, right bronchus intubation, and CO_2 embolism should be kept in mind. Transforaminal, posterolateral procedures and percutaneous spinal fixation are performed in the prone position.

INTRADURAL PATHOLOGY

The minimally invasive technique using endoscope is also employed for spinal tumor resection or even arteriovenous malformation. General endotracheal anesthesia is used for these procedures.

ROBOT-ASSISTED NEUROSURGERY

Minimally invasive robotic surgery helps to enhance the surgeon's skill, provides better access to the surgical area through small incisions, and results in better precision, decreased radiation exposure, less blood loss, less pain, shorter operative times, earlier recovery, and shorter hospital stay. Most neurosurgical robotic systems are designed to assist in stereotactic surgeries. Incorporation of image-processing software integrates the information obtained from preoperative images and intraoperative MRI/CT systems, thus allowing image-guided navigation. This facilitates planning and guides direction of the trajectories to the area of interest in real time. The different types of robots are (a) independent, which operates according to preprogrammed instructions, (b) dependent, where the surgeon completely controls the movement of surgical instruments, and (c) shared-control, which commonly has a passive arm that stabilizes the instruments and moves only when the surgeon chooses. Robotic arm–based technology is used for endoscopic third ventriculostomy (ETV), tumor resection, deep brain stimulation, epilepsy surgery, and minimally invasive spinal surgery. The anesthesiologist should ensure complete immobility of patient, tailor hemodynamic monitoring depending on the comorbidities, monitor closely for any complication, and be ready for emergent undocking of the robot and conversion to open surgery in cases of uncontrollable bleeding.

CONCLUSION

As the overall quality of life has improved and life expectancy has increased over the years, geriatric patients frequently present for different surgical procedures. Minimally invasive neurosurgery in the geriatric population is becoming popular as newer techniques enabling more precision with minimal tissue trauma are continuously evolving. However, these keyhole surgeries should not be considered risk free. The management of anesthesia for coexisting diseases should be similar to any other open surgery. Close vigilant monitoring and prompt management of any sudden complication should be the objective.

REFERENCES

1. Singh H, Essayed WI, Cohen-Gadol A, Zada G, Schwartz TH. Resection of pituitary tumors: Endoscopic versus microscopic. *J Neurooncol*. 2016;130:309–17.
2. Little AS, Kelly D, Milligan J et al. Predictors of sinonasal quality of life and nasal morbidity after fully endoscopic transsphenoidal surgery. *J Neurosurg*. 2015;122:1458–65.
3. Nishioka H. Recent evolution of endoscopic endonasal surgery for treatment of pituitary adenomas. *Neurol Med Chir (Tokyo)*. 2017; 57:151–8.
4. Pledger CL, Elzoghby MA, Oldfield EH et al. Prospective comparison of sinonasal outcomes after microscopic sublabial or endoscopic endonasal transsphenoidal surgery for nonfunctioning pituitary adenomas. *J Neurosurg*. 2016;125:323–33.
5. Salimi A, Sharifi G, Bahrani H et al. Dexmedetomidine could enhance surgical satisfaction in trans-sphenoidal resection of pituitary adenoma. *J Neurosurg Sci*. 2017;61:46–52.
6. Gopalakrishna KN, Dash PK, Chatterjee N, Easwer HV, Ganesamoorthi A. Dexmedetomidine as an anesthetic adjuvant in patients undergoing transsphenoidal resection of pituitary tumor. *J Neurosurg Anesthesiol*. 2015;27:209–15.

7. McAdam D, Muro K, Suresh S. The use of infraorbital nerve block for postoperative pain control after transsphenoidal hypophysectomy. *Reg Anesth Pain Med.* 2005;30:572–3.

8. Chadha R, Padmanabhan V, Rout A, Waikar HD, Mohandas K. Prevention of hypertension during trans-sphenoidal surgery – The effect of bilateral maxillary nerve block with local anaesthetics. *Acta Anaesthesiol Scand.* 1997;4:35–40.

9. Ali AR, Sakr SA, Rahman ASMA. Bilateral sphenopalatine ganglion block as adjuvant to general anaesthesia during endoscopic transnasal resection of pituitary adenoma. *Egypt J Anaesth.* 2010;26:273–80.

10. Aver'ianov DA, Cherebillo V, Shatalov VI, Shchegolev AV. Comparison of stress response severity during intravenous, inhalation and combined anesthesia (inhalation plus local) for pituitary transsphenoidal adenomectomy. *Anesteziol Reanimatol.* 2011 Jul–Aug;(4):10–3.

11. Cafiero T, Cavallo LM, Frangiosa A, Burrelli R, Gargiulo G, Cappabianca P, de Divitiis E. Clinical comparison of remifentanil-sevoflurane vs. remifentanil-propofol for endoscopic endonasal transsphenoidal surgery. *Eur J Anaesthesiol.* 2007;24:441–6.

12. Asemota AO, Ishii M, Brem H, Gallia GL. Comparison of complications, trends, and costs in endoscopic vs microscopic pituitary surgery: Analysis from a US Health Claims Database. *Neurosurgery.* 2017;81:458–72.

13. Li A, Liu W, Cao P, Zheng Y, Bu Z, Zhou T. Endoscopic versus microscopic transsphenoidal surgery in the treatment of pituitary adenoma: A systematic review and meta-analysis. *World Neurosurg.* 2017;101:236–46.

14. Prabhakar H, Rath GP, Bithal PK, Suri A, Dash H. Variations in cerebral haemodynamics during irrigation phase in neuroendoscopic procedures. *Anaesth Intensive Care.* 2007;35:209–12.

15. Fabregas N, Lopez A, Valero R, Careero E, Caral L, Ferrer E. Anesthetic management of surgical endoscopies: Usefulness of monitoring the pressure inside the neuroendoscope. *J Neurosurg Anesthesiol.* 2000;12:21–8.

16. Dewaele F, Kalmar AF, Van Canneyt K, Vereecke H, Absalom A, Caemaert J, Struys MM, Van Roost D. Pressure monitoring during neuroendoscopy: New insights. *Br J Anaesth.* 2011;107:218–24.

17. Wilson TJ, McCoy KE, Al-Holou WN, Molina SL, Smyth MD, Sullivan SE. Comparison of the accuracy and proximal shunt failure rate of freehand placement versus intraoperative guidance in parietooccipital ventricular catheter placement. *Neurosurg Focus.* 2016; 41(3):E10.

18. Wilson TJ, Stetler WR Jr, Al-Holou WN, Sullivan SE. Comparison of the accuracy of ventricular catheter placement using freehand placement, ultrasonic guidance, and stereotactic neuronavigation. *J Neurosurg.* 2013;119:66–70.

19. Phan S, Liao J, Jia F, Maharaj M, Reddy R, Mobbs RJ, Rao PJ, Phan K. Laparotomy vs minimally invasive laparoscopic ventriculoperitoneal shunt placement for hydrocephalus: A systematic review and meta-analysis. *Clin Neurol Neurosurg.* 2016;140:26–32.

20. Figueiredo EG, Deshmukh P, Nakaji P et al. The minipterional craniotomy: Technical description and anatomic assessment. *Neurosurgery.* 2007;61(5 Suppl. 2):256–64, discussion 264.

21. Fischer G, Stadie A, Reisch R et al. The keyhole concept in aneurysm surgery: Results of the past 20 years. *Neurosurgery.* 2011;68(1 Suppl Operative):45–51, discussion 51.

22. Madhugiri VS, Ambekar S, Pandey P, Guthikonda B, Bollam P, Brown B, Ahmed O, Sonig A, Sharma M, Nanda A. The pterional and suprabrow approaches for aneurysm surgery: A systematic review of intraoperative rupture rates in 9488 aneurysms. *World Neurosurg.* 2013;80:836–44.

23. Elias WJ, Durieux ME, Huss D, Frysinger RC. Dexmedetomidine and arousal affect subthalamic neurons. *Mov Disord.* 2008;23:1317–20.

24. Kobayashi K, Imagama S, Ando K et al. Risk factors for delirium after spine surgery in extremely elderly patients aged 80 years or older and review of the literature: Japan Association of Spine Surgeons with Ambition Multicenter Study. *Global Spine J.* 2017;7:560–6.

25. Oichi T, Oshima Y, Chikuda H et al. In-hospital complication rate following microendoscopic versus open lumbar laminectomy: A propensity score-matched analysis. *Spine J.* 2018; 18(10):1815–21.

26. Kim KH. Safe sedation and hypnosis using dexmedetomidine for minimally invasive spine surgery in a prone position. *Korean J Pain.* 2014;27:313–320.

27. Ulutas M, Secer M, Taskapilioglu O et al. General versus epidural anesthesia for lumbar microdiscectomy. *J Clin Neurosci.* 2015;22: 1309–13.

28. Fang G, Ding Z, Song Z. Comparison of the effects of epidural anesthesia and local anesthesia in lumbar transforaminal endoscopic surgery. *Pain Physician.* 2016 19(7):E1001–4.

29. O'Toole JE, Sheikh H, Eichholz KM, Fessler RG, Perez-Cruet MJ. Endoscopic posterior cervical foraminotomy and discectomy. *Neurosurg Clin N Am.* 2006;17:411–22.

30. Newton PO, Marks M, Faro F et al. Use of video-assisted thoracoscopic surgery to reduce perioperative morbidity in scoliosis surgery. *Spine.* 2003;28:S249–54.

31. Lee JM, Lee SK, Lee SJ et al. Comparison of remifentanil with dexmedetomidine for monitored anaesthesia care in elderly patients during vertebroplasty and kyphoplasty. *J Int Med Res.* 2016;44:307–16.

32. Liu L, Cheng S, Lu R et al. Extrapedicular infiltration anesthesia as an improved method of local anesthesia for unipedicular percutaneous vertebroplasty or percutaneous kyphoplasty. *Biomed Res Int.* 2016;2016:5086414.

11

Neurosurgery: Functional neurosurgery

SUPARNA BHARADWAJ, CHRISTINE DY-VALDEZ, AND JASON CHUI

INTRODUCTION

Functional neurosurgery encompasses a variety of surgical interventions that are designed to alter the physiological activity of the central nervous system for functional neurological disorders. Many of these chronic neurological disorders that were once thought to be untreatable are now being successfully managed surgically (Table 11.1). Historically, the surgical principles of functional neurosurgery were to lesion the brain structures, thereby removing abnormal neuronal circuits. Typical examples of these procedures are thalamotomy, pallidotomy, and cingulotomy. However, these lesioning procedures were irreversible and were associated with severe permanent side effects. As such, there was interest in developing a neuromodulation technique that aims to achieve the same functional outcome as lesioning procedures but with less morbidity.

The benefit of deep brain stimulation (DBS) was first described in 1987 as an alternative to the lesioning procedures for Parkinson's disease (1,2). The high reversibility, titratability, and minimal invasiveness of the neuromodulation technique have prompted further investigation in employing neuromodulation to other functional disorders such as dystonia, essential tremors, obsessive-compulsive disorder, epilepsy, and chronic pain. The application of spinal cord and peripheral nerve stimulation in a variety of pain disorders has also been rapidly developed in the same period of time.

Functional neurosurgery in the present day focuses on improving the quality of life of patients who suffer from functional disorders such as neuralgia, movement disorder, and epilepsy surgery. As the name "functional" implies, most patients who present for functional neurosurgery are young to middle-aged who are hoping to return to their normal daily activities following surgery. One exception is patients with movement disorders (e.g., Parkinson's disease) who typically present in an older age group. This chapter discusses the nuances and practical issues of anesthesia for DBS surgery in geriatric patients.

DEEP BRAIN STIMULATION SURGERY

The benefits of DBS have been demonstrated in major clinical trials (3–6) and it has been shown to improve motor function, reduce the side effects of antiparkinsonian medication in patients with advanced Parkinson's disease, as well as produce persistent tremor suppression in patients with essential tremor. At present, DBS is US Food and

Table 11.1 Diseases being treated with functional neurosurgery

Functional neurosurgery has a role for the following diseases:
- Movement disorders
  - Parkinson's disease, essential tremor, dystonia, Tourette syndrome, and hemifacial spasm
  - Spasticity of cerebral origin (multiple sclerosis and spinal cord injury)
- Pain disorders
  - Chronic pain from neuropathic injuries or diseases, as well as malignant causes
  - Trigeminal neuralgia, post-herpetic neuralgia, and nerve injuries
- Epilepsy
- Neuropsychiatric conditions, including obsessive-compulsive disorder and depression

Drug Administration (FDA)-approved for medically refractory Parkinson's disease and essential tremor. The FDA also approved DBS as a humanitarian treatment for primary generalized and segmental dystonia (2003) and obsessive-compulsive disorder (2009). It has also been used off-label for chronic pain, post-traumatic stress disorder (PTSD), refractory epilepsy, and major depression. Other indications for use such as Alzheimer's disease (7), multiple sclerosis (8), minimally conscious or vegetative states (9), and traumatic brain injury are currently under investigation.

The mechanism of DBS is unknown. One postulated hypothesis is that the high-frequency stimulation, typically >100 Hz, to the target nuclei causes cellular hyperpolarization and hence inhibition of its neuronal activity (the so-called "neuronal jamming" phenomenon) (10). This inhibition of firing of the stimulated nucleus results in a simultaneous activation of surrounding fiber pathways and hence a complex modulation in the entire basal ganglia thalamocortical network. This results in improved sensorimotor processing and reduced disease symptoms (2).

The target sites for stimulation depend on the underlying functional disorder and the patient's symptoms. High frequency stimulation of the ventrointermediate nuclei (VIM) of the thalamus produces an effect similar to that of a thalamotomy and is used for patients with essential tremor. In patients with Parkinson's disease, the usual anatomical targets are either subthalamic nuclei (STN) or globus pallidus pars internal (GPi) and the aim is to relieve motor symptoms such as rigidity, bradykinesia, akinesia, and tremor. GPi is also a target for primary generalized dystonia. Other less common target sites for stimulation include the nucleus accumbens for obsessive-compulsive disorder and depression, the posterior thalamic region or periaqueductal gray region for incessant pain, and the anterior thalamic nucleus for epilepsy.

The DBS system consists of three components: the implanted pulse generator (IPG), the lead, and an extension. The IPG is a battery-powered neurostimulator encased in a titanium housing. The lead is a coiled wire insulated in polyurethane with four platinum-iridium electrodes and is placed in one or two different nuclei of the brain. The lead is connected to the IPG by an extension, which is an insulated wire that runs subcutaneously from the head, behind the ear to the IPG, down the side of the neck, to the infraclavicular fossa (or the abdomen in some cases). The stimulation setting of the IPG can be calibrated against the patient's symptom control and side effects. The recent generation of the DBS system has a remote control that allows the patient to turn off the IPG by themselves. The pulse generator's battery usually lasts between 2 and 5 years depending on the stimulation setting.

Patient selection and preparation for DBS

Preoperative evaluation begins with a meticulous patient selection process. The majority of DBS failure is associated with improper patient selection. A multidisciplinary approach including a neurosurgeon, neurologist, and neuropsychiatrist is usually involved to enable an individualized assessment.

The preoperative assessments involve an "off/on" evaluation and a neuropsychological evaluation. During an "off/on" evaluation, a Unified Parkinson's Disease Rating Scale (UPDRS) is used to quantify the severity of parkinsonian symptoms (11). The potential DBS candidate is first evaluated for his UPDRS score 12 hours after stopping his dopaminergic medications (i.e., in the "off" state).

After that, the patient is challenged by a supra-threshold dose of dopaminergic medications (e.g., 200 mg of levodopa or apomorphine), and then reevaluated for the UPDRS score in this "on" state. An optimal surgical candidate should demonstrate at least a 30% improvement in the motor part (Part III) of the UPDRS score, as a positive levodopa response has been considered to be one of the strongest predictors of successful surgical outcomes in DBS for parkinsonian patients (12).

The neuropsychological evaluation is performed in the medication "on" state to evaluate the emotional and cognitive well-being of the patient before the surgery. Patients with a significant cognitive decline (e.g., dementia) often perform poorly after the surgery. In general, patients with dementia who are taking acetylcholinesterase inhibitors and/or memantine are considered to be inappropriate candidates for the DBS procedure. Patients with untreated major depression or anxiety are at risk for poor psychosocial adjustment after the DBS procedure (13).

During preoperative preparation, it is also important to convey to the patient that DBS is not a curative procedure. After the DBS procedure, most patients usually only achieve a similar degree of symptomatic relief to that produced by antiparkinsonian medication. The main benefit of the DBS procedure is to reduce the side effects of antiparkinsonian medication (3–6). The degree to which preoperative expectations are met as well as subjective outcomes of the procedure (13) have been shown to correlate better with patient satisfaction than quantitative improvement in symptom scores (14).

Before the surgery, all patients are required to have a cranial MRI for surgical planning. Anesthesiology is occasionally consulted if the patient fails to complete the preoperative imaging because of significant fluctuating motor symptoms. A low-dose intravenous sedation (e.g., propofol or midazolam) is usually sufficient to abolish the dyskinesia or rigidity that interferes with MRI image acquisition. General anesthesia is seldom required.

Surgical technique of DBS

DBS surgery is best performed by an experienced team with specific expertise in stereotactic and functional neurosurgery. This surgical team usually consists of a neurosurgeon, a neurophysiologist, and a neuroanesthesiologist. DBS surgery involves two stages:

1. Insertion of the electrodes into the deep brain nuclei
2. Internalization of the leads and implantation of the programmable impulse generator

STAGE 1: INSERTION OF THE ELECTRODES INTO THE DEEP BRAIN NUCLEI

In the past few decades, two main approaches have been developed for DBS electrode placement. The first is based on the neurophysiological localization. It typically includes the use of frame-based imaging to visualize brain structures and establish coordinates, microelectrode recordings (MER) and macrostimulation testing in an awake patient. The second method relies completely on real-time interventional MRI (iMRI) guidance for deep brain nuclei localization. This method avoids the intraoperative awake testing/neurophysiological recordings and permits the use of general anesthesia. Although a randomized controlled study has yet to be performed, several cohort studies of iMRI techniques reported comparable efficacy with each neurophysiological technique.

Neurophysiological localization

All patients require a preoperative MRI for surgical planning. This surgical planning is to determine the electrode trajectories based on the patient's anatomy to avoid vessel injury, entry to ventricles, and damage to eloquent brain structures. On the date of surgery, the surgery starts with placement of a rigid head frame, followed by a computed tomography (CT) to establish external triplanar reference coordinates by fusion with the previously acquired preoperative MRI images. Different types of head frames can be used, such as the Cosman-Roberts-Wells frame or the Leksell frame. The choice is driven mainly by the surgeon's preference. Importantly, all these frames limit access to the patient's airway and often result in unique airway challenges for anesthesiologists.

In the operating room, the patient is usually positioned in a semi-sitting position with the stereotactic frame fixed to the operating table. A burr hole is created to allow for electrode insertion. The electrode is inserted to a depth 10–15 mm from the target site. To localize the target deep brain nuclei, an MER technique (i.e., record and amplify the activity of individual neuron cells via the microelectrode) is used. It is typically performed by simultaneously advancing of the microelectrode in 0.25–0.5 mm steps along its trajectory toward the target nuclei while spontaneous neuronal discharges are intermittently recorded. The variations in differing spontaneous deep brain nuclei firing rates and movement-related changes in firing rates are used to characterize the specific brain target (e.g., STN typically has a high-frequency burst pattern). The microelectrode is advanced until no STN activity is seen and the substantia nigra pars reticulata (SNr) activity appears.

The next step is macrostimulation, which can be performed with the same electrodes as those used for MER. While the stimulation is applied, the neurosurgeon performs a physical examination to assess the improvement of cardinal symptoms (e.g., hypokinesia and rigidity) and occurrence of side effects that are due to the stimulation of surrounding structures. Once a satisfactory effect is achieved, a final electrode is implanted under fluoroscopy guidance to replace the microelectrode. The final electrode is secured and the wound is closed. A contralateral DBS lead can be repeated in a similar fashion. A postoperative CT can confirm the position of electrodes and rule out intracerebral hemorrhage.

The neurophysiologic localization technique allows electrode adjustment based on physiology and symptomatology and confirms the effect of DBS in vivo to ensure that implantation is within the motor territories of the intended brain nuclei. However, this technique is time consuming, technically demanding, and often results in multiple electrode adjustment/penetration. Interestingly, a recent study comparing the data of over 28,000 DBS patients from the Centers for Medicare and Medicaid Services (CMS) and the National Surgical Quality Improvement Program (NSQIP) between 2004 and 2013 reported 15.2%–34% rates of revision and removal of the DBS system, in which 48.5% of cases were due to improper targeting or lack of therapeutic effect (15).

Real-time interventional MRI-guided technique

This new approach for implanting DBS electrodes is entirely based on real-time iMRI guidance using a skull-mounted device (SmartFrame; MRI Interventions, Irvine, CA) and a software platform (ClearPoint; MRI Interventions). Typically, the patient is placed under general anesthesia followed by initial MRI imaging for planning and placement of a skull-mounted device. Afterward, the surgeon will determine the target coordinates and align the trajectories of these electrodes using the ClearPoint system. The electrodes are inserted under iMRI navigation.

The MRI unit and the operating room are usually designed to be separated by a sliding door, and the MR machine is accessible to the operating room via a robotic arm attached to the ceiling. Conversely, some surgical centers have a different setup that requires them to transfer the anesthetized patient into the MRI suite for the iMRI. After obtaining MRI images that confirm compliance with the preplanned trajectory, the electrodes were inserted into the target nuclei at an appropriate depth.

Because this iMRI-guided technique avoids the use of a stereotactic head frame in awake patients and does not require the tedious MER or macrostimulation procedure, it is very useful for pediatric patients or patients with severe movement disorders who might not be able to lie still on the operating table. Patients are also not required to discontinue their preoperative antiparkinsonian medication for intraoperative testing. In addition, as the planning, insertion, and confirmation of lead placement takes place in a single procedure, it has a potential benefit of minimizing error from "brain shift" due to cerebrospinal fluid loss during burr hole creation. The intraoperative imaging also allows visual confirmation of electrode positions and early detection of intraoperative complications (e.g., intracerebral hemorrhage) and reduces the number of attempts required for successful electrode placement. Thus far, the initial experience of this iMRI technique is very favorable. The clinical outcomes are comparable to the traditional neurophysiological localization technique, and 98% of patients achieve clinically acceptable placement with a single brain penetration (average accuracy of 0.6–0.8 mm) (16–18).

STAGE II: LEAD AND PULSE GENERATOR INTERNALIZATION

After the electrodes are successfully placed and tested, the stage II procedure includes tunneling the electrodes from the scalp via the side of the neck to an infraclavicular area or abdomen, to be connected to the impulse generator. As with most tunneling procedures, the stage II procedure can be highly stimulating. There is no requirement for the patient to remain awake, and no need for the headframe. After the headframe is removed, general anesthesia can be induced in the usual fashion using either laryngeal mask airway (LMA) or endotracheal intubation, and most patients can be maintained using an inhalational agent.

The stage I and II procedures can be completed on the same day or on two separate occasions (usually 3–14 days apart). The main advantage of the delayed stage II procedure is that time is allowed to better test the beneficial effect of the DBS, since the "microlesion" effect (that caused by the electrode placement) could cause surrounding edema that could mask the patient's symptoms and bias the assessment. A postoperative CT or MRI is usually performed to confirm the anatomical placement of the DBS system and to exclude complications such as intracranial hemorrhage and pneumocephalus.

ANESTHETIC MANAGEMENT OF DBS

Anesthetic evaluation

The anesthetic considerations for patients undergoing DBS procedures are broadly divided into disease-related concerns and procedure-related concerns (Table 11.2). The largely geriatric patient population in DBS procedures also increases the risk of concurrent medical comorbidities, such as hypertension, diabetes, and coronary and cerebral vascular disease.

Patients with Parkinson's disease are an increased risk of aspiration because of the abnormal pharyngeal muscle dysfunction and pooling of saliva from impaired swallowing. Rigidity, bradykinesia, or dyskinesia of the respiratory muscles result in an obstructive lung disease pattern in one-third of patients. Parkinson's disease and antiparkinsonian medication can also cause cardiosympathetic denervation, reduced circulating epinephrine, and

Table 11.2 Anesthetic consideration for DBS

Disease-related considerations

- *Parkinson's disease*
  - *Respiratory system*: Obstructive lung disease pattern (1/3 of patients), pharyngeal muscle dysfunction that increases the risk of aspiration
  - *Autonomic dysfunction*: Orthostatic hypotension
  - *Cardiovascular instability*: Cardiac arrhythmia, hypertension
  - *Adverse effects of antiparkinsonian medication*: Abnormal glucose metabolism (Selegiline), hypotension, orthostatic hypotension, and potential interaction with anesthetic agents
  - Tremor and muscle rigidity, especially during the "off" state, interfere with positioning
  - *Speech impairment and confusion*: Impair cooperation during the surgery
- *Essential tremors*: Bradycardia due to beta-blocker administration
- *Dystonia*
  - Increased risk of hemodynamic instability, laryngospasm, spasmodic dysphonia
  - Commonly associated with neurodegenerative disorders and cerebral palsy—poor communication, growth retardation
- *Epilepsy*: Recurrent seizures, concurrent developmental delay, multiple anti-epileptic medications with potential drug interactions

Surgery-related considerations

- The use of stereotactic head frame limits the access to the airway
- Semi-sitting position increases the risk of venous air embolism
- Lengthy procedure may lead to fatigue and discomfort
- Anesthetic agents easily interfere with microelectrode recordings
- Macrostimulation testing requires an awake and cooperative patient
- Perioperative complications are frequent (e.g., intracranial hemorrhage, stroke, seizures, hypertension, decreased level of consciousness, nausea and vomiting, airway obstruction, respiratory distress)

postganglionic hypersensitivity. Clinically, it often manifests as orthostatic hypotension, autonomic dysfunction, and cardiac arrhythmias. Significant tremors and muscle rigidity during the "off" medication state may interfere with positioning, patient comfort, and intraoperative monitoring. Speech impairment and cognitive impairment may decrease the cooperation during macrostimulation testing.

One major assessment is to determine whether the patient can tolerate the stage I procedure with minimal to no sedation. Intraoperative anxiety may precipitate hypertension, which increases the risk of intracranial hemorrhage (19). Presenting a detailed and thorough description of the procedure to the patient often helps to manage expectations and may alleviate their anxiety. Patients with chronic pain or opioid tolerance may require increased doses of sedatives during the procedure and often increase the complexity of perioperative management.

As airway access is usually restricted in the presence of the stereotactic head frame, a comprehensive airway assessment is required to plan for a multi-stage airway management strategy. An anticipated difficult airway mandates careful administration of sedatives to avoid iatrogenic airway obstruction.

The decision to continue antiparkinsonian medication should be discussed with the neurosurgical team. Most patients are required to stop their usual medication on the morning of the surgery to elicit an "off-medication" state for intraoperative MER and macrostimulation testing. However, in some cases the transient discontinuation of medication might significantly exacerbate the motor symptoms to an extent that precludes safe conduct of the procedure. Therefore, in selected patients it is prudent to continue with a reduced dose of antiparkinsonian medication on the morning of the surgery. Long-acting benzodiazepines and other sedatives (e.g., lorazepam) should be avoided because of the potential interference with the MER and macrostimulation. It is common practice to withhold angiotensin-converting enzyme inhibitors and angiotensin II receptor blockers on the day of the procedure to avoid intraoperative hypotension. This practice, however, was found to be a predictor of increased antihypertensive used intraoperatively (20).

Anesthetic techniques for DBS stage I

Anesthetic techniques for the stage I procedure include monitored anesthesia care (MAC), conscious sedation, and general anesthesia. Most neurosurgical centers standardize their anesthetic techniques (including the choice of the anesthetic drugs) for the DBS procedure. In our institute, we prefer the conscious sedation technique rather than MAC because we found that most patients tolerate the procedure better with sedation, especially during the dissection and closure phases of the procedure; in addition, the presence of an anesthesiologist has greatly facilitated intraoperative crisis management. In our institute, only a minority of patients require general anesthesia due to intolerance of the awake procedure such as severe anxiety, intolerable tremors, dystonia or choreoathetosis in the "off" state, and pediatric patients.

Placement of the stereotactic head frame is usually performed under local/regional anesthetic technique. Scalp block can be accomplished with local anesthetics by blocking the bilateral auriculotemporal, zygomaticotemporal, supraorbital, supratrochlear, occipital, and greater occipital nerves. Subcutaneous infiltration with local anesthetics is used at the pin sites and at the site of incision(s) for the burr hole(s) for electrode insertion. Scalp blocks (supraorbital and greater occipital nerve blocks) have been shown to be less painful than subcutaneous infiltration (21). The local anesthetics frequently used include bupivacaine, ropivacaine, and lidocaine with and without epinephrine. Local anesthetic toxicity resulting in seizures and respiratory and cardiac arrest during DBS procedure has been reported. If the procedure is long, additional infiltration may be required for closure.

MONITORING AND POSITIONING

Intraoperatively, standard monitoring includes aspects such as oxygen saturation, electrocardiogram, noninvasive arterial blood pressure, and end-tidal CO_2. Supplemental oxygen is usually given via nasal prongs with a side port for end-tidal CO_2 monitoring. Patients with severe movement disorders and spasticity might cause difficulty in monitoring. Noninvasive blood pressure monitoring may be erroneous, as pulse oximeter waveforms and values may be unreliable in the presence of spasticity or tremors. Invasive blood pressure monitoring is routinely used in our institute because intraoperative hypertension is associated with intraoperative intracranial hemorrhage (19).

Vigilant monitoring and maintenance of optimal intraoperative blood pressure are vital.

Appropriate positioning is one of the key steps to ensure patient comfort and cooperation. The head and neck are positioned with some degree of flexion at the lower cervical spine and extension at the atlanto-occipital joint to make the airway patent. The legs are slightly flexed and supported below the knees. The use of clear plastic drapes allows direct visualization from the surgical field to the patient (Figure 11.1).

AIRWAY MANAGEMENT

As direct laryngoscopy is often challenging in patients with a stereotactic frame in a semi-sitting position, an airway management plan should be formulated and the ease of initiating a rescue airway intervention (e.g., bag-mask ventilation or insertion of an LMA) should be assessed at the beginning of the procedure. In our institute, we routinely position the anterior bar front curved piece with its convex side up, two fingerbreadths away from the nasal bridge (Figure 11.2). We found that this frame position allows easy bag-mask ventilation and direct laryngoscopy. A recent mannequin study found that the use of LMA and video laryngoscopy achieved higher successful first attempts than direct laryngoscopy (97% for both vs. 93%) in the setting of a stereotactic head frame. The average time of securing the airway device was faster for LMA than intubation with video laryngoscopy (35 sec vs. 55 sec) (22). However, in some cases the airway can only be secured with fiberoptic intubation or after removing the stereotactic frame emergently.

Adequate pain control, attention to temperature control, and avoidance of excessive fluid administration (bladder distension) are also important to

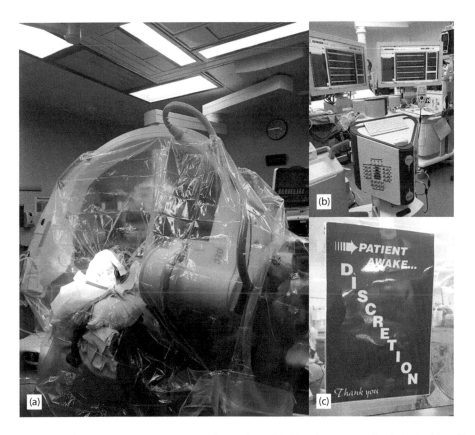

Figure 11.1 A typical operating room setup and position of DBS using neurophysiological localization technique. (a) Transparent drapes are used to allow direct visualization of the patient from the surgical field. Fluoroscopy is used to confirm the final placement of the DBS electrodes. (b) A neurophysiological system used for advancing the microelectrode, microelectrode recording, and macrostimulation. (c) A warning sign of awake patient.

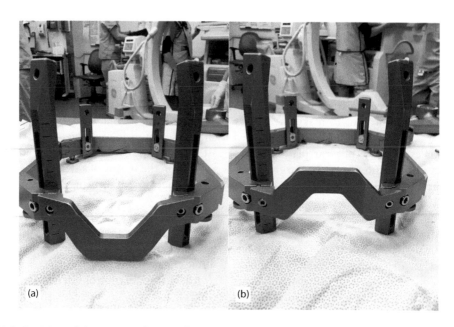

Figure 11.2 Position of the anterior bar on the Leksell frame (a) shows the anterior bar is positioned in a convex side-down position. This anterior bar position usually obstructs the mask ventilation and direct laryngoscopy. (b) Shows the anterior bar is positioned in a convex side-up position. The anterior bar should be at least two finger breadths above the nasal bridge of the patient.

ensure patient comfort. During macrostimulation testing, limb positions are dynamic. One must balance between securing lines and monitors while minimizing restraints of attached cables, as well as thermoregulation with exposed extremities. Patients should be encouraged to void before surgery. In our institution, we routinely use a sheath/condom catheter for patient comfort. Good patient communication, repeated reassurance, and verbal encouragement during the procedure is important in maintaining motivation.

Pharmacological considerations in the DBS procedure

The main anesthetic goal for the implantation of DBS electrodes is to ensure patient comfort while avoiding all drugs that interfere with MER and macrostimulation. The anesthetic drug effects on the various target nuclei (STN vs GPi) differ and are explained by their effect on the GABA receptors. The role of GABA in the pathophysiology of tremor is well described in the neurology literature, especially in the context of essential tremor (23). The anti-tremor effect of GABA agonists in Parkinson's disease has long been observed (24). It was postulated that propofol may act through

the $GABA_A$ receptor in the extra-thalamic tremor pathway (25). There has been more success obtaining MERs from the STN nuclei during anesthesia than from other nuclei such as the GPi (26). GPi neurons are known to receive higher GABA input when compared to STN neurons. Thus, GPi are more readily suppressed by anesthetic drugs, and the MER for the GPi target is often more technically challenging. The anesthetic effects on the activity of VIM nuclei are not clear.

Propofol is one of the most commonly used sedative agents in DBS. Propofol is generally administrated at a rate of 25–50 µg/kg/min (27) or at a target-controlled infusion serum level of 0.35 µg/mL (28), with or without supplementary remifentanil or fentanyl. Propofol is commonly used in most institutes for DBS because it provides titratable sedation and is a familiar agent. However, propofol infusions at 50 µg/kg/min resulted in significantly decreased STN neuronal activity (−23.2%). This suppressive effect was transient, and all STN neuronal activity returned to normal shortly after cessation (27). It is generally recommended to stop propofol infusion 20–30 minutes before the MER. Interestingly, this reversible suppressive effect of propofol can be used to abolish severe tremor and dyskinesia in patients who cannot lie still or who have severe tremor artifacts on the MER. A very low dose of propofol infusion at 20 μg/kg/min is usually sufficient to abolish the tremor and avoid spurious movement while maintaining deep brain nuclei activities on the MER (42). Although most anesthesiologists are familiar with the use of propofol, over-sedation with propofol is frequently seen. The pharmacokinetic property of propofol in patients with Parkinson's disease is altered compared with the general population (28). In clinical practice, there are concerns regarding either the residual suppressive effect of propofol on MER or prolonging the surgery because of a long waiting time to ensure the suppressive effect completely wears off.

Dexmedetomidine has emerged as an attractive alternative for DBS procedures. It has the desirable properties of having a minimal suppressive effect on MER at low doses and a minimal risk of respiratory depression. A low-dose dexmedetomidine infusion at 0.3–0.6 μg/kg/h has been successfully used during DBS in parkinsonian patients with minimal interference with MER and macrostimulation (29,30). A retrospective study of 19 patients found that dexmedetomidine provided better patient satisfaction and reduced the use of intraoperative antihypertensives compared to the absence of anesthetics during DBS (monitored anesthetic care) (29), while another retrospective study showed that the addition of dexmedetomidine to propofol did not reduce the use of antihypertensives (32). Dexmedetomidine has become the sedative agent of choice in many institutes because of its perceived benefits over other agents (31), although the evidence is limited and the number of patients in the studies are small.

Opioids such as fentanyl or remifentanil are frequently used because of their minimal suppressive effects on deep brain nuclei, though high infusion rates of opioids can worsen muscle rigidity and cause respiratory depression. Benzodiazepines should be avoided because of the prolonged suppressive effect on MER and respiratory depression.

In our institute, we do not have a standardized protocol for the sedatives used during DBS. The choice of sedative agent and dosing are largely based on the discretion of the attending anesthesiologist and upon assessment of the individual patient and his/her experience with the agent. However, regardless of the sedative agents chosen,

we routinely cease infusion of sedatives 20–30 minutes before the MER. We have recently published a cohort study (32) comparing the outcome differences between propofol-based, dexmedetomidine-based, and opioid-based sedative regimens in DBS for patients with Parkinson's disease. In our cohort, the choice of sedative agents was not associated with poor surgical outcomes, and they did not prolong the duration of MER or stage I surgery. Thus, we recommend that the choice of anesthetic agents be dictated by the anesthesiologist according to patient factors (e.g., comorbidities), his/her experience with the agent, and local practices.

The depth of anesthesia can be monitored by processed electroencephalography to avoid over-sedation during propofol infusion. Intact STN activities remained equivalent to the awake state in MER if the dose of propofol infusion was titrated to a Bispectral Index (BIS) of >80 (33). However, a small prospective study failed to demonstrate the clinical benefit of faster arousal and cardiopulmonary stability in comparing BIS-guided sedation with standard management (34).

The anesthetic requirement for macrostimulation is to provide an awake and cooperative patient for assessing the patient's symptoms. In our practice, as we routinely discontinue sedative infusion 20–30 minutes before the MER, most patients are completely ready for physical examination at the time of macrostimulation. General anesthesia normally interferes with evaluation of DBS by abolishing clinical symptoms such as tremors and rigidity. Paresthesia or abnormal motor activity associated with stimulation of adjacent structures (internal capsule and medial lemniscus) cannot be assessed properly during general anesthesia.

General anesthesia

General anesthesia for DBS surgery is an important alternative for patients who cannot tolerate conscious sedation due to excessive fear, anxiety, or severe "off-medication" effects. Intraoperative MER is often more challenging under general anesthesia because the suppressive effects of high-dose anesthetics can result in a poorly defined neuronal firing pattern on the MER. Experience in intraoperative MER under general anesthesia is sparse, and neuronal firing patterns are not well characterized.

A few case series have reported successful MER and motor outcomes in parkinsonian patients undergoing STN-DBS using MER localization under general anesthesia (propofol or volatile anesthetics). These case series reported a successful MER under controlled general anesthesia and the MER were able to detect bursting STN patterns in all study cases. Though one of the typical features of STN (widening of background noise baseline in MER) were lost during general anesthesia, the overall motor outcomes and symptom improvement were comparable between general anesthesia and historical controlled data under local anesthesia. It appears that anesthetic suppression is a genuine phenomenon, but under controlled general anesthesia, MER and patient outcomes showed no clinical differences based on non-randomized data (42).

The anesthetic considerations for general anesthesia are similar to the previous description for conscious sedation. The key differences are that (i) intubation is usually performed before the placement of the stereotactic headframe and imaging, and (ii) a controlled light general anesthesia is given during the period of MER. This is often achieved with a combination of low-dose inhalation anesthetic (<0.5 MAC), opioid (such as remifentanil infusion at 0.03–0.06 µg/kg/min), and propofol infusion at 50–75 µg/kg/min. A small case series of five patients reported no changes in MER activities between local anesthesia and general anesthesia using remifentanil at 0.25–1 µg/kg/min and ketamine infusion at 0.5–3 mg/kg/h in the same patient (35). Because of the deliberate reduction of anesthetics, we always inform our patient about the possibility of awareness in the preoperative evaluation. However, there are increasing numbers of neurosurgical centers equipped with iMRI guidance capacity. The need for using controlled general anesthesia for neurophysiological guidance may be less likely to be encountered.

PERIOPERATIVE COMPLICATIONS IN DBS

Intraoperative complications are common in DBS and were reported to occur in 12%–16% of patients (36,37). The incidence of common anesthetic and surgical intraprocedural complications are listed in Table 11.3.

Table 11.3 Perioperative complications of DBS

Complications	Incidence (%)
Agitation and confusion	2.8–5.8
Airway obstruction	0.03–1.1
Respiratory distress	0.02–1.1
Hypertension	3.9–0.4
Nausea and vomiting	0.02–1.7
Seizures	0.8–4.5
Intracranial hemorrhage	0.8–2.8

Source: Chui J et al. *Can J Neurol Sci.* 2017;110:1–8; Venkatraghavan L et al. *J Neurosurg Anesthesiol.* 2006;18(1):64–7; Khatib R et al. *J Neurosurg Anesthesiol.* 2008;20(1):36–40.

Airway and respiratory complications

Airway compromise can occur due to over-sedation or secondary to other complications such as seizures or intracranial hemorrhage. Airway access is usually limited by the stereotactic head frame. It is also commonly observed that many patients have a gradual downward shift of the body during the surgery, resulting in airway obstruction or an awkward posture that might further complicate airway management. Intraoperative arterial desaturation or respiratory failure occurs in 1.6%–2.2% of patients (36,37). Patients with Parkinson's disease are often associated with an obstructive ventilatory pattern and coexisting pulmonary comorbidities secondary to upper airway dysfunction such as retained secretion, atelectasis, or lung infection, and hence have less respiratory reserves. In the event of acute desaturation or acute upper airway obstruction, we should aim to rapidly resume ventilation and avoid excessive spurious movement that might result in brain injury. It is important to communicate with the surgeon during the resuscitation to decide whether there is a need to remove the intracranial electrodes and stereotactic headframe, and to place the patient in a supine position for airway management. A suggested algorithm is summarized in Figure 11.3.

Cardiovascular complications

Hypertension is a common intraoperative complication. In our own cohort, the incidence of this complication was up to 37% (defined as SBP > 160 mmHg) (32). Intraoperative hypertension has been shown

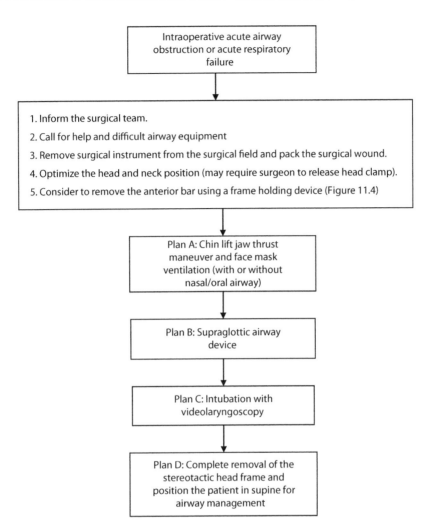

Figure 11.3 A suggested algorithm of intraoperative airway management during DBS.
Note: Supraglottic airway device and stereotactic frame disassembly kit (e.g., screw drive) should be available in the operating room in all cases.

to be associated with intracerebral hemorrhages. A retrospective study found intraoperative hypertensive patients (defined as SBP > 160/90 mmHg) were 11.7 times more likely than normotensive patients to experience intracranial hemorrhage during DBS (10.7% vs. 0.9%, respectively; p = 0.01) (38). Most hypertensive patients can be managed with repeated bolus or infusion of labetalol and/or hydralazine. An infusion of more potent medication such as nitroglycerine and sodium nitroprusside is seldom required. Of interest, transient MER suppression has been seen with metoprolol boluses of blood pressure control in a few cases (43). Perioperative hemodynamic management should take into account the possibility of autonomic dysfunction in patients with Parkinson's disease. Coronary vasospasm has also been reported during DBS (39).

Venous air embolism

The semi-sitting position during DBS increases the risk of venous air embolism, especially in dehydrated patients. The incidence of venous air embolism during DBS was reported around 4.5%. Most air embolisms occur immediately after burr hole creation. It often presents with sudden vigorous coughing, followed by tachycardia, tachypnea, chest discomfort, abrupt change in mental status,

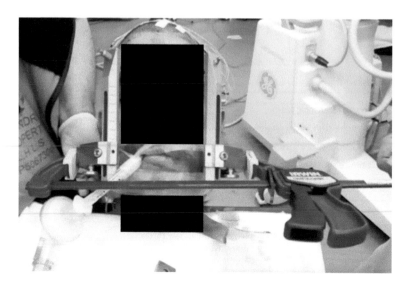

Figure 11.4 A patient presented with acute airway obstruction during surgery. The anterior bar was removed while the Leksell frame was stabilized using a frame-holding device. (Courtesy: The patient was consented for photography for teaching and educational purposes.)

arterial desaturation, and hypotension. Therefore, we usually irrigate the surgical wound (site of burr hole) with copious volumes of saline and apply bone wax or fibrin glue immediately after burr hole creation. It is also recommended to avoid hypovolemia and to caution about the occurrence of venous air embolism in patients with repeated coughing during the procedure (40,41).

Surgical complications

Common surgically related intraoperative complications include seizure, electrode misplacement, intracranial hemorrhage, and akinetic mutism. Seizure occurs in 0.8%–8% of DBS procedures, most commonly during macrostimulation. Most seizures are focal and self-limited after stopping the macrostimulation; only a few patients may require a small bolus of midazolam or propofol to abolish the seizure activity. Intracranial hemorrhage was reported in 0.8%–2.8% of patients (32,36). As the location of electrode insertion is in close proximity to deep-seated eloquent structures (e.g., internal capsule), the feasibility of a rescue surgical intervention is usually limited, and the prognosis is usually unsatisfactory.

CONCLUSION

DBS is an effective, well-established treatment for movement disorders but with considerable intraoperative complications. It is important for anesthesiologists to understand the anesthetic considerations of this increasingly popular procedure. The risks associated with this procedure increase for geriatric patients.

REFERENCES

1. Benabid AL, Pollak P, Louveau A, Henry S, de Rougemont J. Combined (thalamotomy and stimulation) stereotactic surgery of the VIM thalamic nucleus for bilateral Parkinson disease. *Appl Neurophysiol*. 1987;50(1–6): 344–6.
2. Miocinovic S, Somayajula S, Chitnis S, Vitek JL. History, applications, and mechanisms of deep brain stimulation. *JAMA Neurol*. 2013; 70(2):163–71.
3. Deuschl G, Schade-Brittinger C, Krack P et al. A randomized trial of deep-brain stimulation for Parkinson's disease. *N Engl J Med*. 2006; 355(9):896–908.
4. Okun MS, Gallo BV, Mandybur G et al. Subthalamic deep brain stimulation with a constant-current device in Parkinson's disease: An open-label randomised controlled trial. *Lancet Neurol*. 2012;11(2):140–9.
5. Weaver FM, Follett K, Stern M et al. Bilateral deep brain stimulation vs best medical therapy for patients with advanced Parkinson

disease: A randomized controlled trial. *JAMA.* 2009;301(1):63–73.

6. Varma TRK, Fox SH, Eldridge PR et al. Deep brain stimulation of the subthalamic nucleus: Effectiveness in advanced Parkinson's disease patients previously reliant on apomorphine. *J Neurol Neurosurg Psychiatry.* 2003; 74(2):170–4.

7. Laxton AW, Stone S, Lozano AM. The neurosurgical treatment of Alzheimer's disease: A review. *Stereotact Funct Neurosurg.* 2014; 92(5):269–81.

8. Schulder M, Sernas T, Mahalick D, Adler R, Cook S. Thalamic stimulation in patients with multiple sclerosis. *Stereotact Funct Neurosurg.* 1999;72(2–4):196–201.

9. Yamamoto T, Katayama Y, Kobayashi K, Oshima H, Fukaya C, Tsubokawa T. Deep brain stimulation for the treatment of vegetative state. *Eur J Neurosci.* 2010;32(7):1145–51.

10. Benabid AL, Pollak P, Gervason C et al. Long-term suppression of tremor by chronic stimulation of the ventral intermediate thalamic nucleus. *Lancet.* 1991;337(8738):403–6.

11. Movement Disorder Society Task Force on Rating Scales for Parkinson's Disease. The Unified Parkinson's Disease Rating Scale (UPDRS): Status and recommendations. *Mov Disord.* 2003;18(7):738–50.

12. Rodriguez RL, Fernandez HH, Haq I, Okun MS. Pearls in patient selection for deep brain stimulation. *Neurologist.* 2007;13(5):253–60.

13. Maier F, Lewis CJ, Horstkoetter N et al. Patients' expectations of deep brain stimulation, and subjective perceived outcome related to clinical measures in Parkinson's disease: A mixed-method approach. *J Neurol Neurosurg Psychiatry.* 2013;84(11):1273–81.

14. Hasegawa H, Samuel M, Douiri A, Ashkan K. Patients' expectations in subthalamic nucleus deep brain stimulation surgery for Parkinson disease. *World Neurosurg.* 2014;82(6):1295–9.e2.

15. Rolston JD, Englot DJ, Starr PA, Larson PS. An unexpectedly high rate of revisions and removals in deep brain stimulation surgery: Analysis of multiple databases. *Parkinsonism Relat Disord.* 2016;33:72–7.

16. Sidiropoulos C, Rammo R, Merker B et al. Intraoperative MRI for deep brain stimulation lead placement in Parkinson's disease: 1 year

motor and neuropsychological outcomes. *J Neurol.* 2016;263(6):1226–31.

17. Ostrem JL, Ziman N, Galifianakis NB et al. Clinical outcomes using ClearPoint interventional MRI for deep brain stimulation lead placement in Parkinson's disease. *J Neurosurg.* 2016;124(4):908–16.

18. Ostrem JL, Galifianakis NB, Markun LC et al. Clinical outcomes of PD patients having bilateral STN DBS using high-field interventional MR-imaging for lead placement. *Clin Neurol Neurosurg.* 2013;115(6):708–12.

19. Xiaowu H, Xiufeng J, Xiaoping Z et al. Risks of intracranial hemorrhage in patients with Parkinson's disease receiving deep brain stimulation and ablation. *Parkinsonism Relat Disord.* 2010;16(2):96–100.

20. Rajan S, Deogaonkar M, Kaw R et al. Factors predicting incremental administration of antihypertensive boluses during deep brain stimulator placement for Parkinson's disease. *J Clin Neurosci.* 2014;21(10):1790–5.

21. Watson R, Leslie K. Nerve blocks versus subcutaneous infiltration for stereotactic frame placement. *Anesth Analg.* 2001;92(2):424–7.

22. Brockerville M, Unger Z, Rowland NC, Sammartino F, Manninen PH, Venkatraghavan L. Airway management with a stereotactic headframe in situ-a mannequin study. *J Neurosurg Anesthesiol.* 2018;30(1):44–8.

23. Deuschl G, Raethjen J, Hellriegel H, Elble R. Treatment of patients with essential tremor. *Lancet Neurol.* 2011;10(2):148–61.

24. Anderson BJ, Marks PV, Futter ME. Propofol–contrasting effects in movement disorders. *Br J Neurosurg.* 1994;8(3):387–8.

25. Hall SD, Prokic EJ, McAllister CJ et al. GABA-mediated changes in inter-hemispheric beta frequency activity in early-stage Parkinson's disease. *Neuroscience.* 2014;281:68–76.

26. Benarroch EE. Subthalamic nucleus and its connections: Anatomic substrate for the network effects of deep brain stimulation. *Neurology.* 2008;70(21):1991–5.

27. Raz A, Eimerl D, Zaidel A, Bergman H, Israel Z. Propofol decreases neuronal population spiking activity in the subthalamic nucleus of Parkinsonian patients. *Anesth Analg.* 2010; 111(5):1285–9.

28. Fábregas N, Rapado J, Gambús PL et al. Modeling of the sedative and airway

obstruction effects of propofol in patients with Parkinson disease undergoing stereotactic surgery. *Anesthesiology*. 2002;97(6):1378–86.

29. Rozet I, Muangman S, Vavilala MS et al. Clinical experience with dexmedetomidine for implantation of deep brain stimulators in Parkinson's disease. *Anesth Analg*. 2006;103(5):1224–8.

30. Hippard HK, Watcha M, Stocco AJ, Curry D. Preservation of microelectrode recordings with non–GABAergic drugs during deep brain stimulator placement in children. *J Neurosurg Pediatr*. 2014;14(3):279–86.

31. Venkatraghavan L, Luciano M, Manninen P. Review article: Anesthetic management of patients undergoing deep brain stimulator insertion. *Anesth Analg*. 2010;110(4):1138–45.

32. Chui J, Alimiri R, Parrent A, Craen RA. The effects of intraoperative sedation on surgical outcomes of deep brain stimulation surgery. *Can J Neurol Sci*. 2017;110:1–8.

33. Elias WJ, Durieux ME, Huss D, Frysinger RC. Dexmedetomidine and arousal affect subthalamic neurons. *Mov Disord*. 2008;23(9): 1317–20.

34. Schulz U, Keh D, Barner C, Kaisers U, Boemke W. Bispectral index monitoring does not improve anesthesia performance in patients with movement disorders undergoing deep brain stimulating electrode implantation. *Anesth Analg*. 2007;104(6):1481–7, table of contents.

35. Lettieri C, Rinaldo S, Devigili G et al. Deep brain stimulation: Subthalamic nucleus electrophysiological activity in awake and anesthetized patients. *Clin Neurophysiol*. 2012; 123(12):2406–13.

36. Venkatraghavan L, Manninen P, Mak P, Lukitto K, Hodaie M, Lozano A. Anesthesia for functional neurosurgery: Review of complications. *J Neurosurg Anesthesiol*. 2006;18(1):64–7.

37. Khatib R, Ebrahim Z, Rezai A et al. Perioperative events during deep brain stimulation: The experience at Cleveland clinic. *J Neurosurg Anesthesiol*. 2008;20(1):36–40.

38. Gorgulho A, De Salles AAF, Frighetto L, Behnke E. Incidence of hemorrhage associated with electrophysiological studies performed using macroelectrodes and microelectrodes in functional neurosurgery. *J Neurosurg*. 2005;102(5):888–96.

39. Glossop A, Dobbs P. Coronary artery vasospasm during awake deep brain stimulation surgery. *Br J Anaesth*. 2008;101(2):222–4.

40. Suarez S, Ornaque I, Fábregas N, Valero R, Carrero E. Venous air embolism during Parkinson surgery in patients with spontaneous ventilation. *Anesth Analg*. 1999;88(4):793–4.

41. Kumar R, Goyal V, Chauhan RS. Venous air embolism during microelectrode recording in deep brain stimulation surgery in an awake supine patient. *Br J Neurosurg*. 2009;23(4): 446–8.

42. Chui J, Alamri R, Bihari F, Hebb M, Venkatraghavan L. Propofol reduces microelectrode-recording (MER) artifacts caused by Parkinsonian tremor during deep brain stimulation (DBS): A case report. *J Neuroanaesthesiol Crit Care*, 2018;5:21–25

43. Coenen VA, Gielen FL, Castro-Prado F, Abdel Rahman A, Honey CR. Noradrenergic modulation of subthalamic nucleus activity in human: Metoprolol reduces spiking activity in microelectrode recordings during deep brain stimulation surgery for Parkinson's disease. *Acta Neurochir (Wien)*. 2008 Aug;150(8):757–62;

12

Neuromonitoring

LESLIE C. JAMESON AND CLAUDIA F. CLAVIJO

INTRODUCTION

Until recently corrective spine surgery was associated with the treatment of adolescent scoliosis but today, with the increasing geriatric population and advances in surgical techniques, many elderly patients can safely undergo complex axial skeletal and neurosurgical surgery. This change in the population's age distribution means the increased surgical procedures will require more intraoperative neurophysiologic monitoring (IONM) to guide surgical decisions from spinal cord stress to awake intracranial brain mapping (1). The standard studies performed include the summative studies, somatosensory-evoked potentials (SEP), motor-evoked potentials (MEP) and continuous studies, electromyography (EMG), and electroencephalography (EEG). The increase in the elderly population and the number of high-risk surgical interventions needed to maintain their health and mobility is not trivial. In the 1950s, approximately 205 million Americans were older than 60 years of age. By the year 2000, this number increased three times, to approximately 606 million people 60 years and older. Projections suggest that by 2050, the geriatric community will represent approximately 22% of the world population and the individuals over 80 years will be one out of five people (20%) in the over-60 demographic (2,3).

The anesthesiology community must be prepared to manage the progressive changes in physiology, the pathologies and the other particular challenges that this geriatric population presents.

PHYSIOLOGIC CHANGES AND COMMON MEDICAL PATHOLOGIES

Medical disease

> **Tip:** Diabetes mellitus, chronic renal disease, and neurodegenerative disease increase the need for skeletal and neurologic surgery and increase the difficulty in obtaining IONM.

Increase of medical comorbidities is a natural and inevitable process during aging. Consequently, the overall prevalence of chronic diseases increases with every decade of life. According to the American National Council on Aging, 80% of adults 65 years and older (geriatric) have at least one chronic condition, and 68% have two or more chronic conditions (4). Today and in the future, chronic and degenerative diseases including cardiovascular, metabolic, skeletal, and neurodegenerative diseases will dominate

Table 12.1 Common chronic diseases in the elderly and their physiologic impact

Affected systems	Common diseases (prevalence—%)	Effects on the affected organs
Cardiovascular	Hypertension (58%), coronary artery disease (29%), heart failure (14%), peripheral arterial disease (14.5%)	Low perfusion, ischemia, necrosis
Metabolic	Diabetes (27%), Hypercholesterolemia (47%) (5)	Neuropathy (decreased sensation, trauma, amputation) Retinopathy (blindness) Nephropathy
Skeletal	Arthritis (31%)	Inflammation, decreased range of motion, axial instability, falls
Renal	Chronic kidney disease (18%) (6)	Peripheral and autonomic neuropathy, myopathy (decreased sensation, pain, weakness), mineral, bone, and calcific cardiovascular abnormalities (fractures, hypercalcemia, hyperphosphatemia)
Respiratory	COPD (11%)	Limited exercise capacity, deconditioning
Mental and Neurodegenerative	Depression (14%), Alzheimer's and dementia (11%), Parkinson's (0.2%) (1)	Low mobility, uncoordinated gait, falls

Source: Prince MJ et al. Lancet. 2015;385(9967):549–62 (2).
Note: The prevalence and consequences of these diseases in this population has an impact on IONM quality.

(Table 12.1) medical care. These chronic conditions interfere with daily activities and quality of life, some in a very debilitating manner, and diminish the ability to perform IONM. For example, peripheral neuropathy (PN), the most common neuropathic syndrome in diabetes, affects more than 50% of the 472 million diabetic patients globally. Metabolic and vascular factors (prolonged hyperglycemia exposure, cardiovascular comorbidities) are implicated in the development and progression of PN. Loss of nerve fibers as well as microvascular defects in the endoneurial and epineural vessels have been identified in sural nerve biopsies. Common symptoms of PN include sensory loss in a "glove-and-stocking" pattern, pain such as burning, tingling, shooting, or lancing, and paresthesia, decreased proprioception, and decreased sensation to temperature and vibration. Abnormal nerve conduction studies are seen even in early stages. Significant motor deficits can be seen in patients with severe and advanced disease (5). Even with technically optimized IONM, obtaining reliable responses in these patients is challenging.

Chronic kidney disease (CKD) has a prevalence of approximately 15% in developed countries. Patients with CKD frequently have complications of the central and peripheral nervous systems such as stroke, peripheral and autonomic neuropathies, encephalopathy, and cognitive dysfunction (6). The physical disability of CKD is most commonly PN or uremic neuropathy which affects approximately 90% of dialysis patients. Direct damage to the large and small nerve and muscle fibers from uremia is likely the cause of the neuropathy. Recent evidence demonstrated that prolonged hyperkalemia plays a major role in nerve toxicity in a dose-dependent manner. Hyperkalemia produces nerve dysfunction that can be reversed by normalizing potassium levels. Patients with PN report pain and loss of sensation initially in the lower extremities that later progresses to the upper extremities. Motor weakness is seen in advanced stages of PN and in uremic myopathy. While both produce muscle atrophy and weakness, the pattern of distribution is different, with myopathy being more proximal than neuropathy. Autonomic neuropathy is also seen in CKD patients increasing cardiovascular symptoms.

Lack of motor coordination, difficulty walking, and frequent falls are seen often in patients with musculoskeletal, neurological, and metabolic conditions (7). Neurologic tumors, neural degenerative disease, and movement disorders can also require surgical interventions.

Patients with neurologic disease present a challenge for IONM physicians and anesthesiologists during surgical procedures (8). Geriatric patients are often on multiple chronic pain medications including narcotics and antiseizure medications, such as pregabalin and gabapentin. They often have frailty and are at increased risk of perioperative complications due to decreased physiologic reserve. Effective IONM can reduce the risk of neurologic events that will require long-term rehabilitation—time these patients may not have.

Surgical conditions associated with IONM

SPINE

> **Tip:** An unstable spine produces enhanced spinal cord and nerve degeneration. These effects can result in neurologic changes that are associated with failure to be able to obtain IONM.

The spine is not spared the effects of aging. All structures are affected in various degrees and include bone, joints (arthritic inflammation), ligaments, and muscles. The changes are not isolated to one area but include all skeletal components (Table 12.2). Changes in disc height and composition, facet joint structure, canal narrowing

Table 12.2 Common spine and neurosurgical procedures in the geriatric population that may require IONM

Location	Pathology	Interventions

Spine
  Cervical
  Thoracic
  Lumbar
	Degenerative disease
	Structural disease
	  Sacroiliac joint and facet arthropathy
	  Stenosis, spondylolisthesis, spondylolysis
	Metabolic
	  Myelopathy, neuropathy
	Deformity
	  Scoliosis, kyphosis, lordosis, flat back
	Traumatic
	  Fracture, soft tissue damage
	Infections
	  Osteomyelitis, discitis, spinal/epidural
	  abscess, meningitis
	Neoplastic
		Decompression and fusion
		Hardware Instrumentation
		Laminectomy
		Foraminotomy
		Discectomy
		Disc replacement
		Intralaminar implant

Intracranial Disease		
Tumor	Meningioma, pituitary, astrocytoma acoustic neuroma, glioblastoma, medulloblastoma	Biopsy, resection Embolization of tumor
Trauma	Head injuries	Evacuation, burr hole, craniectomy, brain resection

Neurovascular	Aneurysm, arteriovenous malformations,
	  stroke
		Clipping, embolization, clot
		  lysis, resection

Movement Disorders	Parkinson's disease, dystonia, essential tremor, seizure	Deep brain stimulator

Source: Fehlings MG et al. *Spine (Phila Pa 1976)*. 2010;35(9 Suppl):S37–46 (10); Huang CY et al. *Front Aging Neurosci*. 2017;9:96 (12); Papadopoulos EC et al. *Spine J*. 2015;15(5):983–91 (13).

(stenosis), inflammation, hypertrophy, and osteophyte formation result in spine instability (3,9,10). Vertebral bodies suffer sclerosis of the endplates and bone remodeling, with osteophyte formation creating nerve root pain. This often requires surgical intervention with nerve-specific IONM. Spondylolisthesis, a vertebra sliding forward, scoliosis, sideways curve of the spine, and kyphosis (excessive outward curvature of the thoracic spine) all contribute to malalignment and destabilization of the spine, creating pain and instability with aging. Stretch and compression of the spinal cord and nerves results in neurologic dysfunction and difficulty obtaining IONM (Figure 12.1).

Osteoporosis results from endocrine and lifestyle changes. Hormones responsible for bone formation, vitamin D, and calcium absorption all decrease with age. Osteoclastic activity is stimulated by the increase in chemokines (signaling proteins that induce directed chemotaxis). All result

in decreased bone mass density, alteration in the bone architecture, and ultimately an increased risk of vertebral body fractures requiring acute surgical intervention. The prevalence of vertebral fractures that are osteoporotic in nature has been estimated at 39% in geriatric patients (10).

The aging spinal cord experiences changes that increase the difficulty of obtaining IONM. With increased age, there is decreased density of the small myelinated fibers in the corticospinal tract, reduced neurons in the ventral horn (intermediate zone), and a decreased number of large alpha- and medium-size gamma-motor neurons (3,10). Common spinal and spinal cord disorders that need surgical intervention include myelopathy secondary to degenerative cervical disease, central cord syndrome after hyperextension injuries, degenerative scoliosis and kyphosis, vertebral compression fractures, degenerative spondylolisthesis, stenosis, and spinal axial instability, among others (Table 12.2). All degenerative changes in the spinal elements cause spinal canal narrowing, increased venous pressure, and decreased flow of the cerebrospinal fluid. These changes predispose elderly patients to central cord syndrome after hyperextension injuries (3,11).

Central nervous system

> **Tip:** Assessing the patient for neurologic decline, especially hearing and memory, may help the clinician assess the anesthetic management changes needed to support IONM.

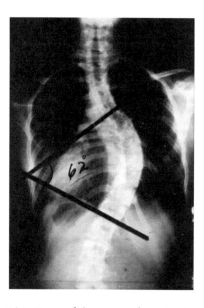

Figure 12.1 X-ray of the spine of an elderly adult with severe scoliosis. Prior to correction, spinal blood vessels and nerves on the outer curve are stretched, reducing the vessel lumen and blood flow. On the inner curve, vessels and nerves are tortuous, causing turbulent blood flow and reduced blood flow in the nerve vasa vasorum. With correction, there is an acute reversal of perfusion conditions. The alteration in anatomy makes IONM, typically SEP, MEP, EMG, important for evaluation of function, adequacy of blood flow, and assessment of the patient's neurologic reserve during surgery. (From author's personal files.)

An aging population requires a disproportionate amount of neurosurgical care. In the mid-1980s, approximately 10% of neurosurgical candidates were older than 70 years, while recent reports indicate this number has increased to approximately 22% (14). Common neurosurgical procedures in this population are described in Table 12.2. It is important to account for the changes produced by age on the central nervous system (CNS). Aging affects all neurologic elements, with the most distressful being the progressive loss of neurons in the cerebral cortex and cortical function. Both the number of neuroreceptors, and the amount of neurotransmitter release, serotonin, acetylcholine, and dopamine, is markedly reduced. Cerebrovascular and cardiac disease produce focal to global reductions in cerebral blood flow, cerebral activity, and function. Neurologic decline manifests as a reduction of perception, memory, and reasoning (15). These changes make cortical recordings of SEP and stimulation of MEP challenging. Neuron loss produces notable decreases in hearing and the ability to obtain an auditory brainstem response (ABR). Specialized intraparenchymal EEG mapping is commonly used for placement of a deep brain stimulator (DBS) to treat movement disorders. Endovascular interventions during stroke, aneurysm occlusion, and AVM embolization often require IONM services to detect hypoperfusion using SEP, MEP, and EEG (Table 12.3).

On the annual Aging, the Central Nervous System and Mobility Conference Series organized by the Gerontological Society of America, The

Table 12.3 Summary of recommended IONM studies for common surgical procedures

Type of Procedure	Recommended monitoring modalities by procedure					
			EMG			
	SEP	MEP	Free Run	Stim	ABR	EEG
Spine skeletal						
Spinal cord	•	•	•	•		
Cauda equina or below (Lumbar Spine)	•	±	•	•		
Head and neck						
Parotid only			•CN7	•CN7		
Neck			•CN7,10, Cv2–4	•CN7,10 Cv2–4		
Thyroid	•	•	•CN10	•CN10		
Cochlear implant			•CN 7		•	
Mastoid			•CN 7		±	
Brain						
Supratentorial						
Motor cortex[a,b] lesion	•	•	•			•
Sensory cortex[a,b] lesion	•	•	•			•
Eloquent "speech"[b] lesion		*				•
Seizure mapping						•
Posterior fossa						
Acoustic neuroma	•		•CN5,7	•	•	
Cerebellopontine angle tumor	•		•CN5,7–9,11,12	•	•	
Other: tumor/vascular	•	±	•	•	±	
Vascular	•	•	•	±	•	
Aortic arch	•					•
Aorta-endovascular	•	•				•
Carotid artery						•
Stroke—intracranial	±	±				•
Metastatic tumor—spine	•	•	•			±

Note: Free-run EMG has the cranial or cervical nerve root added that is often monitored during these procedures. EEG is used to monitor CNS hypoperfusion in vascular surgery and induced seizures in awake craniotomy with supratentorial brain mapping. CN = cranial nerve, Cv = cervical nerve root, ± = preference, * = requires motor function to speak.

[a] Asleep
[b] Awake

National Institute of Aging, and the University of Pittsburgh in 2012, investigators reported that approximately 35% of 70-year-old adults and most of the 85-year-old adults have a gait abnormality due to the consequences of neurological and skeletal aging (16). Gait abnormalities increase the risk of fall, trauma, and hospitalization, often resulting in surgical interventions. The geriatric population compromised about 8.5% of the worldwide population. About 50% of the reported 69,720 primary brain and spinal cord tumors are diagnosed yearly in geriatric individuals (Table 12.2) (11). This group also has a significant burden of metastatic CNS lesions. Surgical treatment can require IONM guidance with either awake or anesthetized for mapping of motor and sensory cortex (cortical MEP, SEP) and assessment of possible seizure foci (EEG) (17).

INTRAOPERATIVE NEUROPHYSIOLOGIC MONITORING TESTS

General principles

> **Tip:** The basis for evoked potentials is a stimulus and a measured response. Activities that would interfere with the stimulus or response measurement should be avoided.

Mitigating surgically related neurologic complications in the elderly depends on optimization of anesthetic management and IONM techniques to allow for early detection of functional changes associated with surgical procedures and physiological events. The most frequently used evoked techniques include MEP, SEP, stimulated electromyography (sEMG), and ABR (18–20). Visual evoked potentials (VEP) are performed in only a few centers and are not addressed in this review. The conceptual basis for all evoked potentials is a stimulus (electricity, sound or light) that activates a neuron, an axon/dendrite, a cochlea, or a retina that then propagates the signal to areas of the sensory, auditory, or visual cortex or muscles. The response can be detected with another electrode array. Other routine studies include measurement of spontaneous activity, EEG, and EMG.

Since the 1980s, IONM has been utilized in adolescent and young adult structural spine surgery and posterior fossa procedures to reduce risk of neurological injury (21). Increased surgical volume in geriatric patients requires IONM services be adapted to allow montoring thus reducing patient risk. The pre-existing comorbid conditions of this population makes providing equivalent neurologic assessment challenging. Table 12.3 summarizes the recommended IONM studies by surgical procedure (22).

> **Tip:** Environmental factors that produce wave-based oscillating interference (i.e., heating element, motor, sound) should be avoided; they disrupt IONM.

Basic measurements for all evoked potentials include latency, time from stimulus to first wave deflection, amplitude, the difference between the maximum negative and positive deflection, and configuration (expected appearance). Latencies are a function of distance from stimulus to recording location. This distance is influenced by patient height, limb length, gender, and pre-existing nerve conduction velocity. Amplitude is determined by the number of neurons, axons, or myofibrils depolarizing simultaneously under the measuring electrode. Increasing stimulation strength increases the potential amplitude by recruiting more neurologic tissue to depolarize. Inherent variation in conduction velocity will decrease amplitude or change the response appearance. Figure 12.2 demonstrates some expected IONM responses in a young adult and a geriatric patient. In the geriatric patient, the normal variation in nerve conduction means the response will be distributed over a longer time, causing a lower peak amplitude and possibly a longer latency and a "smudged" configuration. Presence of comorbid conditions aggravate this situation.

Since each patient serves as their own control, agents of change should be alterations in anesthesia management and surgery actions. All signals must meet a criterion of size and configuration before a change can be detected. Identifying a 50% reduction in amplitude with a 1500 μV

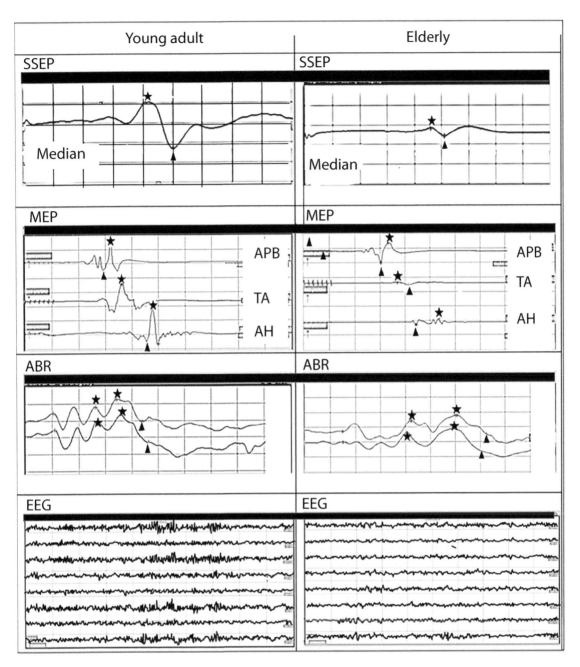

Figure 12.2 Comparison of young adult and geriatric adult IONM responses. The young adult responses demonstrate the expected normal amplitude (star to triangle marker), the latency (distance to red marker), and configuration of the most commonly performed summative tests, SEP, MEP, and ABR. The geriatric adult has in all responses a longer latency, smaller amplitude, and less precise and defined configuration. These characteristics make it more difficult to recognize and interpret change in waveforms as change in neurologic function due to surgical events or other causes. Comparing EEG responses demonstrates reduction in frequency and amplitude of waves in the geriatric adult compared to the young adult. These changes are similar to changes seen with hypoperfusion or hypoxic events. The geriatric patient EEG suggests very deep anesthesia that has been associated with prolonged wake-up and postoperative delirium. *Abbreviations:* APB, abductor polis brevis; TA, tibialis anterior; AH, abductor halicus. (From authors' archives.)

MEP is clearly easier and more reliable than in a 235 µV MEP. Under ideal circumstances, change will only originate from the surgical procedure. Baseline studies, usually the first reproducible response, establish the patient's normal response under operative conditions. While modest variability is normal, change that constitutes a warning for potential injury is an established deviance from baseline studies. This value is determined by each organization and is based on local community and national IONM standards. The standards may vary by age and health of the patient (18,23). When an alert occurs, all members of the surgical, anesthesia, and supporting teams are informed. Each has a role to play in reversing the change, from tailoring anesthesia to moving surgical retractors.

A major problem in all IONM studies is environmental interference—usually oscillating energy waves that are not detected by our senses (i.e., electromagnetic waves, radio waves) but permeate our environment. All responses, summative and continuous, are vulnerable to interference from energy sources such as electrocautery, motors, light, and heating elements. Often grouped together as "60 cycle," they are wave-based oscillating energy that can disrupt IONM detection.

> **Tip:** When compared to a young adult, a geriatric patient has responses that are smaller amplitude, longer latency, and more variable configuration.

Summative and continuous responses measure different functionality. SEP, MEP, and ABR studies are summative. Summative responses require a constant time-locked stimulation that creates a propagating wave of depolarization at a fixed frequency; they will reach the monitoring site within the same time interval. Summation of repetitive responses removes the random background noise (EEG, equipment, electrical interference) and enhances the size of the stimulated response to create a reproducible and reportable signal. Eventually the random activity sums to zero and the desired signal emerges (MEP, ABR, SEP). The number of stimuli to achieve a reliable response will depend on the size of the response relative to the random noise. Myelopathy, neuropathy,

normal aging, patient physiology, anesthesia, and environment factors can create an unreliable or absent response. Summation for MEP requires four to nine stimulation events to recruit enough neurons to produce a single secondary response, muscle contraction, with EMG. The increased MEP variability in configuration demonstrates that different myofilaments contract with each stimulus.

EEG and EMG are continuous spontaneous electrical activity that is of an adequate amplitude and frequency to be primarily detected and analyzed. EEG, EMG, and sEMG are vulnerable to suppression by the same factors that alter summative responses.

SPECIFIC IONM STUDIES

Summative responses

> **Tip:** SEPs are performed more frequently throughout the surgery than MEPs. Consequently, they are more likely to detect a response change even though MEPs are more sensitive to change (24).

Somatosensory evoked potentials are electrophysiologic responses measured over sensory cortex (cortical) or cervical spine (subcortical) and are created by the depolarization of a mixed motor sensory peripheral nerve in the arms (median/ulnar nerve) or legs (posterior tibial/tibial/peroneal nerve). The response is generated by electrical stimulation (20–60 mA) at a frequency between 1.41 and 2.79 Hz. SEP responses are transmitted with through ipsilateral dorsal (posterior) column/medial lemniscus and arrive in the contralateral sensory cortex, left foot to right brain. They convey tactile information, discriminatory touch, vibration, and position/movement sense. During transmission to sensory cortex, sensory pathway has few synapses and better perfusion, making the response more resistant to hypoperfusion events (hypotension, stretch, compression). Needle or contact electrodes produce repetitive nerve SEP stimuli; responses are averaged to produce a summative waveform from sensory cortex. Since the amplitude is very small relative to environmental and physiologic artifact, the response requires

200–500 repetitions to produce a reliable wave-form. The response must be reproducible and have an amplitude of at least 0.3–0.5 µV (Figure 12.2).

A weakness in SEP monitoring is time lag between the neurologic event (potential injury) and identifying a SEP change that occurred due to nerve damage, spinal cord traction, hardware mis-alignment, hypotension, or acute anemia. It may require as long as 16 minutes, much longer than MEP at 1–2 minutes. MEP is usually performed less frequently, relegating it to a confirmatory role in an acute injury. Based on the available evidence, the generally accepted SEP alert that correlates with postoperative neurologic deficit is an ampli-tude decrease of 50% and/or a latency increase of 10% (18,24). These criteria originated with studies of young adults and adolescent patients undergo-ing spine surgery. There are no current alert criteria for elderly adults. SEP remains a nearly universal IONM modality in spinal cord, brain sensory, and cortical monitoring or brainstem tumor resection (Table 12.3).

> **Tip:** MEPs are sensitive to any source of hypoperfusion.

Transcranial motor evoked potentials are a sum-mated response generated by a series of four to nine electrical pulses of between 200 and 600 volts, each 140 µsec, applied over the motor cortex (25). This stimulation will depolarize motor neurons along much of the motor strip. The nerve response is measured by a secondary response of muscle contraction or EMG. Enough myofibrils must con-tract simultaneously to produce a detectible EMG. Any muscle could be measured, but by convention it is most frequently abductor pollicis brevis (APB), tibialis anterior (TA), and abductor hallucis (AH). With direct mapping of the spine or cerebral cor-tex, EMG recordings are recorded from the areas that are assumed to be projections from the motor cortex (Figure 12.2).

Spinal cord motor pathways lie in the anterior column and synapse in the anterior horn. Unlike the better-perfused SEP, the anterior motor path-ways have only a single-vessel blood supply and multiple synapses. Consequently, MEP gray-mat-ter neurons are more sensitive to ischemia than SEP axons located in the dorsal columns. The size

of the contraction reflects the number of axons simultaneously causing the muscle contraction (7). Physiologic changes associated with aging, muscle function, vascular and cardiac disease, hyperten-sion, and skeletal deformity make motor responses more sensitive and more difficult to obtain. MEPs are performed whenever the tissue at risk involves a high probability of neuron injury beginning with the cerebral cortex to the final anterior horn cells. MEP alert criteria have not been universally established throughout the IONM community. University of Colorado IONM requires a signal amplitude of at least 300 µV to be reliable for moni-toring. An alert is a reproducible amplitude reduc-tion of 50% from baseline and first peak latency increase of 20%. MEP is frequently used in vascu-lar surgery such as thoracoabdominal aneurysms, aortic arch procedures (both endovascular and open procedures), and preemptive stroke assess-ment since MEP changes quickly reflect hypoper-fusion (26). Direct cortical stimulation of motor and sensory cortex has unique stimulation param-eters and is very helpful in defining the extent of the tumor (17,27).

> **Tip:** Auditory brainstem responses can be disrupted by the loud ambient noise in the operating room.

Auditory brainstem responses (**ABR or BAEP**) are the summative evoked potential responses obtained by activating the hair cells in the cochlea using high-frequency sound waves (28). The audi-tory pathway creates a series of responses that are propagated from the eighth nerve to the cochlear nucleus and eventually to the auditory cortex. Stimulation is a series of 1000 clicks at a frequency of 11.4 Hz. The sound is 70–90 dB in the "active" ear, and the sound in the inactive ear is 40–60 dB of white noise to prevent ambient sound from interfering with the stimulus. The responses moni-tored during surgery and anesthesia are cochleo-gram and short-latency brainstem responses (Figure 12.2). Mid- and long-latency responses are primarily used for diagnostic audiology in awake patients. Each stimulation requires 10 msec with allows 30–50 repetitions per second. Trigeminal neuralgia, acoustic neuromas, and cerebropontine angle tumors are frequent in geriatric patients with hearing deficits. Reducing the stimulus frequency, increasing the sound volume, and increasing the number of stimuli may allow ABR to be obtained in patients with hearing deficits. The criteria for an alert are the same as for SEP.

Responses are peaks/troughs labeled I through V', with peaks I, III, and V-V' being the most useful for surgical purposes. Wave I is produced by the extracranial portion of the cranial nerve VIII and assures a stimulus is present. Changes in waves II to V/V' specifically identify approximate injury location during posterior fossa surgery. The presence of the V/V' complex, which is not only the largest but also the most reliable response, assures that the signal has traversed through the at-risk region. ABR responses are the most resistant to anesthetic agent depression, but due to size and hearing loss they are the most difficult to obtain and maintain during the procedure (29).

Continuous responses

> **Tip:** EMG responses will be eliminated or significantly affected by the use of neuromuscular blockade. Neuromuscular blockade is not recommended when EMG techniques are needed.

EMG is spontaneous muscle activity and is recorded continuously. EMG can be an evoked potential when a specific nerve is stimulated, resulting in a burst of sEMG activity. Free-run or spontaneous activity is used to detect unintended stimulation of a peripheral mixed motor sensory nerve and will appear as a burst of high-frequency, high-amplitude signal. The surgeon is notified by technical staff or by converting the signal to sound. Peripheral nerve EMG monitoring does not require technical personnel. Surgical personnel frequently use it independently to find facial, trigeminal nerves during head and neck surgery. More sophisticated monitoring in the posterior fossa require IOM technicians and uses a combination of spontaneous and stimulated response of motor cranial nerves V through XII (Table 12.4). EMG and sEMG are very helpful in assessing the integrity of the brainstem during posterior fossa

Table 12.4 Muscle groups monitored during posterior fossa surgery

Cranial nerve	Muscle usually monitored
III	Medial rectus (ocular)
IV	Superior oblique
V	Masseter, temporalis
VI	Lateral rectus
VII	Orbicularis oculi, oris
IX	Stylopharyngeus
X	Vocalis
XI	Trapezius
XII	Palatoglossus (tongue)

surgery (30). Stimulation may be a single pulse or 3–5 pulses/second. Stimulus strength, 0.05–10 mA, is selected depending on the location, size of the nerve, and delicacy of the surrounding tissue. Alerts are single large spikes, a long, high-frequency, repetitive response, or a burst followed by silence when the nerve is cut. Inability to obtain a stimulated response may signal the nerve is permanently injured. In thyroid surgery, it is most often an indication the specialized tracheal tube with embedded electrodes to measure vocal cord EMG is misdirected (31,32). Nondepolarizing neuromuscular blocking agents cannot be used when EMG is required.

> **Tip:** Asymmetrical EEG suggests regional injury such as stroke or surgical hypoperfusion.

Electroencephalography is a continuous recording of electric currents between the pyramidal cells and neurons by scalp electrodes. Understanding the neurophysiology of this process is complex and readily available in other sources (33). EEG recording is primarily used in vascular procedures, carotid endarterectomy, thoracic aorta repair, and in some cardiac procedures (Table 12.3). The normal aging brain loses cortical volume, increases in cerebral spinal fluid, decreases in neurotransmitters, and has an increased in sensitivity to anesthetic drugs. These issues make the EEG lower in amplitude and frequency in the elderly than in younger individuals. Wave changes related to hypotension, ischemia, hypothermia, hypoglycemia, and neurologic

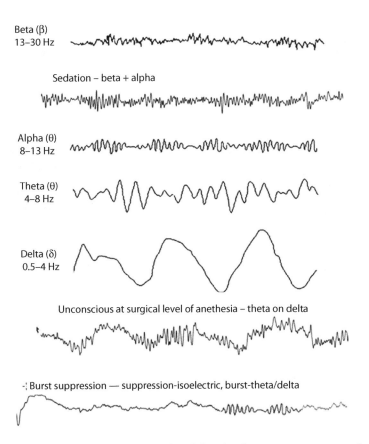

Beta (β)
13–30 Hz

Sedation – beta + alpha

Alpha (θ)
8–13 Hz

Theta (θ)
4–8 Hz

Delta (δ)
0.5–4 Hz

Unconscious at surgical level of anethesia – theta on delta

-¦ Burst suppression — suppression-isoelectric, burst-theta/delta

Figure 12.3 Illustrated EEG waveforms associated with levels of consciousness. Anesthesia consistently produces characteristic EEG activity. This can be recognized with frontal EEG provided by processed EEG monitoring products when the EEG waveform is provided. Most notable is the reduction in frequency (slowing) and decrease in frequency (theta, delta) waves. The presence of delta waves is strongly associated with deep non-REM sleep, deep anesthesia, and events that depress brain activity such as stroke and traumatic brain injury.

disease are similar or identical to those that are found during anesthesia. The signals are slower, decreased in amplitude, and more likely to become completely suppressed. Like all IOM studies, the EEG should appear symmetric in amplitude, frequency, and shape on comparable scalp locations. Figure 12.3 demonstrates four characteristic EEG wave patterns that are used to quantitate the level of brain activity and the change seen with anesthesia. Analytic programs provide spectral edge, compressed spectral array, and bispectral analysis from paired EEG inputs. These analysis techniques assist in identification of regional change. It is necessary to identify regional change during vascular events such as stroke. EEG is most frequently available to all anesthesia providers as processed frontal lobe EEG with proprietary analysis. Determination of

EEG alert is slowing, decreased amplitude, and a 50% reduction in power compared to the same contralateral brain area.

ANESTHESIA AND OUTCOMES

Anesthetic management

Tip: Anesthetic plan should be tailored to the patient's age and comorbidities to provide ideal conditions for IOM. Knowledge of the effects of the different anesthetics on IOM responses is crucial to provide optimal care.

Anesthetic management has a major influence on the ability for the IONM team to provide reliable information to the surgeon. The basic anesthetic drug effect on IONM is long established. Much of this work initially took place more than 20 years ago in a patient population that was young and undergoing scoliosis surgery. Consequently, the general effect of these drugs on IOMN remains uncontested but the degree of impact on the geriatric population remains less well defined. It is outside the scope of this chapter to discuss in detail the effects of anesthetic drugs on IONM; it is readily available elsewhere (35,36). In general, volatile anesthetics (VA) depress all IONM responses, with the most sensitive being MEP, and the least sensitive ABR. MEP responses can be reduced or eliminated with administration of VA creating false alert. False alerts undermine trust in IONM and can cause patient harm; consequently, careful selection and introduction of new drugs during IONM may be crucial to the outcome (37–40). It has been reported that MAC 0.5 or less of VA combined with propofol/narcotic-based total intravenous anesthesia (TIVA) can be used during IONM even in geriatric patients (40). VA MAC for an 80-year-old is approximately 22% lower than a 40-year-old and 30%–45% lower than in a child (41). Without MAC adjustment VA may have an unexpectedly profound effect on IONM and exacerbate physiologic depression present in a myelopathic and neuropathic geriatric patient. Large studies have shown that while balanced technique—VA plus TIVA—can be utilized, there is an increased risk of failure to detect real IONM changes, making it difficult to differentiate anesthetic effect from surgical injury (Figure 12.4).

Intravenous drugs have less effect on IONM. TIVA is the most commonly used technique because it causes the least IONM depression. TIVA dosing (42) is reduced within the geriatric group. Narcotics generally have little IONM effect. Methadone, an NMDA receptor antagonist, may at least briefly

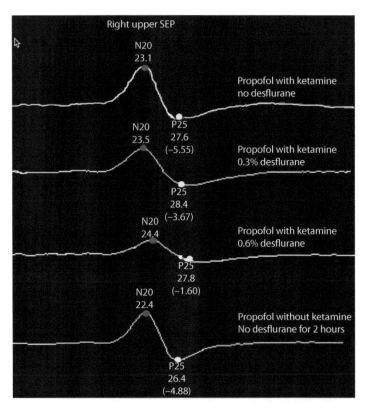

Figure 12.4 Effects of desflurane on SEP response. Planned exposure to desflurane in a middle-aged adult with diabetes and spinal stenosis. Initial responses were large and characteristic of upper extremity SEP response. End-tidal (ET) desflurane 0.3% reduced the response amplitude (red to yellow marks) by 30%. At 0.6% ET desflurane, the latency (red mark) was prolonged and amplitude decreased about 70%. Signals recovered to baseline 2 hours after desflurane was discontinued. (From author's archive.)

decrease MEP responses. Dexmedetomidine at doses below 0.6 mg/kg/h when added to a propofol-based TIVA may decrease MEP even in young adults. One randomized controlled trial was discontinued by the safety monitor due to reductions in responses with propofol and dexmedetomidine TIVA (43). A recent 40-subject trial found no difference in IONM with the same dexmedetomidine protocol in middle-aged adults (44). Notably, the reduction by 50% of MEP amplitude was not significant. As an NMDA antagonist, ketamine provides blood pressure support and analgesia, allows significant reduction in both narcotic and other hypnotic dosing, particularly for the chronic opioid-dependent patient. Ketamine is a mainstay of TIVA combinations.

Adjuvant drugs, lidocaine and magnesium, are often added to reduce perioperative pain while reducing the narcotic risks. There are no studies that define the effect of either lidocaine or magnesium on MEP or depth of anesthesia when administered at the infusion dose currently used for perioperative analgesia. One study found decreased SEP with much higher doses of lidocaine than is currently recommended, and one case report found significant SEP reduction (45,46). There is inadequate information to make a recommendation on whether magnesium should be used or if used at what dosage. Drugs that accumulate effects over long procedures should be introduced with care in patients with large signals.

The elderly tolerate hypoperfusion poorly in any organ system. Spine procedures cause significant physiologic stress with large blood loss, anemia, hypotension, hypothermia, and activation of inflammatory markers. These events impact neurologic function, from change in IONM to postoperative delirium. Maintaining physiologic stability and avoiding hypotension, anemia, hypothermia, and reduced cardiac output improves IONM's ability to identify change caused by surgical actions.

Appropriate therapy can improve postoperative recovery. Figure 12.5 demonstrates the effects of a surgical and anesthetic decision to induce hypotension on a SEP. In most circumstances, the first response to IONM reductions is an increase in blood pressure and perfusion. Anesthetic management that provides the best environment for IONM should be established whenever possible and adjuvant therapies carefully added or avoided even when large responses are present.

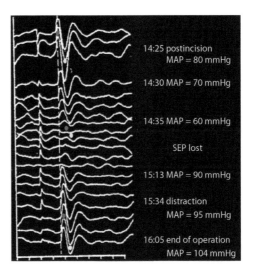

14:25 postincision
MAP = 80 mmHg

14:30 MAP = 70 mmHg

14:35 MAP = 60 mmHg

SEP lost

15:13 MAP = 90 mmHg

15:34 distraction
MAP = 95 mmHg

16:05 end of operation
MAP = 104 mmHg

Figure 12.5 Response of a geriatric patient to controlled hypotension. Controlled hypotension was requested to reduce blood loss in a 67-year-old man with spinal stenosis. Patient's preoperative mean arterial pressure (MAP) was 100 mmHg. This "waterfall" presentation (repeated SEP graphed by time) demonstrated SEP amplitude change (red to yellow marks) as the MAP decreases followed by recovery as MAP is elevated. (From author's archive.)

IONM management principles apply to all surgical procedures. Specialized expertise is necessary to manage patients during craniotomy for posterior fossa surgery or direct cortical mapping in awake or anesthetized patients. The most difficult management is the awake craniotomy. Direct cortical stimulation does not produce discomfort, but the stimulus can propagate and produce superficial or generalized seizure. This event is detected quickly by the IONM technical staff. The surgeon will use cold balanced salt solution to disrupt the seizure while the anesthesiologist will administer a small dose of propofol if needed. Airway management may be necessary. IONM personnel are critical for a safe outcome in these high-risk procedures.

OUTCOMES

Tip: Multimodal IONM is associated with effective interventions in the adult and geriatric surgical population.

IONM is accepted to reduce the incidence of neurologic injury during spine procedures. Similarly, IONM improves neurologic outcome after tumor removal, aneurysm, arteriovenous malformations, endovascular stroke therapy, and metastatic tumor embolization. Vascular surgery procedures that have risk of neurologic injury to the spinal cord and brain such as thoracic aneurysm, aortic arch aneurysm, carotid endarterectomy, and cardiac lesions with circulatory arrest are increasingly requesting IONM studies. Multimodal technique is used in all IONM requested procedures (Table 12.3).

Significant financial resources are required to perform IONM studies, raising the question "Is it worth it?" (24,47,48) Efficacy is not established in all or most procedures. This is based on the reality that while the incidence of severe preventable injury is rare, the devastating nature of the injury is real. Surgical teams and anesthesiologists consider positive outcomes supported by population studies as adequate to consider IOM valuable when making critical decisions.

In one of the few large prospective observational studies in idiopathic scoliosis procedures in adults, successful intervention for IONM loss resulted in no postoperative neurologic deficits. Interventions included elevating blood pressure and modifying hardware placement or traction. Failure to obtain return of IONM response resulted in postoperative deficits (49). Similar findings are reported for geriatric cervical spine procedures, where 12% (14 patients) had MEP changes. Ten resolved with intervention and did not have postoperative deficits. The remaining four had deficits (50). Carotid endarterectomy, posterior fossa surgery, and thyroid/radical neck studies in adult patients report similar findings of similar quality.

Multimodal IONM is associated with effective interventions in the adult and geriatric surgical population.

CONCLUSION

By 2050, 22% of the world will be over 65 years of age. PN and myelopathy are common neurologic disabilities caused by medical and surgical diseases. Diabetes mellitus, chronic renal disease, and neurodegenerative disease increase the difficulty in obtaining IONM. Mitigating neurologic injury during surgery requires multiple studies, SEP, MEP, ABR, EMG, and EEG to decrease the risk

of neurological damage. TIVA remains the most frequently used anesthetic during IONM testing. Volatile anesthetics and adjuvant drugs can have unexpected negative consequences on IONM procedures, particularly MEP. IONM demonstrates that hypoperfusion is a common treatable problem in at-risk patients. There is reasonable evidence that maintaining or regaining a response is associated with normal neurologic outcome. Loss of MEP is associated with postoperative neurologic injury.

REFERENCES

1. Prince MJ, Wu F, Guo Y et al. The burden of disease in older people and implications for health policy and practice. *Lancet.* 2015; 385(9967):549–62.
2. Healthy Aging Team. Top 10 Chronic Conditions in Adults 65+ and What You Can do to Prevent or Manage Them. 2017. 4-6-18; Available at: https://www.ncoa.org/blog/10-common-chronic-diseases-prevention-tips/
3. Fehlings MG, Tetreault L, Nater A et al. The aging of the global population: The changing epidemiology of disease and spinal disorders. *Neurosurgery.* 2015;77(Suppl 4):S1–5.
4. Firman J. 2017-NOCOA-Impact-Report. 2017. 4-4-18; Available at: https://www.ncoa.org/resources document 2.9.2018
5. Tesfaye S, Selvarajah D. Advances in the epidemiology, pathogenesis and management of diabetic peripheral neuropathy. *Diabetes Metab Res Rev.* 2012;28(Suppl 1):8–14.
6. Arnold R, Issar T, Krishnan AV et al. Neurological complications in chronic kidney disease. *JRSM Cardiovasc Dis.* 2016;5: 2048004016677687.
7. Hunter SK, Pereira HM, Keenan KG. The aging neuromuscular system and motor performance. *J Appl Physiol (1985).* 2016;121(4): 982–95.
8. Kukkar A, Bali A, Singh N, Jaggi AS. Implications and mechanism of action of gabapentin in neuropathic pain. *Arch Pharm Res.* 2013;36(3):237–51.
9. Roussouly P, Nnadi C. Sagittal plane deformity: An overview of interpretation and management. *Eur Spine J.* 2010;19(11):1824–36.

10. Fehlings MG, Brodke DS, Norvell DC, Dettori JR. The evidence for intraoperative neurophysiological monitoring in spine surgery: Does it make a difference? *Spine (Phila Pa 1976).* 2010;35(9 Suppl):S37–46.

11. Rosso AL, Studenski SA, Chen WG et al. Aging, the central nervous system, and mobility. *J Gerontol A Biol Sci Med Sci.* 2013;68(11):1379–86.

12. Huang CY, Lin LL, Hwang IS. Age-related differences in reorganization of functional connectivity for a dual task with increasing postural destabilization. *Front Aging Neurosci.* 2017;9:96.

13. Papadopoulos EC, Boachie-Adjei O, Hess WF et al. Early outcomes and complications of posterior vertebral column resection. *Spine J.* 2015;15(5):983–91.

14. Chibbaro S, Di Rocco F, Makiese O et al. Neurosurgery and elderly: Analysis through the years. *Neurosurg Rev.* 2010;34(2):229–34.

15. Leung J. Elderly patients. In: Stoelting RK, Miller R (eds). *Basics of Anesthesia.* 5th ed. Philadelphia PA: Elsevier; 2007. pp. 518–29.

16. Varma VR, Hausdorff JM, Studenski SA et al. Aging, the central nervous system, and mobility in older adults: Interventions. *J Gerontol A Biol Sci Med Sci.* 2016;71(11):1451–8.

17. Eseonu CI, Rincon-Torroella J, ReFaey K et al. Awake craniotomy vs craniotomy under general anesthesia for perirolandic gliomas: Evaluating perioperative complications and extent of resection. *Neurosurgery.* 2017;81(3):481–9.

18. Le Roux P, Menon DK, Citerio G et al. Consensus summary statement of the International Multidisciplinary Consensus Conference on Multimodality Monitoring in Neurocritical Care: A statement for healthcare professionals from the Neurocritical Care Society and the European Society of Intensive Care Medicine. *Neurocrit Care.* 2014;21:S1–26.

19. Kirkman MA, Smith M. Multimodality neuromonitoring. *Anesthesiol Clin.* 2016;34(3):511–23.

20. Staarmann B, O'Neal K, Magner M et al. Sensitivity and specificity of intraoperative neuromonitoring for identifying safety and duration of temporary aneurysm clipping based on vascular territory, a multimodal

strategy. *World Neurosurg.* 2017;100:522–30.

21. York DH, Chabot RJ, Gaines RW. Response variability of somatosensory evoked potentials during scoliosis surgery. *Spine (Phila Pa 1976).* 1987;12(9):864–76.

22. Oya J, Burke JF, Vogel T, Tay B, Chou D, Mummaneni P. The accuracy of multimodality intraoperative neuromonitoring to predict postoperative neurologic deficits following cervical laminoplasty. *World Neurosurg.* 2017;106:17–25.

23. Macdonald DB, Skinner S, Shils J, Yingling C. Intraoperative motor evoked potential monitoring—A position statement by the American Society of Neurophysiological Monitoring. *Clin Neurophysiol.* 2013;124(12):2291–316.

24. Pease M, Gandhoke GS, Kaur J et al. 319 Predictive value of intraoperative neurophysiological monitoring during spine surgery: A prospective analysis of 4489 consecutive patients. *Neurosurgery.* 2016;63(Suppl. 1):192–3.

25. Jameson L. Transcranial motor evoked potentials. In: Koht A, Sloan TB, Toleikis JR (eds). *Monitoring the Nervous System for Anesthesiologists and Other Health Professionals.* Switzerland: Springer; 2017. pp. 19–34.

26. So VC, Poon CC. Intraoperative neuromonitoring in major vascular surgery. *Br J Anaesth.* 2016;117(Suppl. 2):ii13–25.

27. Abalkhail TM, MacDonald DB, AlThubaiti I et al. Intraoperative direct cortical stimulation motor evoked potentials: Stimulus parameter recommendations based on rheobase and chronaxie. *Clin Neurophysiol.* 2017;128(11):2300–8.

28. Seubert C, Herman M. Auditory evoked potentials. In: Koht A, Sloan T, Toleikis J (eds). *Monitoring the Nervous System for Anesthesiologists and Other Health Professionals.* Gewerbesuasse, Switzerland: Springer; 2017. pp. 35–50.

29. Thirumala PD, Kodavatiganti HS, Habeych M et al. Value of multimodality monitoring using brainstem auditory evoked potentials and somatosensory evoked potentials in endoscopic endonasal surgery. *Neurol Res.* 2013;35(6):622–30.

30. Deletis V, Fernandez-Conejero I. Intraoperative monitoring and mapping of

the functional integrity of the brainstem. *J Clin Neurol.* 2016;12(3):262–73.

31. Wong KP, Mak KL, Wong CKH, Lang BHH. Systematic review and meta-analysis on intra-operative neuro-monitoring in high-risk thyroidectomy. *Int J Surg.* 2017;38:21–30.

32. Yang S, Zhou L, Lu Z, Ma B, Ji Q, Wang Y. Systematic review with meta-analysis of intraoperative neuromonitoring during thyroidectomy. *Int J Surg.* 2017;39:104–13.

33. Purdon PL, Sampson A, Pavone KJ, Brown EN. Clinical electroencephalography for anesthesiologists: Part I: Background and basic signatures. *Anesthesiology.* 2015;123(4):937–60.

34. Thirumala PD, Thiagarajan K, Gedela S, Crammond DJ, Balzer JR. Diagnostic accuracy of EEG changes during carotid endarterectomy in predicting perioperative strokes. *J Clin Neurosci.* 2016;25:1–9.

35. Hayashi H, Kawaguchi M, Abe R et al. Evaluation of the applicability of sevoflurane during post-tetanic myogenic motor evoked potential monitoring in patients undergoing spinal surgery. *J Anesth.* 2009;23(2):175–81.

36. Sloan TB. Anesthesia management and intraoperative electrophysiological monitoring. In: Koht A, Sloan TB, Toleikis JR (eds). *Monitoring the Nervous System for Anesthesiologists and Other Health Care Professionals.* Switzerland: Springer; 2017. pp. 317–44.

37. Tamkus A, Rice KS, Kim HL. Intraoperative neuromonitoring alarms: Relationship of the surgeon's decision to intervene (or not) and clinical outcomes in a subset of spinal surgical patients with a new postoperative neurological deficit. *Neurodiagn J.* 2017;57(4): 276–87.

38. Tamkus AA, Rice KS, McCaffrey MT. Perils of intraoperative neurophysiological monitoring: Analysis of "false-negative" results in spine surgeries. *Spine J.* 2018;18(2):276–84.

39. Kim SH, Jin S-J, Karm M-H et al. Comparison of false-negative/positive results of intraoperative evoked potential monitoring between no and partial neuromuscular blockade in patients receiving propofol/remifentanil-based anesthesia during cerebral aneurysm clipping surgery: A retrospective analysis of 685 patients. *Medicine (Baltim).* 2016;95(34):e4725.

40. Hernandez-Palazon J, Izura V, Fuentes-García D et al. Comparison of the effects of propofol and sevoflurane combined with remifentanil on transcranial electric motor-evoked and somatosensory-evoked potential monitoring during brainstem surgery. *J Neurosurg Anesthesiol.* 2015;27(4):282–8.

41. Nickalls RW, Mapleson WW. Age-related iso-MAC charts for isoflurane, sevoflurane and desflurane in man. *Br J Anaesth.* 2003;91(2): 170–4.

42. Higgs M, Hackworth RJ, John K, Riffenburgh R, Tomlin J, Wamsley B. The intraoperative effect of methadone on somatosensory evoked potentials. *J Neurosurg Anesthesiol.* 2017;29(2):168–74.

43. Mahmoud M, Sadhasivam S, Salisbury S et al. Susceptibility of transcranial electric motor-evoked potentials to varying targeted blood levels of dexmedetomidine during spine surgery. *Anesthesiology.* 2010;112(6): 1364–73.

44. Rozet I, Metzner J, Brown M et al. Dexmedetomidine does not affect evoked potentials during spine surgery. *Anesth Analg.* 2015;121(2):492–501.

45. Schubert A, Licina MG, Glaze GM, Paranandi L. Systemic lidocaine and human somatosensory-evoked potentials during sufentanil-isoflurane anaesthesia. *Can J Anaesth.* 1992;39(6):569–75.

46. Chaves-Vischer V, Brustowicz R, Helmers SL. The effect of intravenous lidocaine on intraoperative somatosensory evoked potentials during scoliosis surgery. *Anesth Analg.* 1996;83(5):1122–5.

47. Lu Y, Qureshi SA. Cost-effective studies in spine surgeries: A narrative review. *Spine J.* 2014;14(11):2748–62.

48. Fischer CR, Cassilly R, Dyrszka M et al. Cost-effectiveness of lumbar spondylolisthesis surgery at 2-year follow-up. *Spine Deform.* 2016;4(1):48–54.

49. Buckwalter JA, Yaszay B, Ilgenfritz RM, Bastrom TP, Newton PO. Analysis of intraoperative neuromonitoring events during spinal corrective surgery for idiopathic scoliosis. *Spine Deform.* 2013;1(6):434–38.

50. Lee HJ, Kim IS, Sung JH, Lee SW, Hong JT. Significance of multimodal intraoperative monitoring for the posterior cervical spine surgery. *Clin Neurol Neurosurg.* 2016;143:9–14.

13

Positions in neurosurgery

ZILVINAS ZAKAREVICIUS, MIKHAIL GELFENBEYN, AND IRENE ROZET

INTRODUCTION

Proper positioning of the geriatric patient for neurosurgery is an important task for both surgeon and anesthesiologist. Surgical preference for positioning to access the anatomic target often represents a challenge in an anesthetized, and often paralyzed geriatric patient. Therefore positioning is the joint responsibility of surgeon and anesthesiologist. When positioning a patient, it is important to acknowledge the physiologic and potential pathologic consequences of the specific position.

In this chapter we describe commonly used positions during neurosurgical procedures, their benefits and risks, and preventive measures to minimize position-related complications in geriatric patients.

GENERAL PRINCIPLES

Patient positioning for surgery should be considered and discussed between neurosurgeon and anesthesiologist prior to surgery. Risks and benefits of patient positioning during neurosurgery should be discussed in detail during the *preoperative evaluation* visit by both the surgeon and the anesthesiologist. The patient's questions should be appropriately answered, and discussion should

be documented. Discussion of positioning is now advocated to be included in the written informed consent (1).

In the anesthetized patient, positioning is typically attended to after induction of general anesthesia and necessary vascular (additional peripheral, arterial, and/or central) line placement. Positioning of neurosurgical patients is a complex process, requiring adequate anesthetic depth, maintenance of hemodynamic stability and appropriate oxygenation as well as preservation of monitoring, especially invasive.

MONITORING DURING POSITIONING

Patient positioning should be carefully undertaken utilizing a patient-centered *team approach*. All members of the operating room, including surgeons, anesthesiologists, and nurses, should operate as a single well-integrated and unified team. Preferably, patient positioning should be led by the senior surgeon and the senior anesthesiologist. The plan for positioning should be verbalized, all the equipment (pads, chest roll, arm boards, etc.) should be prepared and ready to go, and help should be called for if needed (e.g., in complex positioning of the obese patient, or with multiple lines in-situ, chest tubes, intracranial pressure [ICP] monitoring) should be made prior to attempting positioning.

Prior to complex positioning, the endotracheal tube should be disconnected from the ventilator tubing to prevent *inadvertent extubation* of the patient. Disconnection of the endotracheal tube should be as brief as possible, especially in patients with low reserve (e.g., advanced age, morbid obesity, severe lung disease). Ventilation with high FiO_2 (80%–100%) for 3–5 minutes prior to disconnection may prevent desaturation during positioning, especially if the patient is positioned from supine to lateral or prone position, or if repositioning is required. Fast reconnection of the endotracheal tube and reestablishing of the capnography is especially helpful when the rest of the monitoring is not recorded.

Positioning often requires disconnection of monitors, creating a dangerous "blackout" state (2). Optimally, this should be avoided, or the time of full disconnection should be shortened. Continuous hemodynamic monitoring during positioning is especially important in frail geriatric patients, who often present with multiple comorbidities, with high risk for hemodynamic instability, low lung functional residual capacity, and higher risks for thromboembolism (e.g., in patients with previous bed rest longer than 7 days or trauma patients). Special considerations should be taken in positioning trauma patients (especially with hemo- or pneumothoraces who are dependent on chest tubes functioning), and after acute subarachnoid hemorrhage, with increased ICP, brain mass, and brain swelling. Therefore pulse oximetry, blood pressure, and ICP should be monitored throughout positioning whenever possible. At least one monitor, preferably an invasive blood pressure, should be considered to be continued throughout the positioning. Chest tubes, if present, should be unclamped.

COMMON POSITIONING-RELATED COMPLICATIONS

The most common positioning-related complications include *pressure sores* and *peripheral nerve injury* (3). Although the overall incidence of peripheral nerve injuries in the general surgical population is believed to be less than 1% (4), when somatosensory evoked potential (SSEP) monitoring is used to monitor nerve ischemia in spine and cranial surgeries, the pooled incidence of peripheral nerve injuries is 2.15%, with the highest of 11% in the prone position (5). According to the Anesthesia Closed Claims Project database, 36% of all peripheral nerve injury claims across all the surgical subspecialties were made for brachial plexus injury, followed by ulnar (30%), median (10%), sciatic (10%), radial (8%), and femoral (4%) nerve injury. Improper positioning or padding was identified as a primary cause, which accounted for 30% of the nerve injuries in this database (5).

Development of peripheral nerve injury is associated with patient's age, diabetes, extremes of weight, alcohol and tobacco use, vascular disease, pre-existing paresthesias, and length of surgery (3).

The recent American Society of Anesthesiologists Practice Advisory (3) recommends preventive strategies for the patient positioning and *protective padding* to decrease risk of perioperative pressure sores and peripheral neuropathies (Table 13.1). Careful padding should be implemented in every case, regardless of whether the patient is

Table 13.1 Immediate interventions for prevention of VAE with detection of air bubbles in the right atrium

Surgeons
1. Irrigation of the operative field with saline
2. Application of the wet gaze
3. Use of gelatin foam
4. Coagulation of the open vessels
5. Waxing of the bone

Anesthesiologists
1. Aspiration from the central line (20 mL syringe should be attached to the CVL during the procedure)
2. Switching ventilation to 100% oxygen
3. Turning the bed into Trendelenburg position to have head at a level of heart or lower
4. Compression of jugular veins
5. Giving intravenous fluids

generally anesthetized or awake/sedated. The general rules involve padding of arm board, use of chest rolls in the lateral position (decreases the risk of upper extremity neuropathy), padding at the elbow (decreases the risk of upper extremity neuropathy), padding to prevent pressure of a hard surface against the peroneal nerve at the fibular head (decreases the risk of peroneal neuropathy). Padding should be applied carefully, because tight padding may increase the risk of perioperative neuropathy.

The mechanism of perioperative peripheral nerve injury is multifactorial. Local mechanical insults on the nerve with stretching, pressure, or transection, and duration of the insult are damaging to the nerve. Other factors include perfusion, inflammation, metabolism, and underlying neuronal reserve. All of these may potentially alter neuronal integrity during the surgery and neuronal health intraoperatively. Prolonged immobilization under anesthesia per se may cause neuronal damage. Despite all the precautions taken during positioning, peripheral nerve injury, especially during prolonged cases, is never 100% predictable or preventable (5).

DOCUMENTATION

Intraoperative patient positioning should be carefully documented. An early *postoperative assessment of nerve function* of extremities should be performed because it may lead to early appropriate diagnosis of peripheral neuropathies.

The majority of neurosurgical procedures are lengthy. Complications in neurosurgery-related positioning include visual loss, venous and paradoxical air embolism, cerebral edema, intracranial bleeding, pneumocephalus, quadriplegia, and macroglossia.

HEAD POSITIONING

Patient positioning for neurosurgeries, including burr holes, craniotomies, and the majority of spine surgeries starts with positioning of the head and neck. Positioning of the head and neck is the initial and most important part of the neurosurgical procedure and requires special consideration.

Knowledge of the neurosurgical approach to head positioning is important to the anesthesiologist and overall perioperative management success. Therefore *preoperative evaluation* of range of motion of the patient's head and neck in elective cases is essential, as it can approximate the patient's tolerance of the desired intraoperative positioning during a lengthy surgery. This is especially important in the geriatric population that is known for high incidence of degenerative spine disease, osteophytes, and limited neck and head motion.

Craniotomy types

The head is positioned depending on the surgical target. Craniotomies are classified into several types depending on the location: frontal, temporal, parietal, occipital, and pterional (6,7). Craniotomy can involve more than one skull bone, e.g., fronto-temporal craniotomy or fronto-temporo-parietal craniotomy. Other types of craniotomy include *burr hole* craniotomy, in which the surgery is carried out through a small hole. This is done for lesions on the surface of the brain. *Stereotactic* craniotomy often requires an enlarged burr hole, where a 3-dimensional coordinates system is used to precisely locate the lesion deep in the brain.

With the development of the functional neurosurgery, *awake craniotomy* is becoming more popular, where the patient is either awake throughout the procedure or can be woken up during the surgery. It is commonly done for functional neurosurgery such as in epilepsy surgeries, or in implantation of deep brain stimulators (e.g., in Parkinson's disease). The neurological assessment in the awake patient is essential.

Head fixation

During head positioning, special attention should be paid to the skeletal fixation of the head with the pin fixation device, providing both immobility of the head and surgical comfort. Application of the Mayfield frame causes a profound sympathetic stimulation with profound tachycardia and hypertension. Infiltration of local anesthetic of the skin at the anticipated pin sites in conjunction with a scalp block with local anesthetic before pinning is strongly recommended in anesthetized patients and is crucial in awake procedures. In the anesthetized patient, deepening of general anesthesia before pinning may be done with a bolus of the intravenous anesthetic (e.g., 50–100 mg of propofol, 150–200 mg of sodium thiopental), which should be given while monitoring hemodynamics. To maintain hemodynamic stability, preventing both hypertensive and tachycardic responses as well as hypotension which potentially may compromise cerebral perfusion pressure (CPP), the anesthetic given should be carefully titrated using standard or invasive blood pressure monitoring.

Risks of using the head holder with pins include bleeding, air embolism (especially in sitting position), and scalp and eye laceration. It is important that the deep level of anesthesia or/and muscular paralyzers are maintained in a patient with pin holder frame. An inadvertent patient movement may cause severe bleeding with scalp laceration, and even cervical cord injury with permanent neurological deficit. Patients should be adequately anesthetized until the head holder is removed. If the surgical procedure is to be done with the patient awake and in a pinhead holder in-situ, local anesthesia at the pin sites (skin and periosteum) and placement of a scalp block must provide substantial analgesia and patient comfort. A regional scalp block post craniotomy is currently considered superior to other techniques for postoperative analgesia (8).

Complications of head and neck positioning

Malpositioning of the head and neck may alter cerebral blood flow in the vertebral and carotid arteries and impair venous outflow from the brain (9). This is particularly dangerous in geriatric patients with inadequate collateral cerebral circulation, osteophytes, and arthritis, potentially causing brainstem and cervical spine ischemia, quadriparesis, or quadriplegia (10).

Hyperflexion may reduce the anterior-posterior size of the hypopharynx, causing ischemia of the base of the tongue leading to pharyngeal and tongue edema. This complication is more common when foreign bodies (transesophageal echocardiography [TEE] probe, oral airway) are used. *Hyperflexion, hyperextension, and hyper-rotation* of the neck and head should be avoided. At least 3–4 cm should be allowed between the chin and chest with the neck and head flexion. The head should not be rotated more than 45° laterally from the body's sagittal axis. If more rotation is needed, lateral rotation of the whole body should be considered, or a supportive chest roll placed under the opposite shoulder. Also, any external pressure on the neck (e.g., with the neck collar fixation device or endotracheal tube [ETT]) and "head-down" position should be avoided because of the potential

impairment of cerebral venous outflow with subsequent brain and airway swelling resulting in poor surgical conditions, enhanced surgical bleeding, and even cerebral hemorrhage or ischemia. Fifteen degrees head-up position is generally optimal during neurosurgery to allow adequate venous drainage. Monitoring of the ICP or jugular bulb pressure (JBP) can be helpful during the head and neck positioning. An increase in ICP and JBP might indicate inadequate head and neck positioning. An increase in JBP by 1–2 cm H_2O, or above CVP, would indicate an obstruction of the venous outflow (11).

Preoperative assessment of the range of motion of the head and neck should be performed in every geriatric patient. An ability to move the neck without signs of neurological deterioration such as paresthesias, pain, and dizziness may guide an appropriate intraoperative head and neck positioning. However, the anesthesiologist should be aware that range of motion in the anesthetized, and especially in the paralyzed patient, may be misleadingly overestimated. As a general rule, hyperflexion, hyperextension, lateral fixation, or rotation should be avoided if feasible. Use of neck radiography and transcranial Doppler should be considered (12,13).

BODY POSITIONING

There are five basic body positions utilized in neurological surgery: supine, lateral, prone, sitting, and three-quarters. Each position has special considerations with respect to desired effects and risks, such as compromise in ventilation and hemodynamic stability.

Supine position

This is the most frequently utilized position in neurosurgery. It allows surgical access to the frontal lobes and anterior portion of the spine. An invasive blood pressure transducer should be positioned and zeroed at the level of the external auditory canal (the skull base). There are three types of supine position utilized in neurosurgery.

1. *Horizontal position:* When the patient is lying on his/her back on a straight surgical table. This position is poorly tolerated by the awake patient even for a short period of time due to suboptimal positioning of the hip and knee joints. Special consideration should include prevention

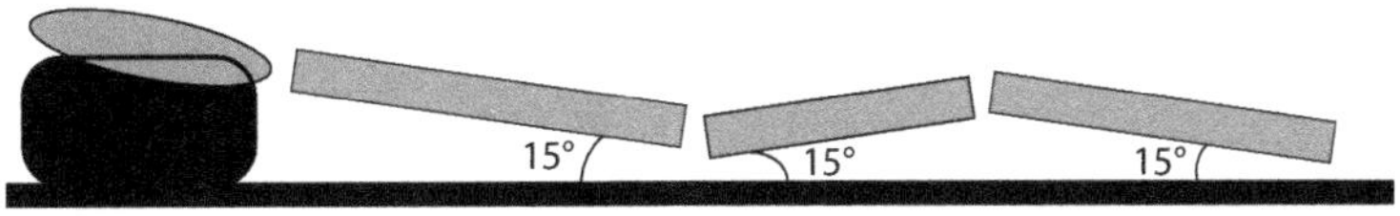

Figure 13.1 Lawn-chair (contoured) position.

of possible skin and peripheral nerve injuries, as well as positioning of the arms.

2. *Lawn chair (contoured) position* (Figure 13.1): This is a modification of the horizontal position, with 15° angulation and flexion at the trunk-thigh-knee. Advantages of this position are more physiological positions of the lumbar spine, hips, and knees, facilitation of venous drainage from the brain secondary to head elevation, and improvement of venous drainage from the lower extremities secondary to elevation of the legs.

3. *Head-up tilt (reverse Trendelenburg) position*: This is a modification of the horizontal position with a 10°–15° surgical table angulation from the horizontal axis. The major advantage of this positioning is improvement of venous drainage from the brain.

ADVANTAGES

The advantages of the supine position include the following: it is the easiest and safest position (does not require endotracheal tube disconnection or invasive monitoring during re-positioning); it provides the best approach to the airway; there is minimal risk for genital and breast injuries and low risk for venous air embolism, pneumocephalus, or vision loss; there is less risk for postoperative upper airway edema or facial soft tissue swelling.

CONCERNS

Anesthesia concerns related to supine position and measurements to prevent them are as follows:

1. Often requires head and neck manipulation to provide surgical comfort. Potentially may impair cerebral venous return leading to brain edema and macroglossia, and nerve damage. Hyperflexion, hyperextension, and rotation more than 45° in relation to body axis should be avoided; head should be elevated to 10°–15°.

2. *Positioning of upper extremities*: To minimize risk of *brachial plexus injury*, the arm should not be abducted more than 90°, and excessive traction down of the shoulders should be avoided (3).

To reduce *ulnar nerve injury*, the upper extremity should be either neutrally positioned or slightly supinated when an arm board is used, to decrease pressure on the postcondylar groove of the humerus; when the arm is tucked at the side, the forearm should stay in a neutral position; flexion of the elbow increases the risk. Although exact methods of prevention of *radial nerve injury* are not clear, the pressure in the spiral groove of the humerus from prolonged contact with a hard surface may increase the risk of radial neuropathy, prolonged pressure on the radial nerve in the spiral groove of the humerus should be avoided, if possible. Periodic assessment of upper extremity position during long surgery should be done, if feasible (3).

3. Vulnerable body pressure points should be protected. Female breasts should be positioned centrally.

4. With the anterior approach to the cervical spine and soft tissue traction for 5 hours or longer, *upper airway edema* is a concern. Avoidance of excessive and/or prolonged surgical traction as well as fluid shifting might be helpful. If there are signs of upper airway swelling, the patient's trachea should not be extubated at the completion of the surgery, and the patient should be transferred to the ICU with the endotracheal tube in-situ.

Lateral position

The lateral position ensures an optimal surgical approach to the temporal and parietal lobes (Figures 13.2 and 13.3).

ADVANTAGES

The advantages of lateral positioning include comfortable approach to patient's airway if the patient is positioned facing anesthesiologist, less risk for postoperative upper airway edema compared with sitting and prone positions, minimal risk for head position-related injuries, minor risk for venous air embolism or pneumocephalus, low

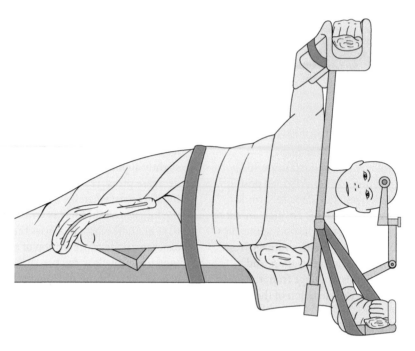

Figure 13.2 Lateral position, head in pins. Dependent arm is hung under the operating table; an upper arm is placed on the arm board.

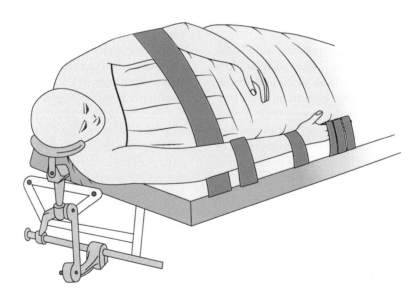

Figure 13.3 Lateral position, head on horseshoe pad. Dependent arm is positioned on the operating table and an arm board, an upper arm is placed over the trunk on the pillow.

risk of visual loss, and minimal risk for breast and genital injuries.

CONCERNS

Anesthesia concerns related to the lateral position and measures to prevent them are as follows:

1. Upper extremity injuries secondary to *brachial plexus* and/or *compression of dependent axillary artery*: Placement of chest axillary roll under the upper chest and away from axilla and avoidance of excessive traction of axilla should be done in every lateral case.

2. Lower extremity injuries related to common peroneal and saphenous nerve injuries: Placement of pillows between knees and ankles as well as avoidance of tubing or catheter presence under or below the legs is recommended.

Prone position

The prone position permits a satisfactory surgical approach to the posterior fossa and the posterior portion of the spine column. Various tables and frames are used in the prone position (Figures 13.4 through 13.7). The choice of frame depends on both surgical and anesthesia preference and should be discussed prior to positioning.

ADVANTAGES

Advantages of the prone position are less risk for venous air embolism (12% of cases) compared with sitting position, less risk for pneumocephalus and quadriplegia compared with sitting position, less risk for cerebral ischemic injuries and preservation of cerebral perfusion pressure when invasive blood pressure monitoring transducer is placed and zeroed at the level of external auditory canal (the skull base) rather than at the level of atrium.

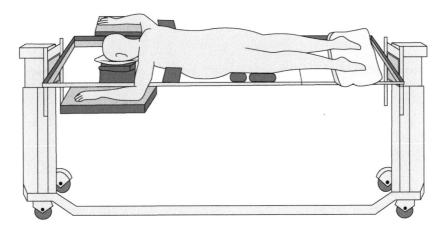

Figure 13.4 Prone position: Jackson frame. Patients with stable spine can be positioned on the Jackson frame directly from supine position. Patients with unstable spine can be positioned on the Jackson table with the following steps: Step 1—supine position on the Jackson table; Step 2—Jackson frame is put over the patient, the thoracic pad is adjusted to support shoulders and thoracic cage, two side pelvic pads are adjusted to the pelvis, and two other side pads are adjusted to support the thighs; the patient is compressed between the table and the frame; Step 3—flipping 180° into prone position; Step 4—after the flipping into prone position has been completed and the Jackson table has been removed from the patient's back, the patient is lying on the Jackson frame. The patient's abdomen hangs free, pelvis is supported, legs are supported and are positioned at the heart level, and the head may be positioned on a foam pillow or headrest or may be fixed with the Mayfield frame.

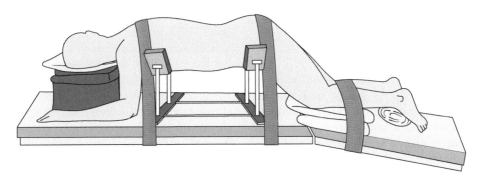

Figure 13.5 Prone position: Relton Hall frame. Positioning on the Relton Hall frame: abdomen hangs free, pelvis is supported, legs are positioned below the heart, head is positioned on the foam pillow or headrest.

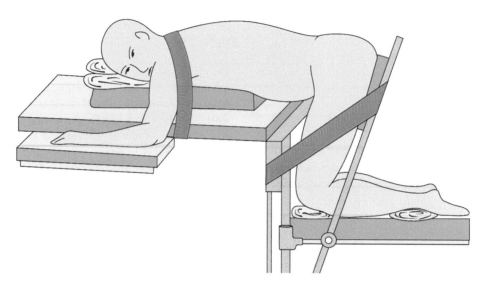

Figure 13.6 Prone position: Andrews frame. Positioning on the Andrews frame: abdomen hangs free, pelvis is partially supported, legs are positioned below the heart, head is positioned on the foam pillow or headrest.

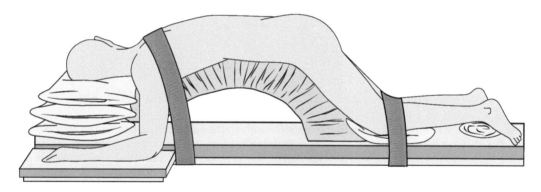

Figure 13.7 Prone position: Wilson frame. Positioning on the Wilson frame: abdomen is partially compressed, pelvis is partially supported, legs are positioned below the trunk, head is positioned on the pillow.

CONCERNS

Anesthesia concerns related to prone position and measures to prevent are as follows.

Monitors

Proper placement requires disconnection of the patient from the ventilator and monitoring devices. Preoxygenation before positioning is recommended, as it may prevent desaturation. Pulse oximetry and/or arterial line should be left in place wherever possible. Limited airway access and copious oral secretions during the long prone procedure may weaken *fixation of the endotracheal tube.* While securing endotracheal tube, additional adhesives with tape should be considered. Judicious use of the cotton tie for fixation of the ETT in combination with tape, adhesive glue, and adhesive dressing (such as Tegaderm™) covering the tape, may be used. Periodical check that the tie is not interfering with surgical field and not compromising venous outflow is essential; the tie should be cut with any suspicion of increased pressure on the neck. To reduce oral secretions, a small dose of intravenous glycopyrrolate (0.2–0.3 mg) may be considered, particularly in patients with copious oral secretions in the beginning of the case (e.g., in heavy tobacco smokers). Free access to the airway, tubing, and connections is essential.

Lung mechanics and gas exchange

In the awake patient, *lung mechanics and gas exchange* in the lungs are optimal regardless of positioning because of perfectly matched ventilation and perfusion across the lungs (14,15). In contrast, anesthesia, muscle paralysis, and positive pressure mechanical ventilation inevitably cause ventilation-perfusion mismatch. In anesthetized prone position, however, *ventilation-perfusion matching* is better than in supine position predominantly due to (i) more even distribution of the perfusion because of higher pulmonary blood flow in the dorsal parts of the normal lungs compared to the ventral parts, and (ii) decrease of gravitational pressure of the abdomen improving respiratory mechanics by the released pressure on the diaphragm with subsequent increase in lung volume, functional residual capacity, and transpulmonary pressure (16,17). Therefore, a Jackson table supporting the chest and the pelvis but leaving the abdominal wall free is the best table for optimal gas exchange in the lungs and venous return to the heart (Figure 13.4). Aside from the surgical preference, use of the Jackson table and frame should be considered in patients undergoing prolonged surgery with potential risk of respiratory compromise, such as respiratory disease or morbid obesity.

Postoperative visual loss

Postoperative visual loss (POVL) is a rare complication of the prone position that predominantly (89% of POVL) occurs due to an ischemic optic neuropathy (ION). Although the incidence of POVL has not been reported higher than 0.2%, it represents the most devastating complication of modern spine surgery (18,19). The highest risk of ION is in patients undergoing prolonged major prone spine surgery such as scoliosis correction and posterior lumbar fusion (18,19).

ION usually develops bilaterally and is associated with anesthetic duration greater than 6 hours, blood loss (more than 1000 mL), and blood transfusion (20). ION is also associated with other conditions, including diabetes, hypertension, smoking, atherosclerosis, anemia, ulcerative colitis, preexisting renal disease, sex, and obesity (19,21). The pathophysiology of ION is multifactorial and poorly understood, as it was shown not to be related to direct compression on the optic globe or any other specific prone position-related factor. ION has been reported to occur in patients who

were placed on different frames and tables (Wilson frame, Jackson table, etc.) and with various head-supporting devises (Mayfield pinning, foam and gel pad), and independently whether or not regular eye check was documented during the surgery.

The current hypothesis of ION suggests hypoperfusion and decreased oxygen delivery to the optic nerve resulting from the decrease in the perfusion pressure of the nerve due to increased venous pressure and venous congestion. This hypothesis is partly supported by the fact that positioning on the Wilson frame (Figure 13.7), where the upper trunk and head are lower than the heart, was found to be an independent risk factor for ION (21). Another important intraoperative risk factor for ION supporting the venous congestion hypothesis is inadequate colloid administration during prolonged spine surgery, as it was shown that patients receiving predominantly crystalloids had a higher risk for ION (22). The only intraoperative measures proven to prevent ION are (i) avoidance of head positioning below the heart level, and (ii) use of colloids rather than crystalloids during long spine cases. Preferably, the Wilson table should be avoided in the long spine cases; if unavoidable, the table should be elevated into the reverse Trendelenburg, to position the head at least at the level of the heart, or higher to at least 10° from supine.

The latest ASA practice advisory for the prevention of perioperative visual loss associated with spine surgery was published in 2012 (23). The American Society of Anesthesiologists (ASA) advisory recommends (i) positioning the head level at or higher than the heart, (ii) consideration of staged spine procedures (to decrease surgical time and blood loss), and (iii) use of colloids along with crystalloids to maintain intravascular volume in patients who have substantial blood loss (23). The French Society of Anesthesia and Intensive Care (SFAR) in conjunction with the French Ophthalmology Society and the French-Speaking Intensive Care Society recently published their guidelines for eye protection in anesthesia and intensive care prevention of ION in prone spine surgery. The guidelines recommend elevation of the head and avoidance of hypotension, severe anemia, and hypovolemia in patients with risk factors (obese, male, hypertensive, and vascular risk factors) (24). However, the guidelines do not provide a specific lower limit of blood pressure or hemoglobin. The difference in methodology used for the development of guidelines probably led to some differences in ASA and SFAR recommendations.

The incidence of perioperative ION in prone spine surgery has decreased between 1998 and 2012 (25). This is probably due to modifications of the historical practice with the abandonment of the Wilson frame, careful positioning of the head with elevation above the heart, the trend to decrease surgical time with staging of long surgeries with risk of the massive bleeding, and popularization of minimally invasive procedures (26).

Central retinal artery occlusion (CRAO) is another rare cause of POVL, which is known to be related to direct or indirect pressure on the globe (16). Clinical features include unilateral periorbital and scleral swelling; fundoscopic examination reveals the hallmark "cherry red spot." It has never been reported in patients using the Mayfield frame. The incidence of CRAO has remained constant (25).

The best POVL management options include high level of suspicion, postoperative vision assessment as soon as the patient is awake, and if any concern remains an urgent ophthalmologic consultation should be obtained.

In summary, practical measures to prevent POVL in the prone position include (i) avoidance any external pressure on eyes, rechecking eyes every 30 min, (ii) aggressive treatment of profound arterial hypotension (probably less than 85 mmHg systolic for normotensive patients or within 20% of the patient's baseline level), (iii) avoidance of severe anemia (no lower threshold for blood transfusion is recommended to date), and (iv) avoidance of prolonged head-down position leading to venous congestion. Postoperative vision assessment should be performed as soon as the patient is awake; if any concern remains, an urgent ophthalmologic consultation should be obtained.

Brachial plexus injury

Excessive traction and hyperextension of shoulders and arms should be restricted. However, in the prone position more than 90° of arm abduction can be tolerated.

Risk of upper airway and tongue (macroglossia) swelling and cranial nerve damage

Judicious use of intravenous fluids and avoidance of excessive head flexion may minimize the risk of macroglossia. At least 2–3 finger-breadths of thyromental distance should be allowed. Unnecessary foreign bodies in the pharynx (TEE probe, oral airway) should be avoided if possible. Properly-sized oral and/or nasogastric tube is usually safe.

Venous air embolism

To minimize venous air embolism risk, limit steep head-up position. Optimal head-up position is 10°–15°.

Sitting position

The sitting position provides the best surgical exposure and anatomic orientation to the posterior fossa and the posterior area of the cervical spine.

ADVANTAGES

Advantages of the sitting position include low ICP, good cerebral-spinous fluid and venous outflow, minimal bleeding, reduced risk for cranial nerve damage, and less need for diuretic therapy and blood transfusions. The sitting position also provides easy airway access, absence of risk for visual loss, and excellent expiratory and ventilatory conditions.

Due to a high risk of historical mortality from venous air embolism with the classical sitting position (Figure 13.8), the modern neurosurgical approach to posterior fossa and posterior cervical spine surgeries recommends a modified semi-recumbent (or semi-sitting) position (27) (Figure 13.9).

CONCERNS

Anesthesia concerns related to sitting position and measures to prevent them are as follows.

Venous air embolism

Venous air embolism (VAE) is an unavoidable consequence of the sitting position, where the surgical field is located much above the right atrium. As a magnitude of the right atrial pressure (normal central venous pressure [CVP]) cannot approach a value of the distance between the level of the heart and the level of the surgical opening, the venous pressure at the surgical field is inevitably negative compared to CVP. The pressure difference creates a "siphon effect," sucking air into the venous circulation, particularly into the noncollapsible capillary venous circulation of the skull and venous sinuses.

A reported incidence of intraoperative VAE in patients in both the classical and semi-sitting position depends on the degree of the VAE and

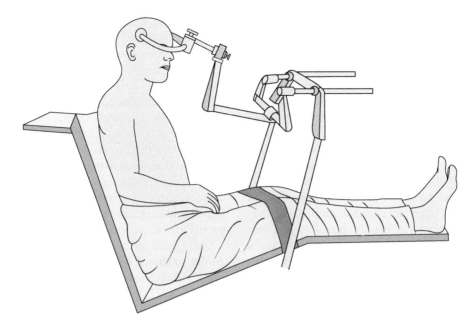

Figure 13.8 Sitting position: Classic sitting position.

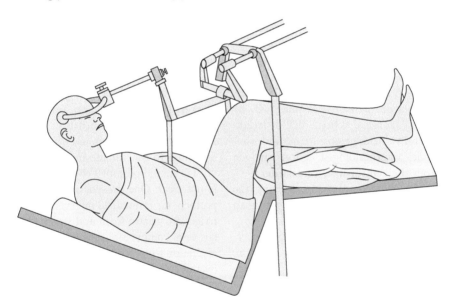

Figure 13.9 Modified (semi-recumbent or semi-sitting) sitting position: Trunk is lowered compared to sitting position, head level is above the heart but much less than in sitting position, hips are flexed at least at 90°, knees are flexed and at the level of the head.

monitoring used, ranging between 2%–76% when monitored with TEE (27–29). Currently, there is no uniform grading system of the VAE; it varies between studies and ranges between clinically insignificant microbubbles identified by precordial Doppler or TEE to various degrees of decrease of end-tidal carbon dioxide, and to profound hemodynamic instability due to massive air embolism leading to abrupt decrease of preload and cardiac output (30). Schmitt and Hemmerling (31) reported 80% (in 13 out of 18 patients) incidence of VAE just with the positive end-expiratory pressure (PEEP) release at the end of the surgery while the patients were still in the sitting position and/or with repositioning to the supine position. Clinically significant VAE should be considered when intervention is required to prevent further hemodynamic instability. In this regard, continuous intraoperative monitoring of the right atrium air should be essential either with precordial Doppler or TEE during the sitting position, as well as invasive blood pressure monitoring. Use of TEE is recommended by the ASA Practice Guidelines for Perioperative Transesophageal Echocardiography for venous air embolism and patent foramen ovale in neurosurgery (Category B2 evidence) (32).

Compared to TEE, precordial transthoracic Doppler does not require special training; it is non-invasive, inexpensive, readily available, and easy to use. Optimal placement of the precordial probe should be guided by detecting the highest pitch over the chest with the intravenous injection of agitated saline. The classical positioning of the probe is at the right upper sternal border. A central line preferably with a multi-orifice catheter should be placed after induction of anesthesia into the right atrium to assure air aspiration, if needed. Correct placement of the catheter may be verified by intravenous electrocardiography, chest radiography, or TEE.

Detection of air bubbles by precordial Doppler or TEE should be treated immediately by both surgeon and anesthesiologist, especially if this is accompanied by a decrease in end-tidal CO_2 by 3 mm Hg or more. Surgical actions include irrigation of the operative field, gelatin foam, and waxing of the bone; anesthesiologist actions include aspiration from the central line, ventilation with $FiO_2 = 1$, jugular vein compression, moving the patient into Trendelenburg position, and giving an intravenous fluid bolus (Table 13.1).

Maintaining normovolemia and adequate perfusion pressure is essential in the sitting position. While maintaining normovolemia, fluid boluses prior to positioning into sitting from supine are recommended (27,33). The beneficial effect of intravenous boluses of colloids (6% hydroxyethyl starch [HES]) compared to Ringer lactate in maintaining hemodynamic stability during the sitting position was demonstrated (33) and should be considered in hypovolemic patients. Judicious use of colloids with slow titration guided by the invasive hemodynamic monitoring (CVP, systolic pressure variation) or TEE should be applied in patients with congestive heart failure in whom hypervolemia may be of concern. Vasoactive medications and inotropes should be used as appropriate. If a patient is

normovolemic, intravenous boluses of ephedrine (5–20 mg) and phenylephrine (50–100 μg) and continuous infusion of phenylephrine may be used to maintain cerebral perfusion mean pressure not lower than 60 mmHg. However, since assessment of cerebral autoregulation in anesthetized patients is not routinely evaluated, an exact number for the lower limit of autoregulation is unknown. Ideally, intraoperative fluid management should be goal-directed and adjusted to the preoperatively assessed cerebral autoregulation. At least two inotropes (norepinephrine, dopamine, dobutamine, epinephrine) should be readily available for cardiovascular support in massive VAE.

During the sitting position, *positive pressure ventilation* should be applied to maintain normocarbia. Application of PEEP above physiological level of 4 cm H_2O may prevent VAE, but it should not be applied in patients with PFO, where it may exaggerate right-to-left shunt and mitigate paradoxical air embolism.

To prevent paradoxical air embolism, every patient should be evaluated for the presence of patent foramen ovale (PFO) before surgery in the sitting position. Optimally, a preoperative test should be done in a conscious patient, using echocardiography (TEE or transthoracic echocardiography) or transcranial Doppler (TCD) (13,34), and some authors advocate for PFO repair prior to neurosurgery (35). However, PFO is often assessed in anesthetized patients after induction to general anesthesia. Whether a finding of PFO should prompt a change in the surgical plan is not clear. One prospective study utilizing strict protocol for immediate interventions (surgical fluid irrigation, gelatin foam and waxing the bone, jugular vein compressions, ventilation with $FiO_2 = 1$, aspiration from central venous line [CVL]) reported overall 10% if incidence of any VAE (1–7 events per patient) with 2% of clinically significant VAE, and no paradoxical air embolism (36).

In summary, preventive measures for venous air embolism and paradoxical air embolism include adequate monitoring with precordial Doppler or TEE, CVL, adequate hydration with crystalloids and colloids before the induction and positioning to maintain adequate circulating blood volume.

Postoperative pneumocephalus and tension pneumocephalus

Pneumocephalus is defined as the presence of air within any of the intracranial compartments. The mechanism of pneumocephalus is under pressure compared with the outside atmospheric pressure, when in most circumstances a valve mechanism allows air to enter the skull but prevents it from escaping, thus creating a pressure differential. While *simple pneumocephalus* occurs nearly in all patients after sitting neurosurgery and is typically asymptomatic and requires no treatment, *tension pneumocephalus* is rare (about 3%) (37). Clinical deterioration of the patient is usually abrupt due to increased ICP secondary to pneumocephalus, and requires immediate surgical decompression. Clinical signs of postoperative tension pneumocephalus include delayed awakening, new neurological deficit, headache, and signs of increased ICP. Consider immediate head computerized tomography (CT) for differential diagnosis. Twist drill hole and dural puncture for decompression may be considered for treatment if needed.

As volume of pneumocephalus might be increased by nitrous oxide (N_2O), if N_2O is used during the surgery it should be discontinued 20–30 minutes *before* closure of the scull. Pneumocephalus can also develop without the use of N_2O and may persist for weeks after surgery. The majority of patients with asymptomatic pneumocephalus can be treated conservatively. About one-third of patients undergoing neurosurgery in the sitting position, however, may develop transient lethargy with supratentorial pneumocephalus (27); more recent data suggest a 3% incidence of clinically significant pneumocephalus (38).

Quadriplegia

Quadriplegia is a rare and devastating complication resulting from cervical spine ischemia, but other conditions such as cerebral palsy and stroke can cause a similar-appearing paralysis. Elderly patients and patients with cervical spine defects or vascular pathologies have a higher risk. Another risk factor is head and neck hyperflexion. In geriatric patients, preoperative assessment of neck and head stability, including imaging (radiography, CT, TCD) may be advocated (8, 12). During positioning, sufficient distance between the chin and neck (at least two finger-breadths) is recommended to avoid neck hyperflexion.

Turning the patient from supine to the sitting position

This maneuver often causes hemodynamic instability due to decreased venous return, leading to decreased stroke volume with subsequent decrease in mean systemic and pulmonary arterial pressure and increase in systemic and pulmonary resistance (39). Jugular veins are usually collapsed, and venous outflow is dependent on the vertebral circulation (40). Although cerebral oxygenation may initially decrease, reflecting decrease of cardiac output (41), cerebral oxygenation normalizes with stabilization of hemodynamics (42). If osmotherapy is required, the preference should be given to hypertonic saline due to less diuretic effect (43) and better preservation of cardiac output compared to mannitol (44). Maintenance of normovolemia, fluid boluses, use of compression devices on the legs (45), and slow, incremental adjustment of table position may prevent an abrupt hemodynamic instability.

Swelling and cranial nerve damage

To prevent *swelling of upper airway, tongue (macroglossia), and cranial nerve damage*, excessive head flexion should be avoided. At least 2–3 finger-breadths of thyromental distance should be maintained. Unnecessary foreign bodies in the pharynx (TEE probe, oral airway) may mitigate obstruction of the venous outflow and should be avoided if possible. Properly-sized oral and/or nasogastric tube is not a concern.

Peripheral nerve injuries

Prolonged sitting position can be damaging to the common peroneal and sciatic nerve. As the sciatic nerve crosses both hip and knee joints, to minimize *sciatic nerve injury*, excessive flexion of the knee and extension of the hip should be avoided (3). The buttock gel pad prevents excessive pressure on the sciatic nerve.

Impairment of brain perfusion

Invasive blood pressure transducer should be zeroed at the level of the circle of Willis. The blood pressure transducer shall be positioned and zeroed at the level of external auditory canal (the skull base) rather at the level of the atrium, to reflect and maintain adequate cerebral perfusion. Maintain CPP at 60 mmHg.

Three-quarters position

This position resembles the lateral position and is utilized for posterior fossa and parieto-occipital region access (Figure 13.9).

ADVANTAGES

Advantages of this position include lower risk of venous air embolism compared with sitting position, and acceptable airway access.

CONCERNS

A major anesthesia concern related to the three-quarter position is brachial plexus injury due to both compression of brachial plexus on the dependent side and stretching of the non-dependent shoulder toward the legs for better surgical exposure. Placement of an axillary roll under the upper chest and away from axilla may prevent injury. Excessive traction of the non-dependent shoulder should be avoided. Other risks are similar to those of the lateral position.

SUMMARY

Positioning of geriatric patients for neurosurgery is an important component of perioperative care. It requires preoperative discussion of risks and benefits and cooperation between the anesthesia and surgical teams. Patient positioning includes multiple technical and physiological challenges. Recognition of potential dangers of patient positioning and proper application of preventive measures decreases risks of perioperative complications. A careful patient-centered team approach to patient positioning will have a significant impact on perioperative management and will improve perioperative morbidity.

REFERENCES

1. Chan SW, Tulloch E, Cooper ES, Smith A, Wojcik W, Norman JE. Montgomery and informed consent: Where are we now? BMJ. 2017 May 12;357.
2. Drummond JC, Patel PM. Neurosurgical anaesthesia. In Miller RD (ed) Anesthesia. 7th ed. Philadelphia: Churchill Livingstone; 2010. pp. 2045–88.
3. Practice Advisory for the Prevention of Perioperative Peripheral Neuropathies 2018. An updated report by the American Society of Anesthesiologists Task Force on prevention of perioperative peripheral neuropathies. Anesthesiology. 2018;128:11–26.
4. Welch MB, Brummett CM, Welch TD, Tremper KK, Shanks AM, Guglani P, Mashour GA. Perioperative peripheral nerve injuries: A retrospective study of 380,680 cases during a 10-year period at a single institution. Anesthesiology. 2009 Sep;111(3):490–7.
5. Chui J, Murkin JM, Posner KL, Domino KB. Perioperative peripheral nerve injury after general anesthesia: A qualitative systematic review. Anesth Analg. 2018;127(1):134–43.
6. Clutterbuck R, Tamargo R. Surgical positioning and exposures for cranial procedures. In Winn HR (ed) Yomans Neurological Surgery. 5th ed. Philadelphia: Sounders, Elsevier Inc.; 2004. pp. 623–45.
7. Goodkin R, Mesiwala A. General principles on operative positioning. In Winn HR (ed) Yomans Neurological Surgery. 5th ed. Philadelphia: Sounders, Elsevier Inc.; 2004. pp. 595–621.
8. Akhigbe T, Zolnourian A. Use of regional scalp block for pain management after craniotomy: Review of literature and critical appraisal of evidence. J Clin Neurosci. 2017 Nov;45:44–7.
9. Toole JF. Effects of change of head, limb and body position on cephalic circulation. N Engl J Med. 1968;279:307–11.
10. Vandam L. Positioning of patients for operation. In Rogers M, Tinker J, Covino B (eds) Principles and Practice of Anesthesiology. St. Louis: Mosby-Year Book, Inc.; 1993. pp. 703–18.
11. Rozet I, Vavilala MS. Risk and benefit of patient positioning during neurosurgical care. Anesthesiol Clin. 2007 Sep;25(3):631–53.
12. Ammirati M, Lamki TT, Shaw AB, Forde B, Nakano I, Mani M. A streamlined protocol for the use of the semi-sitting position in neurosurgery: A report on 48 consecutive procedures. J Clin Neurosci. 2013 Jan;20(1):32–4.
13. Fudickar A, Leiendecker J, Köhling A, Hedderich J, Steinfath M, Bein B. Transcranial Doppler sonography as a potential screening tool for preanaesthetic evaluation: A prospective observational study. Eur J Anaesthesiol. 2012 Oct;29(10):471–6.
14. Glenny RW, Robertson HT. Spatial distribution of ventilation and perfusion: Mechanisms and regulation. Compr Physiol. 2011 Jan;1(1): 375–95.
15. Petersson J, Glenny RW. Gas exchange and ventilation-perfusion relationships in the lung. Eur Respir J. 2014 Oct;44(4):1023–41.

16. Johnson NJ, Luks AM, Glenny RW. Gas exchange in the prone posture. *Respir Care.* 2017 Aug;62(8):1097–110.

17. Kumaresan A, Gerber R, Mueller A, Loring SH, Talmor D. Effects of prone positioning on transpulmonary pressures and end-expiratory volumes in patients without lung disease. *Anesthesiology.* 2018 Jun;128(6):1187–92.

18. Holy SE, Tsai JH, McAllister RK et al. Perioperative ischemic optic neuropathy. A case control analysis of 126,666 surgical procedures at a single institution. *Anesthesiology.* 2009;110:246–53.

19. Patil CG, Lad EM, Lad SP et al. Visual loss after spine surgery: A population-based study. *Spine.* 2008;33:1491–6.

20. Lee LA, Roth S, Posner KL et al. The American Society of Anesthesiologists Postoperative Visual Loss Registry. Analysis of 93 spine surgery cases with postoperative visual loss. *Anesthesiology.* 2006;105:652–9.

21. The Postoperative Visual Loss Study Group. Risk factors associated with ischemic optic neuropathy after spinal fusion surgery. *Anesthesiology.* 2012;116:15–24.

22. Ozcan MS, Praetel C, Bhatti MT et al. The effect of body inclination during prone positioning on intraocular pressure in awake volunteers: A comparison of two operating tables. *Anesth Analg.* 2004;99:1152–8.

23. Roth S, Connis RT, Domino KB et al. Practice advisory for perioperative visual loss associated with spine surgery. An updated report by the American Society of Anesthesiologists Task Force on Perioperative Visual Loss. *Anesthesiology.* 2012;116:274–85[19].

24. French Society for Anesthesia and Intensive Care (SFAR), French Ophthalmology Society (SFO), French-speaking Intensive Care Society (SRLF) Expert guidelines. Eye protection in anaesthesia and intensive care. *Anaesth Crit Care Pain Med.* 2017;36(6):411–8.

25. Rubin DS, Parakati I, Lee LA et al. Perioperative visual loss in spine fusion surgery: Ischemic optic neuropathy in the United States from 1998 to 2012 in the National Inpatient Sample. *Anesthesiology.* 2016;125:457–64.

26. Todd MM. News. Good. But why is the incidence of postoperative ischemic optic neuropathy falling? *Anesthesiology.* 2016;125: 445–8.

27. Jadik S, Wissing H, Friedrich K, Beck J, Seifert V, Raabe A. A standardized protocol for the prevention of clinically relevant venous air embolism during neurosurgical interventions in the semisitting position. *Neurosurgery.* 2009 Mar;64(3):533–8.

28. Papadopoulos G, Kuhly P, Brock M, Rudolph KH, Link J, Eyrich K. Venous and paradoxical air embolism in the sitting position. A prospective study with transoesophageal echocardiography. *Acta Neurochir (Wien).* 1994; 126:140–3.

29. Stendel R, Gramm HJ, Schröder K, Lober C, Brock M. Transcranial Doppler ultrasonography as a screening technique for detection of a patent foramen ovale before surgery in the sitting position. *Anesthesiology.* 2000;93: 971–5.

30. Gracia I, Fabregas N. Craniotomy in sitting position: Anesthesiology management. *Curr Opin Anaesthesiol.* 2014 Oct;27(5):474–83.

31. Schmitt HJ, Hemmerling TM. Venous air emboli occur during release of positive end-expiratory pressure and repositioning after sitting position surgery. *Anesth Analg.* 2002 Feb;94(2):400–3.

32. Practice Guidelines for Perioperative Transesophageal Echocardiography. An updated report by the American Society of Anesthesiologists and the Society of Cardiovascular Anesthesiologists Task Force on Transesophageal Echocardiography. *Anesthesiology.* 2010;112(5):1084–96.

33. Lindroos ACB, Niiya T, Silvasti-Lundell M et al. Stroke volume-directed administration of hydroxyethyl starch or Ringer's acetate in sitting position during craniotomy. *Acta Anaesthesiol Scand.* 2013;57:729–36.

34. Jürgens S, Basu S. The sitting position in anaesthesia: Old and new. *Eur J Anaesthesiol.* 2014 May;31(5):285–7.

35. Fathi AR, Eshtehardi P, Meier B. Patent foramen ovale and neurosurgery in sitting position: A systematic review. *Br J Anaesth.* 2009 May;102(5):588–96.

36. Feigl GC, Decker K, Wurms M, Krischek B, Ritz R, Unertl K, Tatagiba M. Neurosurgical procedures in the semisitting position: Evaluation of the risk of paradoxical venous air embolism in patients with a patent foramen ovale. *World Neurosurg.* 2014 Jan;81(1):159–64.

37. Duke DA, Lynch JJ, Harner SG et al. Venous air embolism in sitting and supine patients undergoing vestibular schwannoma resection. *Neurosurgery*. 1998;42:1282–6.

38. Hervías A, Valero R, Hurtado P, Gracia I, Perelló L, Tercero FJ, González JJ, Fàbregas N. [Detection of venous air embolism and patent foramen ovale in neurosurgery patients in sitting position]. *Neurocirugia (Astur)*. 2014 May–Jun;25(3):108–15.

39. Tsaousi GG, Karakoulas KA, Amaniti EN, Soultati ID, Zouka MD, Vasilakos DG. Correlation of central venous-arterial and mixed venous-arterial carbon dioxide tension gradient with cardiac output during neurosurgical procedures in the sitting position. *Eur J Anaesthesiol*. 2010 Oct;27(10):882–9.

40. Cirovic S, Walsh C, Fraser WD et al. The effect of posture and positive pressure breathing on the hemodynamics of the internal jugular vein. *Aviat Space Environ Med*. 2003;74:125–31.

41. Closhen D, Berres M, Werner C, Engelhard K, Schramm P. Influence of beach chair position on cerebral oxygen saturation: A comparison of INVOS and FORE-SIGHT cerebral oximeter. *J Neurosurg Anesthesiol*. 2013 Oct;25(4):414–9.

42. Schramm P, Tzanova I, Hagen F, Berres M, Closhen D, Pestel G, Engelhard K. Cerebral oxygen saturation and cardiac output during anaesthesia in sitting position for neurosurgical procedures: A prospective observational study. *Br J Anaesth*. 2016;117(4):482–8.

43. Rozet I, Tontisirin N, Muangman S, Vavilala MS, Souter MJ, Lee LA, Kincaid MS, Britz GW, Lam AM. Effect of equiosmolar solutions of mannitol versus hypertonic saline on intraoperative brain relaxation and electrolyte balance. *Anesthesiology*. 2007 Nov;107(5):697–704.

44. Tsaousi G, Stazi E, Cinicola M, Bilotta F. Cardiac output changes after osmotic therapy in neurosurgical and neurocritical care patients: A systematic review of the clinical literature. *Br J Clin Pharmacol*. 2018 Apr; 84(4):636–648.

45. Kwak HJ, Lee D, Lee YW, Yu GY, Shinn HK, Kim JY. The intermittent sequential compression device on the lower extremities attenuates the decrease in regional cerebral oxygen saturation during sitting position under sevoflurane anesthesia. *J Neurosurg Anesthesiol*. 2011 Jan;23(1):1–5.

14

Neurotrauma: Geriatric neurotrauma

ALAN J. KOVAR AND ABHIJIT LELE

INTRODUCTION

According to the Centers for Disease Control (CDC), geriatric patients are those above the age of 65 years (1). Patients above the age of 60 years constitute approximately 962 million population in 2017, twice the number as in 1980 (382 million), with projected numbers on the incline for the coming decades (2).

This chapter is dedicated to detailed discussion about epidemiology, pathophysiology, and management of traumatic brain injury (TBI) specific to the geriatric population.

EPIDEMIOLOGY

Traumatic brain injury is a world health burden. Of all the age groups that sustain TBI, the highest incidence is in those 65 years or older, and is consistently high in United States and higher-income countries (3). Traumatic brain injury is a major source of morbidity and mortality in patients above 65 years of age, and is responsible for more than 80,000 emergency visits, of which 75% require hospitalization, amounting to more than $2 billion in healthcare-associated costs annually in United States alone (4). Annual treatment cost of TBI in those 65 or older ranges from $73,000 to $78,000 per patient (3). Age-adjusted rates of TBI for patients 65 years and older are 155.9 per 100,000 population, of which 73.4% have mild injuries (5). The proportion of patients with moderate (23.5%) and severe disabilities (9.7%), and in-hospital mortality (12%) is high (5). The majority of the oldest patients with TBI are female and white (3). Table 14.1 highlights key differences between elderly and young patients with TBI.

Mechanism of injury

Falls (aka, low-level, same-level, or ground level) account for a large proportion of TBI in the elderly (7). According to the CDC, fall-related TBIs among persons aged ≥75 years accounted for 17.9% of the increase in the number of TBI-related emergency department (ED) visits (8), and fall-related TBI (FRTBI) in ages 65 and above can make up anywhere from 37.4% to 89.2% of all TBI-related admissions (7,9).

In a study of TBI in Australia, while overall hospitalization rates of TBI increased by 7.2% per year, the rates of FRTBI increased by 8.4%, with a concomitant increase in non-fall-related TBI by only 2.1% per year (7). Patients who fall are also

Table 14.1 Differences between elderly and young traumatic brain injury (TBI) in the United States

Age (years)	Death rate for TBI[a]	Top etiology for TBI	Hospitalizations for TBI[a]	ED visits for TBI[a]
25–44	14.6	Self-inflicted	65.3	470.0
45–64	17.6	Self-inflicted	79.4	328.2
65+	45.2	Unintentional falls	294.0	603.3

Source: Rates of TBI-related hospitalizations by age group. [Webpage]. 2016; https://www.cdc.gov/traumaticbraininjury/data/rates_hosp_byage.html. Accessed 3/6/2018, 2018. (6)
Abbreviations: TBI, traumatic brain injury; ED, emergency department.
[a] Rates per 100,000 US population.

more likely to have significant comorbidities (often more than three) than those associated with motor vehicle-related TBI (5). Within the geriatric population, falls on same level resulting in TBI, which most commonly occur at home (72.5%), also increase with advancing age (7).

PATHOPHYSIOLOGY

The most common type of injuries seen on computerized tomography (CT) of the head in elderly patients with FRTBI are subdural hemorrhage (45%) (Figure 14.1) (3), concussive injury, and subarachnoid hemorrhage (7). The proportion of

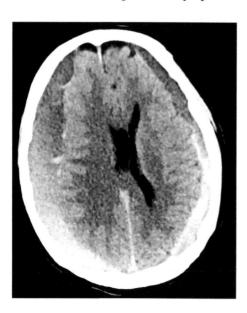

Figure 14.1 Mixed density bilateral subdural hematoma in a 76-year-old patient on warfarin for chronic atrial fibrillation who presented after a ground-level fall.

extradural hematoma decreases with age, while that of subdural hematoma and resultant midline shift increases with age (3). CT lesions are common (57%), despite a reassuring Glasgow Coma Scale (GCS) of 15 (3).

SYSTEMIC IMPLICATIONS

Medical comorbidities are common among this population, and 99% of patients in one study from the UK had at least one comorbidity (3). The most common comorbid conditions are hypertension (38%), cardiac arrhythmias (18%), fluid and electrolyte disorders (17%), diabetes mellitus (15%), and congestive heart failure (13%) (5). Nearly one in five patients older than 65 who were admitted to level I trauma centers with head injuries were on warfarin, and this has been independently shown to be associated with worse outcomes (10).

Unfortunately, age is an independent predictor of poor outcome in the TBI population (11). In a study conducted in Japan, unfavorable outcomes were associated with the Charleston Comorbidities Index, despite reassuring GCS of 13–15 (12).

Table 14.2 highlights important physiological changes associated with aging.

MANAGEMENT

The management of TBI in general is aimed at preservation of cerebral perfusion pressure, cerebral blood flow, and reduction in incidence and severity of secondary brain insults. However, no evidence-based national or international guidelines for management of geriatric neurotrauma exist.

Table 14.2 Cerebral physiologic changes with aging

Category	Description
Structural	Reduction in temporal, cerebellar, and hippocampal volume
Memory	Cognitive decline and reduction in episodic memory
Neurotransmission	Decrease in dopamine, serotonin, and monoamine oxidase
Blood–brain barrier	Increased permeability
Vascular	Thickening of arterial intima, increased vascular resistance, and perfusion pressure in cerebrum
Cerebral metabolic demand for oxygen ($CMRO_2$)	Possible reduction in $CMRO_2$ in frontal lobes
Autoregulation	Shift in the autoregulation curve to the right Increased risk for ischemic conditions under "young" normotensive conditions

Source: Peters R. *Postgrad Med J.* 2006;82(964):84–8; Farrall AJ, Wardlaw JM. *Neurobiol Aging.* 2009;30(3):337–52; Trollor JN, Valenzuela MJ. *Aust N Z J Psychiatry.* 2001;35(6):788–805; Alvis BD, Hughes CG. *Anesthesiol Clin.* 2015;33(3):447–56. (13–16)

Triage to highest level trauma center

Elderly patients with TBI may present with higher GCS than their younger counterparts (17). Hence, triage of patients based on early CT image findings (18) and to the highest trauma level centers, with attention to timely reversal of anticoagulants and neurosurgical consultation, cannot be overemphasized (19). Compared to younger patients, those aged 65 or older are three times more likely to receive a CT head in the emergency department and four times more likely to be admitted to the intensive care unit (ICU) (3). In a study of 437 patients with GCS 15, 21.7% had a change in management (either surgical management, medication change, additional imaging, or ICU admission) after CT results (20).

Data from Florida and New York show that older patients are chronically under-triaged from 15%–80% of the time, as they are often deemed "non-urgent," and exhibit longer wait times potentially leading to delayed definitive care (21). Based on results from a study using the National Trauma Data Bank (1999–2008), across all levels of injury, since patients older than 60 years of age have a higher mortality, age above 60 years may be a criterion for the highest level of trauma activation even with injury severity score of 0–15 (22), as geriatric patients with TBI often present with reassuring GCS compared to younger patients with similar injury severity (3).

Preservation of neuronal function

In order to reduce the risk of cerebral hypoperfusion, changes in cerebral physiology that occur with age warrant discussion. It is believed that with advancing age, there is shift to the right in cerebral perfusion pressure curve, as well as changes in cerebral arteriolar tone (reference). The 4th edition of the Brain Trauma Foundation Guidelines recommend maintaining systolic blood pressure at ≥ 100 mmHg for patients 50–69 years old or at ≥ 110 mmHg or above for patients 15–49 or over 70 years old to decrease mortality and improve outcomes (23).

Neuromonitoring

Extensive evidence to support or refute the benefit of intracranial pressure monitoring in the elderly patient population is lacking. Based on the prevalence of intracranial pressure monitoring reported in studies on patients reported to the National Trauma Data Bank, elderly patients as a group are less likely to receive monitoring compared to those of younger age.

Using an intraventricular catheter, intracranial pressure monitoring may be associated with reduction in in-hospital mortality and improved 6-month outcomes in those aged 65 or older based on a single-center prospective observational study (24).

Elderly patients with TBI are likely to receive a low prevalence of ICP monitoring compared to younger patients. They demonstrate lower ICP and higher Cerebral Perfusion Pressure (CPP) profiles but have worse vascular pressure reactivity and autoregulation abnormalities compared to the younger population (3).

Neurosurgical intervention

In a study of 3194 patients enrolled between 1998 and 2011 in the Japan Neurotrauma Data Bank, 54% of all patients aged 65 years or older were given surgical management (craniectomy, craniotomy, or burr-hole evacuation). Compared to the younger age group, those 65 years or older had more favorable outcomes at 6 months (18% vs 7%), and less mortality (62% vs 81%). The most severely injured (GCS 3–5) had more unfavorable outcomes (96% vs 79%), and more mortality (87% vs 57%) compared to those with GCS 6–15 (25).

Geriatric trauma patients have a higher incidence of pulmonary and infectious complications postoperatively. There is an obvious need for more geriatric specific clinical evidence and management guidelines to help identify which patients would benefit from aggressive versus conservative management (3).

Trauma care bundle

As much as the focus of attention is to preserve cerebrovascular function, it is paramount that there be provision for use of geriatric trauma bundles to reduce falls, aspiration, and delirium during hospitalization (26). The interventions included in these bundles may include daily tether review, daily test of attention and assessment of delirium twice a day, mobilization of patients from bed to chair twice a day, minimization of daytime napping, encouraging meals out of bed as much as possible to minimize aspiration risk, minimizing fall risk through use of chair, bed alarms, low beds, ambulatory aids, and assistance with toileting, medication review using Beer's criteria, and encouraging activities of daily living as much as possible (26).

OUTCOMES

Outcomes data for geriatric neurotrauma are confounded by indication and physician opinion of a patient's prognosis, which may bias treatment decisions.

According to study conducted using a 15-state TBI surveillance system, Coronado et al. demonstrated that despite mild injury being predominant (73.4%), and while 61.2% make a good recovery, the overall mortality for patients 65 years and older is 12% and only gets worse with advancing age: 9.5% in 65–75 years, 12% in 75–84 years, and 14.6% in ≥85 years of age (27), with a concomitant reduction in discharge to home (5). In a study of elderly TBI in the UK, despite most patients sustaining moderate-severe TBI, over 50% made a good recovery (28).

Compared to patients between 18 and 44 years of age, patients between 65 and 79 have a 2.58-fold increase and patients ≥80 have a 3.92-fold increase in in-hospital mortality (29).

On a sample of 97 elderly patients aged ≥70 years in Sweden, Herou et al. demonstrated that mortality was associated with severity of TBI: GCS 10–15: 6%, GCS 6–0: 67%, and GCS 3–5: 100% (30). High-energy trauma, one pupil fixed and dilated, and more extensive intracranial pathology was associated with increased mortality, and there was no correlation between presence of warfarin, more advanced age, or degree of midline shift and mortality (30). Even though a significant portion of patients sustaining TBI may take aspirin or clopidogrel, which have shown to worsen TBI-related mortality (31), platelet transfusion use in this population has not been shown to reduce mortality (32).

Older patients with TBI have significantly higher rates of rehospitalization, home healthcare, and hours of unpaid visits from family/friends (3).

Older adults are at higher risk for post-traumatic epilepsy, and TBI may be a risk for both ischemic or hemorrhagic strokes; TBI is also a risk factor for dementia and Parkinson's disease (3), and a history of TBI in older men is associated with increased risk of depression and cognitive impairment (33).

Since elderly patients show a potential to achieve functional goals even after TBI, their consideration for rehabilitation should ideally be free of age bias (34).

PREVENTION

Since falls are a predominant mechanism of injury, injury prevention has been largely through maintenance of bone health, treatment of osteoporosis, vitamin D supplementation, and use of hip protectors (7). Medication review to reduce side effects such as orthostatic hypotension, periodic eye examinations, evaluation of the home environment, and protective headgear are possible approaches to reduce incidence of TBI (7). In addition, improvement in safety of both hospitals and skilled nursing facilities has the potential to reduce fall-related TBI in the future (35).

SUMMARY

Elderly patients are at high risk for traumatic brain injury, in-hospital mortality, and poor functional outcomes. Age-based triaging to the highest level of trauma center, care focused on the needs of the elderly, using evidence as opposed to propagation of self-fulfilling strategies, allow for optimal care of this extremely vulnerable population. Future areas of work include formulating evidence-based geriatric neurotrauma guidelines.

REFERENCES

1. Klein RJ, Schoenborn CA. Age adjustment using the 2000 projected U.S. population. *Healthy People 2010 Stat Notes*. 2001;(20): 1–10.

2. United Nations, Department of Economic and Social Affairs, Population Division. *World Population Ageing 2017 - Highlights*. (ST/ESA/SER.A/397). 2017.

3. Gardner RC, Dams-O'Connor K, Morrissey MR, Manley GT. Geriatric traumatic brain injury: Epidemiology, outcomes, knowledge gaps, and future directions. *J Neurotrauma*. 2018. [Epub ahead of print]

4. Thompson HJ, McCormick WC, Kagan SH. Traumatic brain injury in older adults: Epidemiology, outcomes, and future implications. *J Am Geriatr Soc*. 2006;54(10):1590–5.

5. Coronado VG, Thomas KE, Sattin RW, Johnson RL. The CDC traumatic brain injury surveillance system: Characteristics of persons aged 65 years and older hospitalized with a TBI. *J Head Trauma Rehabil*. 2005;20(3): 215–28.

6. Rates of TBI-related Hospitalizations by Age Group. [Webpage]. 2016; https://www.cdc.gov/traumaticbraininjury/data/rates_hosp_byage.html. Accessed 3/6/2018, 2018.

7. Harvey LA, Close JC. Traumatic brain injury in older adults: Characteristics, causes and consequences. *Injury*. 2012;43(11):1821–6.

8. Taylor CA, Bell JM, Breiding MJ. Traumatic brain injury-related emergency department visits, hospitalizations, and deaths—United States, 2007 and 2013. *Morb Mortal Wkly Rep*. 2017;66(9):1.

9. Teo DB, Wong HC, Yeo AW, Lai YW, Choo EL, Merchant RA. Characteristics of fall-related traumatic brain injury in older adults. *Intern Med J*. 2018;48(9):1048–55.

10. Pieracci FM, Eachempati SR, Shou J, Hydo LJ, Barie PS. Degree of anticoagulation, but not warfarin use itself, predicts adverse outcomes after traumatic brain injury in elderly trauma patients. *J Trauma*. 2007;63(3):525–30.

11. Mosenthal AC, Lavery RF, Addis M et al. Isolated traumatic brain injury: Age is an independent predictor of mortality and early outcome. *J Trauma*. 2002;52(5):907–11.

12. Okazaki T, Hifumi T, Kawakita K et al. Association between comorbidities, nutritional status, and anticlotting drugs and neurologic outcomes in geriatric patients with traumatic brain injury. *World Neurosurg*. 2016; 93:336–40.

13. Peters R. Ageing and the brain. *Postgrad Med J*. 2006;82(964):84–8.

14. Farrall AJ, Wardlaw JM. Blood-brain barrier: Ageing and microvascular disease--systematic review and meta-analysis. *Neurobiol Aging*. 2009;30(3):337–52.

15. Trollor JN, Valenzuela MJ. Brain ageing in the new millennium. *Aust N Z J Psychiatry*. 2001;35(6):788–805.

16. Alvis BD, Hughes CG. Physiology considerations in geriatric patients. *Anesthesiol Clin*. 2015;33(3):447–56.

17. Kehoe A, Rennie S, Smith JE. Glasgow Coma Scale is unreliable for the prediction of severe head injury in elderly trauma patients. *Emerg Med J*. 2015;32(8):613–5.

18. Reynolds FD, Dietz PA, Higgins D, Whitaker TS. Time to deterioration of the elderly, anticoagulated, minor head injury patient who presents without evidence of neurologic abnormality. *J Trauma*. 2003;54(3):492–6.

19. Wasserman EB, Shah MN, Jones CM et al. Identification of a neurologic scale that optimizes EMS detection of older adult

traumatic brain injury patients who require transport to a trauma center. *Prehosp Emerg Care*. 2015;19(2):202–12.

20. Sartin R, Kim C, Dissanaike S. Discussion of: "Is routine head CT indicated in awake stable older patients after a ground level fall?" *Am J Surg*. 2017;214(6):1055–8.

21. Wolf L. Triage and early recognition of significant head injury in the geriatric trauma patient. *J Emerg Nurs*. 2006;32(4):357–9.

22. Shifflette VK, Lorenzo M, Mangram AJ, Truitt MS, Amos JD, Dunn EL. Should age be a factor to change from a level II to a level I trauma activation? *J Trauma*. 2010;69(1):88–92.

23. Carney N, Totten AM, O'Reilly C et al. Guidelines for the management of severe traumatic brain injury, fourth edition. *Neurosurgery*. 2017;80(1):6–15.

24. You W, Feng J, Tang Q et al. Intraventricular intracranial pressure monitoring improves the outcome of older adults with severe traumatic brain injury: An observational, prospective study. *BMC Anesthesiol*. 2016; 16(1):35.

25. Shimoda K, Maeda T, Tado M, Yoshino A, Katayama Y, Bullock MR. Outcome and surgical management for geriatric traumatic brain injury: Analysis of 888 cases registered in the Japan Neurotrauma Data Bank. *World Neurosurg*. 2014;82(6):1300–6.

26. Mattison ML, Catic A, Davis RB et al. A standardized, bundled approach to providing geriatric-focused acute care. *J Am Geriatr Soc*. 2014;62(5):936–42.

27. Mak CH, Wong SK, Wong GK et al. Traumatic brain injury in the elderly: Is it as bad as we think? *Curr Transl Geriatr Exp Gerontol Rep*. 2012;1:171–8.

28. Hawley C, Sakr M, Scapinello S, Salvo J, Wrenn P. Traumatic brain injuries in older adults—6 years of data for one UK trauma centre: Retrospective analysis of prospectively collected data. *Emergency Med J*. 2017; 34(8):509–16.

29. Krishnamoorthy V, Vavilala MS, Mills B, Rowhani-Rahbar A. Demographic and clinical risk factors associated with hospital mortality after isolated severe traumatic brain injury: A cohort study. *J Intensive Care*. 2015;3:46.

30. Herou E, Romner B, Tomasevic G. Acute traumatic brain injury: Mortality in the elderly. *World Neurosurg*. 2015;83(6):996–1001.

31. Ohm C, Mina A, Howells G, Bair H, Bendick P. Effects of antiplatelet agents on outcomes for elderly patients with traumatic intracranial hemorrhage. *J Trauma*. 2005;58(3):518–22.

32. Downey DM, Monson B, Butler KL et al. Does platelet administration affect mortality in elderly head-injured patients taking antiplatelet medications? *Am Surg*. 2009;75(11): 1100–3.

33. Almeida OP, Hankey GJ, Yeap BB, Golledge J, Flicker L. Prevalence, associated factors, mood and cognitive outcomes of traumatic brain injury in later life: The health in men study (HIMS). *Int J Geriatr Psychiatry*. 2015; 30(12):1215–23.

34. Frankel JE, Marwitz JH, Cifu DX, Kreutzer JS, Englander J, Rosenthal M. A follow-up study of older adults with traumatic brain injury: Taking into account decreasing length of stay. *Arch Phys Med Rehabil*. 2006;87(1):57–62.

35. Haring RS, Narang K, Canner JK et al. Traumatic brain injury in the elderly: Morbidity and mortality trends and risk factors. *J Surg Res*. 2015;195(1):1–9.

15

Neurointensive care: Postoperative management

SWAGATA TRIPATHY

INTRODUCTION

The population of elderly people is increasing with an increase in life expectancy, leading to an increase in the number of surgeries in the elderly. There is a progressive decline in function and ability to respond to extrinsic or intrinsic stimuli due to age-related changes at the structural, functional, and molecular levels. Therefore, elderly patients undergoing surgery are at higher risk of postoperative complications due to physiological decline, multiple comorbidities, polypharmacy, cognitive dysfunction, and frailty (1). Postoperative complications result in increased morbidity and mortality and poor surgical outcomes. This may be even more pertinent in the case of neurosurgery and postoperative neurocritical care in the elderly, with an increase of more than 70% admission in elderly patients showing greater severity of illness and comorbidities over the past decade (2).

PHYSIOLOGY OF THE ELDERLY

Nervous system

The prefrontal cortex of the brain is affected by aging, which leads to cognitive changes. There is

gradual decrease in dopamine levels in the brain with increasing age. As the blood—brain barrier becomes more permeable with increasing age, there is increased passage of inflammatory mediators from plasma into the central nervous system. These alter neuronal activity by modulating synthesis of neurotransmitters and their receptors. All these factors contribute to cognitive dysfunction during the postoperative period (3).

Cardiovascular system

In old age there is an increase in systolic blood pressure and decrease in diastolic blood pressure due to arterial stiffness. There is increased sympathetic nervous system activity leading to increased systemic vascular resistance. This leads to left ventricular hypertrophy, which causes prolonged myocardial contraction leading to decrease in ventricular relaxation time, decreased coronary blood flow, and diastolic dysfunction in the elderly. There is decreased ability to buffer changes in blood volume and blood distribution due to venous stiffening, so there is limited blood volume reservoir. The response of the beta-receptor to stimulation is reduced with aging, so there is a decrease in heart rate and contractile response to hypotension, exercise, and catecholamines. There is reduced heart rate variability and ability to control a constant cardiac output due to impaired baroreflex and vagal tone. There is impairment of flow in microvasculature due to decreased bioavailability of nitric oxide in the elderly. All these physiological changes in old age lead to greater blood pressure lability and risk of organ ischemia (3,4).

Respiratory system

With increasing age there is a reduction in elastic recoil of lungs, increasing lung compliance, and decrease in compliance of the chest wall. The functional residual capacity and residual volume gradually increase with aging. As the total lung capacity remains constant, there is decrease in vital capacity. Also, with aging there is a gradual decline in arterial oxygenation. There is reduced tidal volume and higher respiratory rate in the elderly in comparison to younger subjects. Response to hypoxia and hypercapnia decreases in old age. Cough reflex and swallowing also decline with aging. All these changes in old age cause increased work of breathing, atelectasis, infection, and risk of aspiration (2). The closing volume increases, leading to mismatch in ventilation/perfusion during tidal breathing in the supine position (3,4).

Gastrointestinal system

A decrease in the amplitude of esophageal contractions and number of peristaltic movements in old age leads to a delayed gastric emptying time in comparison to younger individuals. There is decrease in gastric acid secretion and intrinsic factor due to atrophic gastritis, leading to decreased calcium absorption. With increasing age, the volume of liver and hepatic blood flow decrease, affecting drug metabolism. This increases the risk of adverse drug reactions (3,4).

Renal system

There is a decline in renal function as age increases. Males are affected more than females due to vascular changes and the effect of androgen. There is decline in creatinine clearance, glomerular filtration rate, ability to dilute or concentrate urine, and a decrease in responsiveness and autoregulation of volume status and plasma

renin activity. All these affect the pharmacokinetics of drugs used perioperatively; elderly patients are more prone to postoperative acute kidney injury (3,4)

Fluid and electrolytes

Many elderly patients may be dehydrated on admission to hospital. Baseline fluid and electrolyte status may be deranged due to preexisting organ dysfunction or medications such as diuretics.

Hematological/immunological systems

Anemia is common in elderly surgical patients. There is a decline in immune system function with increasing age, leading to risk of infection and delayed wound healing.

Endocrine system

There is a decrease in insulin production and increased insulin resistance in old age, affecting glycemic control in the perioperative period.

Musculoskeletal system

In old age there is decreased muscle mass and osteoporotic changes. This increases the risk of fractures, thromboembolism, and pressure sores and impairs rehabilitation.

Pain

There is a decrease in β-endorphins content, γ-aminobutyric acid synthesis, serotonin receptors, and speed of nociceptive processing with increasing age (5). The function of the C and Aδ fibers, which transmit the pain sensation, also declines. The pain threshold is slightly raised with aging in experimental models (6).

CHALLENGES IN GERIATRIC POSTOPERATIVE CARE

Postoperative delirium (POD)

Delirium is an acute disturbance of attention and awareness with additional changes in cognition that tend to fluctuate over time. The consequences of delirium are longer ICU and hospital stay and long-term cognitive function deterioration. Nurses and medical personnel are slow to detect delirium in the postoperative unit despite use of the screening tools (7). The delirium can be due to preoperative, intra-operative, or postoperative causes. Postoperatively causes of delirium may be hypoxia, hypocarbia, hypotension, pain, sepsis, drugs, electrolyte and metabolite imbalance, and embolism (6).

Cognitive dysfunction

Postoperative cognitive dysfunction (POCD) may follow surgery and affects the elderly more often. It increases morbidity and mortality. Though still not understood completely, the patient's preoperative cognitive status and inflammatory processes influence the onset, degree, and duration of POCD. The role and influence of the type of surgery, anesthetic modality, or depth of anesthesia is still debated (8–10).

Pain

In the elderly, pain is managed inadequately due to poor assessment, difficulty in communication, and limited clinical guidelines (11). Inadequate postoperative pain control leads to increased morbidity, delirium, cardiorespiratory complications, and failure to mobilize. In the absence of cognitive impairment, pain can be assessed by asking, using an intensity rating scale such as the Numeric Rating Scale (0 no pain, 1–3 mild pain, 4–6 moderate pain, 7–10 severe pain), Verbal Descriptor Scale (none, mild, moderate, severe) or Visual Analogue Scale. Pain assessment can be difficult if the patient is having severe cognitive impairment. A multimodal approach for assessing pain should be done using the McGill Pain Questionnaire, brief pain inventory, or geriatric pain measure. In the presence of cognitive impairment, physiological observation, facial expressions, body movements, verbalizations, changes in interpersonal interactions, activity/routines and/or mental status can assess pain in the elderly. These should be used in combination (5).

Glycemic control

Poor glycemic control in the preoperative period has been associated with increased risk of infections.

Administration of insulin decreases this risk (12). The recommendation for diabetic patients for strict blood sugar control, however, is not clear as these patients are susceptible to episodes of hypoglycemia which may affect outcomes. A modest approach (controlling to <200 mg/dL, and for those with diabetes only) may be appropriate as advised by two expert panels focused on older surgical patients (13–15).

Maintenance of renal function

Elderly patients more commonly have comorbidities and age-related reduction in renal functions. The reduced muscle mass, decreased production of creatinine, and prolonged immobility in the elderly result in a delay in detection of acute kidney injury (AKI) in the postoperative period. There is limited evidence regarding the risk stratification and prevention of AKI in this age group by the use of panels of injury biomarkers, renal vasodilators, or ischemic preconditioning. Steps taken to prevent episodes of intraoperative hypotension and a judicious fluid balance have a role in renal protection in the elderly. Nephrotoxic drugs and use of osmotic diuretics, as is common in neurosurgery patients, has to be done with close monitoring and extreme caution. As fluid overload is harmful in many ways in the elderly (perpetuating AKI, acute lung injury, poor wound healing, gut dysfunction, etc.), early institution of continuous renal replacement to prevent fluid overload in patients who are unresponsive to diuretics or have an upward creeping fluid balance may be considered (16,17).

Infection and sepsis

Geriatric patients with sepsis have a high mortality rate. In a recent large study, age greater than 75, increased comorbidities, and postoperative sepsis were found to be independent risk factors affecting post ICU discharge mortality up to 1 year (18). The APACHE II, early serum lactate level, and N-terminal prohormone of brain natriuretic peptide levels in combination are important predictors of mortality (19). The C-reactive protein level is an important indicator of acute infection, especially in sepsis (20).

Malnutrition

Malnutrition is a frequent problem in elderly patients. Multifactorial causes affect the nutrition status and have a great effect on the morbidity and mortality of these patients after surgical procedures, both in the ICU and after discharge (21). We found malnutrition to be an independent predictor of mortality even after 1 year of discharge from the ICU in elderly patients (22). Various screening and assessment tools to detect preexisting malnutrition and patients who are at high risk of malnutrition are available, including questionnaires, anthropometric measurements, laboratory parameters, devices to measure body composition, and measures of muscle strength, and may be used to guide interventions in the postoperative period (23).

Postoperative pressure ulcers

Geriatric patients are at a high risk of developing pressure ulcers (24). The change in subcutaneous fat and muscle distribution, greater sedentary habits, and predisposition to poor nutrition are among the many risk factors for the same. Pressure ulcers in the postoperative period increase the morbidly and mortality (24). A low Braden Scale score (<13) and diabetes have shown to predict pressure ulcer risk in the elderly postoperative population. Patients with these factors may benefit from aggressive preventive care (25).

CURRENT RECOMMENDATIONS AND GUIDELINES

The recommendations to reduce postoperative complications in geriatric patients begin with intraoperative measures to prevent or reduce the exposure to the risk factors for the same.

Preoperative interventions to decrease postoperative complications

1. *Risk stratification for developing deep vein thrombosis (DVT)*: All geriatric patients after neurosurgery are at high risk for developing DVT. All these patients should therefore be stratified for DVT and bleeding risk. A structured approach and plan is needed, which may vary according to institute protocols. Drug dosage and duration should be determined based on the patient's risk profile. Different

scoring tools are available for use, without evidence of clear benefit of one over another (26). The recommended prophylaxis for craniotomy or spinal cord surgery is to initiate mechanical thromboprophylaxis in the intraoperative and postoperative periods. Once the risk of bleeding decreases, low molecular weight heparin or unfractionated heparin may be started (27).

2. *Titration of ongoing medications*: Elderly patients, especially those scheduled for neurosurgery, may be taking many different groups of medications (prescription or over-the-counter), supplements, vitamins, and herbal agents. These should be reviewed carefully. Nonessential medications should be stopped to prevent drug interactions and drug errors in the postoperative period. Drugs that have a potential for withdrawal or are essential (cardiac, thyroid, diabetes, parkinsonism drugs, etc.) should be continued (28).

Intraoperative interventions to decrease postoperative complications

1. *Preventing postoperative pulmonary complications*: Perioperative pulmonary aspiration can lead to serious postoperative complications (29). Various strategies can be implemented in the intraoperative period to prevent postoperative pulmonary complications (30).
   a. Regional analgesia, scalp blocks, and other nerve blocks should be used wherever possible.
   b. Short-acting muscle relaxants should be used where possible.
   c. Adequate reversal from neuromuscular blockage prior to extubation should be ensured.

2. *Prevention of pressure ulcers*: Pressure ulcers are common in elderly patients. Risk factors for pressure ulcers include abnormal positioning due to spasticity or contracture, advanced age, chronic moisture, edema, cardiovascular/neurologic or orthopedic disease, incontinence, limited mobility, loss of sensation, and immunosuppression, among others (31,32). Studies have shown that use of a scoring tool to assess the risk of developing pressure ulcer may be better than clinical judgment alone (33–35). Proper positioning and

padding of bony prominences should be ensured to maintain skin integrity and limit pressure on peripheral nerves.

3. *Prevention of intraoperative hypothermia*: The elderly are predisposed to hypothermia due to altered thermoregulation from decreased muscle mass, metabolic rate, and vascular reactivity. Hypothermia begins in the operating room due the direct suppression of thermoregulation by anesthetic agents and indirect effects causing vasodilation (36,37). Surgical site infections, cardiac events, immunosuppression, coagulopathy, and increased oxygen consumption due to shivering may all result as a complication of hypothermia (38,39). Warm IV fluids and body warmers should be used in older patients who are undergoing procedures longer than 30 minutes to avoid hypothermia (40).

4. *Risk stratification for postoperative nausea vomiting (PONV)*: PONV is an important complication in the postoperative period and results in poor patient satisfaction, prolonged time in the post-anesthesia care unit, and unplanned hospital admission in surgical outpatients. Although older age is not a risk factor for PONV, use of general anesthesia and prolonged surgery is. In the elderly patient after neurosurgery, there is a real risk for increase in intracranial pressure. Several tools are available to assist with objective assessment of risk of PONV, including the Apfel and Kolvuranta tools (41,42). Some drugs used for prophylaxis of PONV may not be suitable for the elderly patient (43).

Postoperative interventions to decrease complications

Building checklists to guide management of the geriatric postoperative patient is recommended. The checklist allows a complete evaluation of the patient. A sample is presented in Table 15.1. The common and problematic postoperative complications in geriatric patients are discussed here.

POSTOPERATIVE DELIRIUM

Delirium is a significant age-related postoperative complication. Characterized by an acute decline in cognitive function and attention, it is distinct from chronic cognitive decline and dementia. Risk factors include age >65 years, dementia, poor eyesight or hearing, infection, and severe illness (e.g., ICU admission).

Preoperative diagnosis of dementia allows risk stratification and has implications in diagnosing delirium postoperatively. It is associated with inferior surgical outcomes, longer hospital length of stay, functional decline, higher mortality, and higher resource utilization (44–46).

Routine screening of delirium in elderly patients may result in overdiagnosis and inappropriate treatment; current evidence regarding routine screening is conflicting (47–49). Proper evaluation is also very challenging in the post-neurosurgery patient, as the patient has to undergo an assessment to confirm a disturbance of consciousness and acute change in cognition due to a physiologic derangement (e.g., hypoxia, electrolyte abnormality) (48). There are three subtypes of delirium: hypoactive delirium (lack of awareness and lethargy), hyperactive delirium (patient is combative or agitated), and a mixed subtype (49).

To diagnose delirium, at-risk patients or patients with suspected cognitive impairment should undergo an assessment confirming the following: disturbance of consciousness, a change in cognition, acute onset, and evidence from the history that this is due to physiologic derangement (e.g., hypoxia, hypoglycemia, electrolyte abnormality, acid-base abnormality) (49).

Several validated tools are currently available to evaluate for and diagnose delirium. One of the most widely used instruments is the Confusion Assessment Method (CAM). The CAM-ICU can be used in mechanically ventilated patients who cannot speak (50).

Up to 30% of POD can be prevented. Some strategies are laid out in Table 15.2 (51).

Management of POD in the geriatric patient should focus on multicomponent nonpharmacologic interventions. Pharmacologic interventions should be reserved for patients who put themselves or others at risk with hyperactive delirium.

Short-term, low-dose melatonin to reduce the incidence of delirium in older patients admitted to an acute medical unit may be beneficial, but further research is required before it can be recommended for routine use (52). To decrease the risk of delirium in mechanically ventilated patients, dexmedetomidine should be considered

Table 15.1 Area of evaluation

	Checklist for management strategy
Mentation for delirium/ cognitive impairment	• Adequate assessment and control of pain ongoing? • Substance abuse and withdrawal ruled out? • Indwelling catheters removed where possible? • Physical and mental orientation aided (for e.g., with family at bedside, sleep protocol, noise control in ICU, avoidance of restraints, early ambulation, allow newspapers, music, etc.)? • Psychoactive drugs (such as benzodiazepines, anticholinergics, etc.) and potentially inappropriate medications (for example, Beers Criteria medications) avoided? • Hearing and vision aids reinstituted as soon as possible? • Clinical psychologist visits to be considered early? (risk of depressive delirium/depression is high)
Pulmonary complications	• Early and routine chest physiotherapy ongoing? • Incentive spirometry trained and performed appropriately? • Swallow test done? Appropriate route of nutrition delivery (to prevent aspiration) considered? • Pneumonia prevention bundles (head end elevation, oral hygiene, etc.) in place? • Early mobilization/ambulation being considered?
Patient safety—risk of falls Acute pain management	• Protocols for fall prevention being followed? • Vision, hearing, and walking aids accessible? • Appropriate treatment of delirium? Site, nature of pain, and other related history taken? • Individualized pain control with minimally sedative drugs? • Age- and physiology-appropriate drug dose? • Multimodal approach? • Ongoing education regarding safe and effective use of institutional treatment options?
Preventing urinary tract infections	Catheter care bundles in place? Barrier precautions and hand hygiene in place? Foley catheter indication documented?
Preventing pressure ulcers	Frequent change in position done and documented? Friction and shear minimized? Adequate nutrition? Regular dressing being done?
Nutrition	Patient moving toward resuming normal diet? Dentures available and fitting well? Diet supplementation indicated?

as a sedative alternative to benzodiazepines and propofol (53). Haloperidol is not recommended if there is preexisting Parkinson's disease or Lewy body dementia (52).

A recent study with small number of cases showed that rivastigmine patch used perioperatively reduced the incidence of POD in older patients with cognitive impairment (54).

• The present guidelines suggest haloperidol starting at 0.5–1 mg PO/IM. IV route is not recommended due to increased risk of prolonged

Table 15.2 Preventing delirium in postoperative patients—strategies

Educating healthcare professionals about delirium
Nonpharmacologic interventions such as:

- Increased family presence
- Early mobilization—intermittent removal of tethers such as patient monitors, urinary and nasogastric tubes, etc.
- Cognitive rehabilitation—clock in the room, access to newspapers, etc.
- Sleep hygiene
- Visual and hearing aids
- Nutrition and fluid repletion
- Pain management
- Appropriate medication usage
- Adequate oxygenation
- Bowel care

Table 15.3 Universal fall precautions

- Patient should be allowed time to familiarize with the environment
- A nurse "call bell" and personal belongings should be close at hand
- Fall-proof bathrooms, anti-skid flooring, and handrails for support should be available
- Hospital bed position should be adjustable and have lock-brakes
- Wheelchair wheels should be locked when stationary
- Footwear should be non-slip and of correct size
- Night light or supplemental lighting use
- Visual and hearing aids should be provided as needed
- Room should be clutter-free and floor should be dry
- Patient shifting and positioning should be done with optimal number of personnel and equipment

QT interval (when dose is >35 g/day). Dose should be doubled if ineffective upon reevaluation after 15–30 minutes.

- The following can also be used:
  - Risperidone
  - Olanzapine
  - Quetiapine
  - Ziprasidone

FALLS

Multiple factors can predispose the geriatric patient to falls after neurosurgery. Gait abnormalities due to neurologic and muscular pathology, weakness, decreased vision, dehydration (leading to orthostatic hypotension and head reeling), etc. all put these patients at risk for falls. For elderly postoperative patients who are able to mobilize, universal fall precautions should be in place without hampering early mobilization, ambulation, and physiotherapy (Table 15.3) (55).

FUNCTIONAL DECLINE

Elderly patients are at high risk for functional decline following surgery and hospitalization. Less than 50% recover preadmission levels of functioning at 1 year of discharge. The risk factors are many—advanced age, frailty, cognitive impairment, poor mobility, depression, and the presence of other geriatric syndromes (falls, incontinence, pressure ulcers). Interventions to prevent functional decline encompass all other strategies of

postoperative care as mentioned previously, along with adoption of "geriatric models of care."

There are various models of care designed for the specific needs of the elderly patient. These aim at preventing age-related complications—"geriatric syndromes"—and addressing hospital characteristics that may increase their risk (56).

Implementation of these models may also reduce costs, morbidity, and patient satisfaction. Major components of these models include:

- Geriatric care education to care providers
- Greater involvement of patient and family in establishing treatment goals
- Multidisciplinary care with targeted prevention and management of risk factors
- Evidence-based interventions
- Early transition to lower levels of care

FRAILTY IN GERIATRIC CARE

Frailty is defined as a state of vulnerability with reduced physiological reserves affecting the capacity to maintain or regain homeostasis when exposed to stressors, such as surgery, that place patients at increased risk of adverse health outcomes (57). Frailty has multiple causes, such as physical, psychological, social, or any combination of these. It may include loss of muscle mass and strength, reduced energy and exercise tolerance, cognitive impairment, decreased physiological reserve, and reduced ability to recover from acute stress. Risk factors for frailty are advanced age, functional decline, poor nutrition and/or weight loss, polypharmacy, poverty and/or isolation, and medical and/or psychiatric comorbidity (58). Frailty is associated with an increased risk of adverse outcome (59). A recent meta-analysis found that frailty was associated with increased risk for negative health outcomes such as hospitalization, loss of activities of daily living, premature mortality, physical limitation, and falls and fractures (60). A higher modified frailty index (mFI) has been associated with a higher risk of postoperative complications in patients undergoing spine and cranial neurosurgeries (61,62). The frailty index may provide an additional tool to improve perioperative risk stratification (63,64).

CONCLUSIONS

Postoperative complications in the geriatric patient worsen the outcome. Anticipating and planning for prevention of these complications begins with risk stratification in the preoperative period and runs seamlessly through the intraoperative into the postoperative area. Many age-related postoperative complications share common risk factors. Multicomponent interventions for preventing these complications have been developed and implemented successfully. These interventions employ education, setting treatment goals, evidence-based practice, multidisciplinary care, good communication, and proper planning for discharge.

REFERENCES

1. Griffiths R, Beech F, Brown A et al. Guidelines: Peri-operative care of the elderly. *Anaesthesia.* 2014;69:81–98.
2. González-Bonet LG, Tarazona-Santabalbina FJ, Lizán Tudela L. [Neurosurgery in the elderly patient: Geriatric neurosurgery]. *Neurocirugia (Astur).* 2016;27(4):155–66.
3. Alvis BD, Hughes CG. Physiology considerations in the geriatric patient. *Anesthesiol Clin.* 2015;33(3):447–56.
4. Kanonidou Z, Karystianou G. Anesthesia for the elderly. *Hippokratia.* 2007;11(4):175–7.
5. Schofield PA. The assessment and management of peri-operative pain in older adults. *Anaesthesia.* 2014;69(Suppl. 1):54–60.
6. Garg R, Hariharan U. Postoperative issues in geriatric anaesthesia, continuing medical care of the elderly. *Ann Gerontol Geriatric Res.* 2014;1(4):1016.
7. Numan T, Boogaard MV, Kamper AM et al. Recognition of delirium in postoperative elderly patients: A multicenter study. *J Am Geriatr Soc.* 2017;65:1932–8.
8. Khalil S, Roussel J, Schubert A, Emory L. Postoperative cognitive dysfunction: An updated review. *J Neurol Neurophysiol.* 2015;6:290.
9. Evered L, Scott DA, Silbert B, Maruff P. Postoperative cognitive dysfunction is independent of type of surgery and anesthetic. *Anesth Analg.* 2011;112:5.
10. Riedel B, Browne K, Silbert B. Cerebral protection: Inflammation, endothelial dysfunction, and postoperative cognitive dysfunction. *Curr Opin Anesthesiol.* 2014;27:89–97.
11. Wioletta MD, Sebastian D, Andrzej B. Perception of barriers to postoperative pain management in elderly patients in Polish hospitals—A multicentre study. *J Nurs Manag.* 2016;24:1049–59.
12. Kwon S, Thompson R, Dellinger P, Yanez D, Farrohki E, Flum D. Importance of perioperative glycemic control in general surgery: A report from the Surgical Care and Outcomes Assessment Program. *Ann Surg.* 2013 Jan; 257(1):8–14.
13. Lee P, Min L, Mody L. Perioperative glucose control and infection risk in older surgical patients. *Curr Geriatr Rep.* 2014;3(1):48–55.
14. McGory ML, Kao KK, Shekelle PG et al. Developing quality indicators for elderly surgical patients. *Ann Surg.* 2009;250:338–47.
15. Arora VM, McGory ML, Fung CH. Quality indicators for hospitalization and surgery in vulnerable elders. *J Am Geriatr Soc.* 2007; 55(Suppl. 2):S347–58.

16. Chao CT, Tsai HB, Lin YF, Ko WJ. Acute kidney injury in the elderly: Only the tip of the iceberg. *J Clin Gerontol Geriatr*. 2014 Mar 1;5(1):7–12.

17. Mårtensson J, Bellomo R. Perioperative renal failure in elderly patients. *Curr Opin Anaesthesiol*. 2015;28:123–30.

18. Ou L, Chen J, Hillman K, Flabouris A, Parr M, Assareh H, Bellomo R. The impact of postoperative sepsis on mortality after hospital discharge among elective surgical patients: A population-based cohort study. *Crit Care*. 2017;21:34.

19. Wang H, Li Z, Yin M et al. Combination of Acute Physiology and Chronic Health Evaluation II score, early lactate area, and N-terminal prohormone of brain natriuretic peptide levels as a predictor of mortality in geriatric patients with septic shock. *J Crit Care*. 2015;30:304–9.

20. Ticinesi A, Lauretani F, Nouvenne A et al. C-reactive protein (CRP) measurement in geriatric patients hospitalized for acute infection. *Eur J Intern Med*. 2017;37:7–12.

21. van Wissen J, Bakker N, Heus C, Houdijk APJ. Preoperative nutrition in elderly patients and postoperative outcome. In: Rajendram R, Preedy VR, Patel VB (eds). *Diet and Nutrition in Critical Care*. New York, NY: Springer; 2015, 741-52.

22. Tripathy S, Mishra JC, Dash SC. Critically ill elderly patients in a developing world—Mortality and functional outcome at 1 year: A prospective single-center study. *J Crit Care*. 2014;29:474–e7.

23. Tripathy S, Mishra JC. Assessing nutrition in the critically ill elderly patient: A comparison of two screening tools. *Indian J Crit Care Med*. 2015;19(9):518–22.

24. Jaul E, Menzel J. Pressure ulcers in the elderly, as a public health problem. *J Gen Practice*. 2014;2:174.

25. Gherghina V, Cindea I, Balcan A, Costea D, Popescu R. Predicting the risk of pressure ulcers in elderly patients in the postoperative period: 18AP3-5. *Eur J Anaesthesiol*. 2014; 31:266–7.

26. Gould MK, Garcia DA, Wren SM et al. Prevention of VTE in nonorthopaedic surgical patients. *Antithrombotic Therapy and Prevention of Thrombosis*. 9th ed: American College of Chest Physicians Evidence-Based Clinical Practice Guidelines. *Chest*. 2012; 141(2 Suppl):e227S–77S.

27. Optimal Perioperative Management of the Geriatric Surgical Patient. ACS NSQIP/AGS Best Practices Guideline.

28. Chow WB, Rosenthal RA, Merkow RP et al. Optimal preoperative assessment of the geriatric surgical patient: A best practices guideline from the American College of Surgeons National Surgical Quality Improvement Program and the American Geriatrics Society. *J Am Coll Surg*. 2012;215(4):453–66.

29. Sakai T, Planinsic RM, Quinlan JJ, Handley LJ, Kim TY, Hilmi IA. The incidence and outcome of perioperative pulmonary aspiration in a university hospital: A 4-year retrospective analysis. *Anesth Analg*. 2006;103(4):941–7.

30. Warner MA, Warner ME, Weber JG. Clinical significance of pulmonary aspiration during the perioperative period. *Anesthesiology*. 1993;78(1):56–62.

31. Schoonhoven L, Defloor T, van der Tweel I, Buskens E, Grypdonck MH. Risk indicators for pressure ulcers during surgery. *Appl Nurs Res*. 2002;15(3):163–73.

32. Cox J. Predictors of pressure ulcers in adult critical care patients. *Am J Crit Care*. 2011; 20(5):364–75.

33. Bergstrom N, Braden BJ, Laguzza A, Holman V. The Braden Scale for predicting pressure sore risk. *Nurs Res*. 1987;36(4):205–10.

34. Thorn CC, Smith M, Aziz O, Holme TC. The Waterlow score for risk assessment in surgical patients. *Ann R Coll Surg Engl*. 2013;95(1): 52–6.

35. Pancorbo-Hidalgo PL, Garcia-Fernandez FP, Lopez-Medina IM, Alvarez-Nieto C. Risk assessment scales for pressure ulcer prevention: A systematic review. *J Adv Nurs*. 2006; 54(1):94–110.

36. LacKamp A, Seiber F. Physiologic response to anesthesia in the elderly. In: Rosenthal R, Zenilman M, Katlic M (eds). *Principles and Practice of Geriatric Surgery*. New York: Springer; 2011. p. 300.

37. Esnaola NF, Cole DJ. Perioperative normothermia during major surgery: Is it important? *Adv Surg*. 2011;45:249–63.

38. Forbes SS, Eskicioglu C, Nathens AB et al. Evidence-based guidelines for prevention of perioperative hypothermia. *J Am Coll Surg.* 2009 ;209(4):492–503.e491.

39. Frank SM, Fleisher LA, Breslow MJ et al. Perioperative maintenance of normothermia reduces the incidence of morbid cardiac events: A randomized clinical trial. *JAMA.* 1997;277(14):1127–34.

40. Lawson L, Bridges EJ, Ballou I et al. Accuracy and precision of noninvasive temperature measurement in adult intensive care patients. *Am J Crit Care.* 2007;16(5):485–96.

41. Apfel CC, Laara E, Kolvuranta M, Greim CA, Roewer N. A simplified risk score for predicting postoperative nausea and vomiting: Conclusions from cross-validations between two centers. *Anesthesiology.* 1999;91(3): 693–700.

42. American Society of Peri Anesthesia Nurses. ASPAN's evidence-based clinical practice guideline for the prevention and/or management of PONV/PDNV. *J Perianesth Nurs.* 2006;21(4):230–50.

43. The American Geriatrics Society 2012 Beers Criteria Update Expert Panel. American Geriatrics Society updated Beers Criteria for potentially inappropriate medication use in older adults. *J Am Geriatr Soc.* 2012;60(4): 616–31.

44. Robinson TN, Raeburn CD, Tran ZV, Angles EM, Brenner LA, Moss M. Postoperative delirium in the elderly: Risk factors and outcomes. *Ann Surg.* 2009;249(1):173–8.

45. Witlox J, Eurelings LM, de Jonghe JM, Kalisvaart KJ, Eikelenboom P, van Gool WA. Delirium in elderly patients and the risk of postdischarge mortality, institutionalization, and dementia: A meta-analysis. *JAMA.* 2010; 304(4):443–51.

46. Greer N, Rossom R, Anderson P, MacDonald R, Tacklind J, Rutks I. *Delirium: Screening, Prevention, and Diagnosis–A Systematic Reiew of the Evidence [Internet].* Washington (DC): Department of Veterans Affairs (US); 2011.

47. Young J, Murthy L, Westby M, Akunne A, O'Mahony R. Diagnosis, prevention, and management of delirium: Summary of NICE guidance. *BMJ.* 2010;341:c3704.

48. Robinson TN, Eiseman B. Postoperative delirium in the elderly: Diagnosis and management. *Clin Interv Aging.* 2008;3(2):351–5.

49. American Psychiatric Association. *Diagnostic and Statistical Manual of Mental Disorders.* 5th ed. Washington, DC: American Psychiatric Association; 2013.

50. Inouye SK, van Dyck CH, Alessi CA, Balkin S, Siegal AP, Horwitz RI. Clarifying confusion: The confusion assessment method. A new method for detection of delirium. *Ann Intern Med.* 1990;113(12):941–8.

51. Siddiqi N, Holt R, Britton AM, Holmes J. Interventions for preventing delirium in hospitalised patients. *Cochrane Database Syst Rev.* 2007;2007(2).

52. Choy SW, Yeoh AC, Lee ZZ, Srikanth V, Moran C. Melatonin and the prevention and management of delirium: A scoping study. *Front Med.* 2017;4:242.

53. Lee C, Lee CH, Lee G, Lee M, Hwang J. The effect of the timing and dose of dexmedetomidine on postoperative delirium in elderly patients after laparoscopic major non-cardiac surgery: A double blind randomized controlled study. *J Clin Anesth.* 2018;47:27–32.

54. Youn YC, Shin HW, Choi BS et al. Rivastigmine patch reduces the incidence of postoperative delirium in older patients with cognitive impairment. *Int J Geriatr Psychiatry.* 2017;32: 1079–84.

55. AHRQ. Preventing Falls in Hospitals: A Toolkit for Improving Quality of Care. AHRQ Publication No. 13-0015-EF 2013. Available at: http://www.ahrq.gov/research/ltc/fallpx-toolkit/index.html

56. Capezuti E, Boltz M, Kim H. Geriatric models of care. In: Rosenthal R, Zenilman M, Katlic M (eds). *Principles and Practice of Geriatric Surgery.* New York: Springer; 2011. pp. 253–66.

57. Wahl TS, Graham LA, Hawn MT et al. Association of the modified frailty index with 30-day surgical readmission. *JAMA Surg.* 2017;152: 749–57.

58. BCGuidelines.ca. Frailty in Older Adults – Early Identification and Management, 2017. Available at: bcpsqc.ca/clinical-improvement/48-6/practice-statements (accessed May 7, 2018).

59. Cesari M, Prince M, Thiyagarajan JA et al. Frailty: An emerging public health priority. *J Am Med Dir Assoc.* 2016;17:188–92.

60. Vermeiren S, Vella-Azzopardi R, Beckwée D et al. Frailty and the prediction of negative health outcomes: A meta-analysis. *J Am Med Dir Assoc.* 2016;17:1163.e1–17.

61. Ali R, Schwalb JM, Nerenz DR, Antoine HJ, Rubinfeld I. Use of the modified frailty index to predict 30-day morbidity and mortality from spine surgery. *J Neurosurg: Spine.* 2016; 25:537–41.

62. Tomlinson SB, Piper K, Kimmell KT, Vates GE. Preoperative frailty score for 30-day morbidity and mortality after cranial neurosurgery. *World Neurosurg.* 2017;107: 959–65.

63. Makary MA, Segev DL, Pronovost PJ et al. Frailty as a predictor of surgical outcomes in older patients. *J Am Coll Surg.* 2010;210: 901–8.

64. Partridge S, Harari D, Martin FC, Dhesi JK. The impact of pre-operative comprehensive geriatric assessment on postoperative outcomes in older patients undergoing scheduled surgery: A systematic review. *Anaesthesia.* 2014;69(Suppl. 1):8–16.

16

Neurointensive care: Sedation and analgesia in the ICU

MARC ALAIN BABI

INTRODUCTION

Sedation and analgesia are essential components of the multidisciplinary care management of the critically ill patients in the intensive care unit (ICU). Distress secondary to pain, anxiety, fear, or delirium is fairly common among patients admitted to ICUs and is even more pronounced in elderly patients.

In general, it is useful to consider sedation as having three components: anxiolysis, hypnosis, and analgesia. Many of the sedative-analgesic medications exert their desired effect by affecting one or more of the above components. Nonetheless, before the initiation of a sedative-analgesic medication, the treating physician has to identify the cause of distress in their patients, and treat it accordingly. Anxiety, pain, and delirium are the core clinical components and target of sedative-analgesics in the ICU.

- *Anxiety* is defined as a sustained state of increased autonomic arousal in response to threat or perceived threat (1).
- *Pain* is fairly common in patients admitted to the ICU, and is due to either their primary disease process or in response to routine ICU patient care, such as suctioning, repositioning, recent surgery, invasive lines, endotracheal tube, etc. The assessment and treatment of pain should be considered as a priority in patients admitted to the ICU.
- *Delirium* is defined as an organic syndrome characterized by acute and reversible impairment of consciousness, with periods of hyper- and hyposympathetic activation (1–3). Delirium may be associated with the underlying disease leading to ICU admission. Delirium frequently occurs in ICU patients and is more common in the elderly population. Studies quote the rate of delirium in up to 80% of patients admitted to intensive care units (3,4).

NONPHARMACEUTICAL STRATEGIES

Nonpharmacological strategies to manage agitation should begin with therapies targeting the cause of distress in the patient. This may include reassurance, frequent orientation, frequent communication with the patient, regular family visits, and establishment of wake-sleep cycles and quiet ICU hours (4–6). One trial randomly assigned patients who were mechanically ventilated to receive either a strategy of no sedation followed by continuous verbal reassuring versus continuous sedation using pharmacological agents (6). The trial found that patients managed with a strategy of no sedation had a decrease in ICU length of stay, decrease in hospital length of stay, and decrease in the risk of delirium. In addition, there was no difference in post-traumatic stress disorder, quality of life, or depression in the two groups (6).

PHARMACOLOGICAL AGENTS

In general, sedative-analgesic medication are indicated when treatment of the cause of the distress and nonpharmacological interventions cannot sufficiently control agitation, pain, or delirium. Available agents that are commonly used in the ICU include benzodiazepine such as diazepam, lorazepam, midazolam, opioid analgesics such as fentanyl, hydromorphone, and morphine sulfate, propofol, dexmedetomidine, ketamine, and antipsychotics (haloperidol, quetiapine, and ziprasidone).

SELECTING AN AGENT

No specific sedative-analgesic is superior to another to warrant its use universally in all clinical scenarios. The optimal agent must be tailored to the specific patient's characteristics and in the appropriate clinical context. Important considerations should include the etiology of the patient's distress, expected duration of therapy, medical comorbidities, and potential adverse side effects (7,8). Pharmacokinetic variables such as body weight, renal and hepatic function, and body−fat

ratio should also be considered whenever a sedative-analgesic agent is selected.

ADMINISTRATION

Mounting evidence suggest that continuous infusions of analgesic-sedatives prolong ICU stay and mechanical ventilation (6–8). Current practices and society guidelines therefore favor intermittent bolus doses with frequent interruptions and daily awakening, or dose minimization titrated to light level of sedation (7,8).

MAINTENANCE

The maintenance of a pharmacological sedation requires frequent assessments to determine whether the specific sedative-analgesic agent has achieved its desired therapeutic goal. In addition, assessment of physiological state, laboratory values, and hemodynamic monitoring is essential due to the potential side effects of sedative-analgesics.

Numerous scoring and scale systems to assess pain, sedation, consciousness, and delirium have been developed and are used during the initiation and maintenance of sedative-analgesic medication in the ICU (9). However, one of the major limitations of such scoring systems is that a reference standard does not exist (10).

Current guidelines support the use of the Richmond Agitation-Sedation Scale (RASS) (Table 16.1) (11) and the Riker Sedation-Agitation Scale (SAS). Other alternative scoring systems include the Motor Activity Assessment Scale

Table 16.1 Richmond Agitation-Sedation Scale

Scale	State	Description
+4	Combative	Overtly combative or violent, immediate danger to staff
+3	Very agitated	Pulls on or removes tubes or catheters, aggressive behavior toward staff
+2	Agitated	Frequent nonpurposeful movement or patient-ventilator dyssynchrony
+1	Restless	Anxious or apprehensive but movements not aggressive or vigorous
0	Alert and calm	
−1	Drowsy	Not fully alert, sustained (>10 seconds) awakening, eye contact to voice
−2	Light sedation	Briefly (<10 seconds) awakens with eye contact to voice
−3	Moderate sedation	Any movement (but no eye contact) to voice
−4	Deep sedation	No response to voice, any movement to physical stimulation
−5	Unarousable	No response to voice or physical stimulation

(MAAS), The Minnesota Sedation Assessment Tool (MSAT), and the Ramsay Sedation Scale (10–14).

Withdrawal of medication

When pharmacological agents are no longer needed, the sequence and the rate of discontinuation of the sedative-analgesic mediation must be determined. In general, for patients on multiple medications, the opioid medication should be tapered last so as to prevent pain in an awake patient. However, the rate of reduction should be individualized. Abrupt discontinuation should be avoided given the risk of dependence, tolerance, and/or rebound pain. However, when such agents have been used for short-term periods (i.e., less than 5 days), then it may be appropriate to abruptly discontinue such agents. A gradual reduction (10%–25% per day) may be necessary if the sedative-analgesic agent has been used for longer period of time (15–17).

SPECIFIC AGENTS

Opioid analgesics

Morphine sulfate, fentanyl, and hydromorphone are the most commonly used intravenous opioid analgesics in critically ill patients. Oral opioids such as oxycodone, methadone, and oral morphine are also used when enteral or oral routes of administration are preferred (18,19). All opioids are characterized by their risk of tolerance, dependence, and their lack of amnestic properties. However, they have similar analgesic and sedative properties when administered in equipotent doses (20). Current guidelines of the Society of Critical Care Medicine suggest the administration of intravenous opioids for the management of agitation in mechanically ventilated ICU patients (7).

However, practitioners should be alert to the potential drug–drug interactions in the ICU. Numerous drugs have the potential to interact with opioids. For example, benzodiazepines enhance the central nervous system and respiratory depressant effects of opioids (7,20). Other drugs may interact with opioids by the alteration of the cytochrome P450 system. This includes the commonly used antifungal agents of the azole family (i.e., fluconazole, itraconazole, ketoconazole, voriconazole), macrolide antibiotics, and rifamycin antibiotics (7,19–21).

Nonopioid analgesics

Acetaminophen, nonsteroidal anti-inflammatory agents (NSAIDs), and ketamine may all be used as alternatives or in synergy with opioid analgesics. Anti-epileptic medications such as pregabalin, gabapentin, and carbamazepine may also be used, particularly to treat neuropathic pain or central pain syndromes.

Propofol

Propofol is an intravenous anesthetic that works by activating the central gamma-aminobutyric acid receptor (GABA) alpha receptors and modulating the hypothalamic sleep centers.

Propofol is a highly lipophilic agent and has amnestic, anxiolytic, anticonvulsant, respiratory depressant, and muscle relaxant effects (22–24). The onset of action of propofol is rapid—typically less than a minute due to its highly lipophilic effects, therefore facilitating its passage through the blood–brain barrier (22–26).

The duration of effect is typically 2–20 minutes during short-term use. The short duration of propofol is due to its rapid metabolism by the liver to minimally active metabolites which are then renally excreted (24–26). However, propofol has a large volume of distribution and is highly protein bound. Therefore, different body–fat ratio and disease states affecting hepatic and renal function alter its metabolism, clearance, and distribution (25,26).

The most common side effect of propofol is hypotension. This is often observed in a dose-dependent manner, and almost universally experienced in doses greater than 1 mg/kg intravenous boluses. Other adverse side effects include bradycardia, cardiac arrhythmias, myoclonus, meningismus, respiratory acidosis, hypertriglyceridemia, green or white discoloration of the urine, and anaphylaxis (26–30).

One of the dreaded complications of propofol is propofol infusion syndrome (PRIS). PRIS is a rare complication of prolonged and high doses of propofol (30,31). Characteristics of PRIS include hypotension, refractory bradycardia, metabolic and respiratory acidosis, acute renal failure, rhabdomyolysis, hyperlipidemia, multiple organ failure, and total hemodynamic collapse. It is fatal if not recognized and treated. Treatment consists of discontinuation of the propofol infusion and supportive care as well as treatment of secondary abnormalities.

Dexmedetomidine

Dexmedetomidine is a selective centrally acting alpha 2 agonist. It has anxiolytics and mild analgesic and sedative properties. Unlike propofol, dexmedetomidine does not depress consciousness or respiratory drive. The US and Food and Drug Administration (FDA) approved product information indicates that dexmedetomidine is indicated for the initial sedation of mechanically ventilated patients for up to 24 hours (32,33). No conclusive data on mortality benefit has been reported from the use of dexmedetomidine in critically ill patients (32–34). Potential adverse side effects observed with dexmedetomidine include hypotension, hypertension, nausea, bradycardia, and atrial fibrillation (33–35). Cardiogenic shock has also been reported in one case study (36). The usual dosing of dexmedetomidine is 0.2–0.8 μg/kg/hour. Doses over 1.5 μg/kg/hour do not appear to add to its clinical efficacy (36–38). Dexmedetomidine is metabolized in the liver by the cytochrome P450 system. Antihypertensive agents that may further lower blood pressure with the concurrent use of dexmedetomidine should therefore be cautiously administered or modified during concurrent infusions of dexmedetomidine (34–40).

Benzodiazepines

Benzodiazepines work by binding to specific receptors in the GABA receptor complex, which in turn enhances the binding of this inhibitory neurotransmitter (41,42). The most commonly used benzodiazepines in the ICU are midazolam, lorazepam, and diazepam (42). The potency of benzodiazepines is determined by its binding affinity for the GABA receptor complex (40,42). Benzodiazepines can be administered intravenously, orally, or intramuscularly.

Anxiolysis is generally achieved at lower dose, whereas higher doses result in sedation, muscle relaxation, respiratory and central nervous system depression, and cardiovascular depression. Concurrent administration of benzodiazepines with opioids further potentiates their respiratory and cardiovascular depressive effects, and therefore caution should be exercised (38,40–42).

Benzodiazepines are equally efficacious when administered in equipotent doses (40). However, they differ in potency, rapidity of action, and duration of effect. For example, lorazepam has the highest binding affinity to the GABA receptor complex and therefore the greatest potency (38,41). In addition, how rapidly a benzodiazepine crosses the blood–brain barrier dictates its onset of action (41). Lorazepam is the least lipophilic agent compared to midazolam or diazepam, and therefore has a slower onset of action compared to midazolam and diazepam. Lastly, the duration of effect of benzodiazepine is influenced by the presence of its active metabolites, and patient factors such as age, body weight, hepatic function, renal function, and drug interaction (41–44).

Midazolam has a short duration of effect (2–4 hours) when given in short term due to its rapid hepatic clearance. It is metabolized by the hepatic cytochrome P450 system. Lorazepam has a longer duration of action compared to midazolam, approximately double that of midazolam. It is generally a good choice for longer-term sedation, given its low risk of drug–drug interaction (45). Diazepam has a short duration of effect (generally up to 1 hour) when administered for short-term periods. However, tolerance does occur in all benzodiazepines when continuous infusions are administered. This may reflect change in volume of distribution, binding affinity, or distribution in the density (44,45).

Prolonged administration of benzodiazepines, particularly continuous infusion, may lead to delirium in critically ill patients. Numerous studies have identified the administration of benzodiazepine in critically ill patients and mechanically ventilated patients as an independent risk factor for delirium (4,46–48).

Numerous drugs that are commonly used in the ICU can also interact with benzodiazepines. In particular, drugs that suppress the central nervous system such as opiates may further potentiate the central nervous system–depressing effect of benzodiazepines. Similarly, drugs that interact at the level of the cytochrome P450 system alter the metabolism of benzodiazepines. For example, the azole antifungals, macrolide antibiotics, carbamazepine, rifamycin antibiotics, and hydantoin anticonvulsants all alter the metabolism of benzodiazepines through interaction with the CYP3A4 system (4,37,38,40–48). Nonetheless, lorazepam has the lowest susceptibility to interaction with drugs that inhibit or induce cytochrome P450, as it undergoes extensive glucuronidation in the liver compared to midazolam or diazepam (4,47,48).

Ketamine

Ketamine noncompetitively blocks glutamate N-methyl-D-aspartate (NMDA) receptors as well as other effects at the muscarinic and nicotinic receptor level (7,49). In turn, ketamine produces dissociative anesthesia with minimal respiratory-depressing effect. Ketamine is rarely used in the ICU. However, unlabeled use of ketamine in the ICU may include its use as adjunctive medication during procedural sedation and analgesia, or as an adjunct to opioid analgesia (7).

Ketamine produces a dissociative analgesia in which patients remain conscious with intact breathing, intact brainstem reflexes, and minimal cardiovascular depression (7,49,50). Therefore its use may be attractive in the setting when decrease of systemic blood pressure may be particularly deleterious (i.e., patients with elevated intracranial pressure or systemic shock). Ketamine has also mild bronchodilatory activity (50). However, its use is limited by its psychoactive profile and side effects—notably, agitation, delirium, confusion, and hallucinations. Additional adverse side effects include significant elevation in blood pressure, potential elevation in intracranial pressure, and excessive salivation (50,51).

Antipsychotics

Antipsychotics are widely used in the ICU, especially to treat hyperactive delirium. Some of the commonly used antipsychotics include haloperidol as well as the atypical antipsychotics such as quetiapine, olanzapine, and risperidone.

While there is some evidence of the effective use of antipsychotics to treat delirium in the ICU, there is paucity of data that compare outcome on safety and efficacy on the use of antipsychotics compared to each other.

Other antipsychotics exert their effect by blocking dopamine and other neurotransmitters such as norepinephrine and serotonin. However, their precise mechanism of action in treating delirium in the ICU remains unclear (52).

Haloperidol is one of the most widely used antipsychotics in the ICU. Haloperidol causes a dose-dependent response. It has an onset of action of 10–20 minutes after its infusion and a duration of effect up to 12 hours. It is highly protein bound with a large volume of distribution, and is metabolized by the liver through the cytochrome P450 (CYP3A4 and CYP2D6). It also undergoes glucuronidation (53–58).

Adverse side effects include cardiac side effects—notably, prolongation in QTc interval, which may lead to fatal cardiac arrhythmias such as polymorphic ventricular cardiac tachycardia and torsade de pointes (59,60). Other side effects include acute dystonic reaction, tardive dyskinesia, akathisia, parkinsonism, and neuroleptic malignant syndrome (58–62). The latter is a life-threatening consideration characterized by a distinct clinical syndrome of mental status change, rigidity, fever, and dysautonomia. It may be fatal if not recognized and treated. Treatment includes stopping the causative agent, supportive care, and administration of dantrolene, bromocriptine, or lorazepam (61–64).

Haloperidol interacts with drugs that interact at the level of the CYP3A4 system. This includes systemic azole antifungals, cyclosporine medication, and rifamycins. In addition, caution needs to be exhibited when haloperidol is administered with medication that may prolong the QTc segment. This includes amiodarone, methadone, ondansetron, erythromycin, and metoclopramide (58–64).

CONCLUSION

In summary, there is no specific sedative-analgesic agent that is superior to other agents and that warrants its use universally in critically ill patients. As a result, the selection of a specific agent must be individualized according to the patient's clinical characteristics, appropriate clinical situation, and disease-specific context. The etiology of distress, delirium, pain, expected duration of illness, potential of drug–drug interaction, desired depth of sedation, and pharmacokinetics of the specific agent are some of the essential factors that should guide the selection of a particular agent or combination of agents. Once therapeutic goal is achieved, then the depth of sedation and analgesia should be frequently reassessed and adjusted accordingly. Finally, the end goal of sedation should be clearly defined, and perhaps be the first step set forward when selecting a specific sedative-analgesic agent.

REFERENCES

1. Hansen-Flaschen J. Improving patient tolerance of mechanical ventilation. Challenges ahead. *Crit Care Clin.* 1994;10:659.
2. Milbrandt EB, Deppen S, Harrison PL et al. Costs associated with delirium in mechanically ventilated patients. *Crit Care Med.* 2004; 32:955.
3. McNicoll L, Pisani MA, Zhang Y et al. Delirium in the intensive care unit: Occurrence and clinical course in older patients. *J Am Geriatr Soc.* 2003;51:591.
4. Ely EW, Shintani A, Truman B et al. Delirium as a predictor of mortality in mechanically ventilated patients in the intensive care unit. *JAMA.* 2004;291:1753.
5. Fontaine DK. Nonpharmacologic management of patient distress during mechanical ventilation. *Crit Care Clin.* 1994;10:695.
6. Strøm T, Stylsvig M, Toft P. Long-term psychological effects of a no-sedation protocol in critically ill patients. *Crit Care.* 2011;15: R293.
7. Barr J, Fraser GL, Puntillo K et al. Clinical practice guidelines for the management of pain, agitation, and delirium in adult patients in the intensive care unit. *Crit Care Med.* 2013; 41:263.
8. Griffiths J, Hatch RA, Bishop J et al. An exploration of social and economic outcome and associated health-related quality of life after critical illness in general intensive care unit survivors: A 12-month follow-up study. *Crit Care.* 2013;17:R100.
9. Roberts DJ, Haroon B, Hall RI. Sedation for critically ill or injured adults in the intensive care unit: A shifting paradigm. *Drugs.* 2012; 72:1881.
10. Wittbrodt ET. The ideal sedation assessment tool: An elusive instrument. *Crit Care Med.* 1999;27:1384.
11. Sessler CN, Gosnell MS, Grap MJ et al. The Richmond Agitation-Sedation Scale: Validity and reliability in adult intensive care unit patients. *Am J Respir Crit Care Med.* 2002; 166:1338.
12. Ambuel B, Hamlett KW, Marx CM, Blumer JL. Assessing distress in pediatric intensive care environments: The COMFORT scale. *J Pediatr Psychol.* 1992;17:95.
13. Olleveant N, Humphris G, Roe B. A reliability study of the modified new Sheffield Sedation Scale. *Nurs Crit Care.* 1998;3:83.
14. Ramsay MA, Savege TM, Simpson BR, Goodwin R. Controlled sedation with alphaxalone-alphadolone. *Br Med J.* 1974;2:656.
15. Kher S, Roberts RJ, Garpestad E et al. Development, implementation, and evaluation of an institutional daily awakening and spontaneous breathing trial protocol: A quality improvement project. *J Intensive Care Med.* 2013;28:189.
16. Hager DN, Dinglas VD, Subhas S et al. Reducing deep sedation and delirium in acute lung injury patients: A quality improvement project. *Crit Care Med.* 2013;41:1435.
17. Mehta S, Burry L, Cook D et al. Daily sedation interruption in mechanically ventilated critically ill patients cared for with a sedation protocol: A randomized controlled trial. *JAMA.* 2012;308:1985.
18. Rivosecchi RM, Rice MJ, Smithburger PL et al. An evidence based systematic review of remifentanil associated opioid-induced hyperalgesia. *Expert Opin Drug Saf.* 2014; 13:587.
19. Ishii H, Petrenko AB, Kohno T, Baba H. No evidence for the development of acute analgesic tolerance during and hyperalgesia after prolonged remifentanil administration in mice. *Mol Pain.* 2013;9:11.
20. Salpeter SR, Buckley JS, Bruera E. The use of very-low-dose methadone for palliative pain control and the prevention of opioid hyperalgesia. *J Palliat Med.* 2013;16:616.
21. Nelson LE, Guo TZ, Lu J et al. The sedative component of anesthesia is mediated by GABA(A) receptors in an endogenous sleep pathway. *Nat Neurosci.* 2002;5:979.
22. Deambrogio V, Gatti G, Mongio F et al. A case of superficial lymph node tuberculosis. *Minerva Med.* 1991;82:507.
23. Zecharia AY, Nelson LE, Gent TC et al. The involvement of hypothalamic sleep pathways in general anesthesia: Testing the hypothesis using the GABAA receptor beta3N265M knock-in mouse. *J Neurosci.* 2009;29:2177.
24. Jurd R, Arras M, Lambert S et al. General anesthetic actions *in vivo* strongly attenuated by a point mutation in the GABA(A) receptor beta3 subunit. *FASEB J.* 2003;17:250.

25. Asserhøj LL, Mosbech H, Krøigaard M, Garvey LH. No evidence for contraindications to the use of propofol in adults allergic to egg, soy or peanut†. *Br J Anaesth.* 2016;116:77.

26. Carrasco G, Molina R, Costa J et al. Propofol vs midazolam in short-, medium-, and long-term sedation of critically ill patients. A cost-benefit analysis. *Chest.* 1993;103:557, anesthetic, propofol. *N Engl J Med.* 1995; 333:147.

27. Mirenda J. Prolonged propofol sedation in the critical care unit. *Crit Care Med.* 1995;23:1304.

28. Blakey SA, Hixson-Wallace JA. Clinical significance of rare and benign side effects: Propofol and green urine. *Pharmacotherapy.* 2000;20:1120.

29. Nates J, Avidan A, Gozal Y, Gertel M. Appearance of white urine during propofol anesthesia. *Anesth Analg.* 1995;81:210.

30. Pothineni NV, Hayes K, Deshmukh A, Paydak H. Propofol-related infusion syndrome: Rare and fatal. *Am J Ther.* 2015;22:e33.

31. Wong JM. Propofol infusion syndrome. *Am J Ther.* 2010;17:487.

32. Shehabi Y, Ruettimann U, Adamson H et al. Dexmedetomidine infusion for more than 24 hours in critically ill patients: Sedative and cardiovascular effects. *Intensive Care Med.* 2004;30:2188.

33. Buck ML, Willson DF. Use of dexmedetomidine in the pediatric intensive care unit. *Pharmacotherapy.* 2008;28:51.

34. Jakob SM, Ruokonen E, Grounds RM et al. Dexmedetomidine vs midazolam or propofol for sedation during prolonged mechanical ventilation: Two randomized controlled trials. *JAMA.* 2012;307:1151.

35. Riker RR, Shehabi Y, Bokesch PM et al. Dexmedetomidine vs midazolam for sedation of critically ill patients: A randomized trial. *JAMA.* 2009;301:489.

36. Sichrovsky TC, Mittal S, Steinberg JS. Dexmedetomidine sedation leading to refractory cardiogenic shock. *Anesth Analg.* 2008;106:1784.

37. Patanwala AE, Erstad BL. Comparison of dexmedetomidine versus propofol on hospital costs and length of stay. *J Intensive Care Med.* 2016;31:466.

38. Kawazoe Y, Miyamoto K, Morimoto T et al. Effect of dexmedetomidine on mortality and ventilator-free days in patients requiring mechanical ventilation with sepsis: A randomized clinical trial. *JAMA.* 2017;317:1321.

39. Adams R, Brown GT, Davidson M et al. Efficacy of dexmedetomidine compared with midazolam for sedation in adult intensive care patients: A systematic review. *Br J Anaesth.* 2013;111:703.

40. Pandharipande PP, Pun BT, Herr DL et al. Effect of sedation with dexmedetomidine vs lorazepam on acute brain dysfunction in mechanically ventilated patients: The MENDS randomized controlled trial. *JAMA.* 2007;298:2644.

41. Möhler H, Richards JG. The benzodiazepine receptor: A pharmacological control element of brain function. *Eur J Anaesthesiol Suppl.* 1988;2:15.

42. Arendt RM, Greenblatt DJ, deJong RH et al. In vitro correlates of benzodiazepine cerebrospinal fluid uptake, pharmacodynamic action and peripheral distribution. *J Pharmacol Exp Ther.* 1983;227:98.

43. Ziegler WH, Schalch E, Leishman B, Eckert M. Comparison of the effects of intravenously administered midazolam, triazolam and their hydroxy metabolites. *Br J Clin Pharmacol.* 1983;16(Suppl 1):63S.

44. Greenblatt DJ. Clinical pharmacokinetics of oxazepam and lorazepam. *Clin Pharmacokinet.* 1981;6:89.

45. Jacobi J, Fraser GL, Coursin DB et al. Clinical practice guidelines for the sustained use of sedatives and analgesics in the critically ill adult. *Crit Care Med.* 2002;30:119.

46. Pandharipande P, Shintani A, Peterson J et al. Lorazepam is an independent risk factor for transitioning to delirium in intensive care unit patients. *Anesthesiology.* 2006;104:21.

47. Jones C, Bäckman C, Capuzzo M et al. Precipitants of post-traumatic stress disorder following intensive care: A hypothesis generating study of diversity in care. *Intensive Care Med.* 2007;33:978.

48. Pisani MA, Murphy TE, Araujo KL et al. Benzodiazepine and opioid use and the duration of intensive care unit delirium in an older population. *Crit Care Med.* 2009;37:177.

49. Kundra P, Velayudhan S, Krishnamachari S, Gupta SL. Oral ketamine and dexmedetomidine in adults' burns wound dressing—A

randomized double blind cross over study. *Burns*. 2013;39:1150.

50. Norambuena C, Yañez J, Flores V et al. Oral ketamine and midazolam for pediatric burn patients: A prospective, randomized, double-blind study. *J Pediatr Surg*. 2013;48:629.

51. Patanwala AE, Martin JR, Erstad BL. Ketamine for analgosedation in the intensive care unit: A systematic review. *J Intensive Care Med*. 2017;32:387.

52. van den Boogaard M, Slooter AJC, Brüggemann RJM et al. Effect of haloperidol on survival among critically ill adults with a high risk of delirium: The reduce randomized clinical trial. *JAMA*. 2018;319:680.

53. Riker RR, Fraser GL, Cox PM. Continuous infusion of haloperidol controls agitation in critically ill patients. *Crit Care Med*. 1994; 22:433.

54. Fernandez F, Holmes VF, Adams F, Kavanaugh JJ. Treatment of severe, refractory agitation with a haloperidol drip. *J Clin Psychiatry*. 1988;49:239.

55. Seneff MG, Mathews RA. Use of haloperidol infusions to control delirium in critically ill adults. *Ann Pharmacother*. 1995;29:690.

56. Mac Sweeney R, Barber V, Page V et al. A national survey of the management of delirium in UK intensive care units. *QJM*. 2010; 103:243.

57. Fish DN. Treatment of delirium in the critically ill patient. *Clin Pharm*. 1991;10:456.

58. Stern TA. The management of depression and anxiety following myocardial infarction. *Mt Sinai J Med*. 1985;52:623.

59. Metzger E, Friedman R. Prolongation of the corrected QT and torsades de pointes cardiac arrhythmia associated with intravenous haloperidol in the medically ill. *J Clin Psychopharmacol*. 1993;13:128.

60. Wilt JL, Minnema AM, Johnson RF, Rosenblum AM. Torsade de pointes associated with the use of intravenous haloperidol. *Ann Intern Med*. 1993;119:391.

61. Shalev A, Hermesh H, Munitz H. Mortality from neuroleptic malignant syndrome. *J Clin Psychiatry*. 1989;50:18.

62. Modi S, Dharaiya D, Schultz L, Varelas P. Neuroleptic malignant syndrome: Complications, outcomes, and mortality. *Neurocrit Care*. 2016;24:97.

63. Levenson JL. Neuroleptic malignant syndrome. *Am J Psychiatry*. 1985;142:1137.

64. Bizek KS. Optimizing sedation in critically ill, mechanically ventilated patients. *Crit Care Nurs Clin North Am* 1995;7:315.

17

Neurointensive care: Postoperative cognitive dysfunction

ANASTASIA BOROZDINA, EGA QEVA, AND FEDERICO BILOTTA

Happiness does not lie in happiness, but in the achievement of it.

Fyodor Dostoevsky

INTRODUCTION

Postoperative cognitive dysfunction (POCD) is a postoperative neurological complication associated with memory impairment, thinking, attention, insight, language comprehension, social integration, and other aspects of central nervous function. It may be diagnosed days to weeks after surgery and may last months or chronically complicate cognitive status after the surgery, accelerating progression into dementia such as Alzheimer's disease (AD) (1). Even though this condition is often reversible, it decreases the patient's quality of life and increases the cost of hospitalization and out-of-hospital care. Therefore, this possible postoperative complication must be well framed and focalized in order to improve the prognosis of surgical patients and reduce medical resources needed.

The main risk factors for development of POCD are advanced age, preexisting cognitive impairment (often present in elderly patients),

multimorbidity, and lower education level (2). In accordance with this fact, occurrence of POCD is an emerging epidemic in countries that are experiencing a growth in aging population, the so-called "Baby Boomer generation," represented by people who were born after World War II. Overall, better life conditions and general world consolidation made it possible for this generation to become "older boomers." Even if POCD is strongly associated with anesthesia and surgery, no studies have been able to demonstrate type of anesthesia and anesthetics as independent risk factors, while the benefits of intraoperative monitoring of anesthetic depth and cerebral oxygenation have been confirmed (3). Since surgeons are facing an increasing number of older patients, age-relative complications and aspects of perioperative care are becoming a trending topic in many medical specialties, and especially in perioperative medicine (4).

The elderly brain is more vulnerable due to decrease of cognitive reserve, preexisting cerebrovascular dysfunction, or degenerative disease (5). Moreover, perioperative stress, inflammation response, and multimorbidity could contribute to development of transit cognitive deficit in the early postoperative period (6). Important changes occurring in drug metabolism and pharmacodynamics promote increased half-time elimination and altered drug sensitivity. Careful monitoring of depth of anesthesia is required in order to minimize the risk of overdosing of many anesthetic agents (7). Higher pain thresholds in older patients, because of a reduction of myelinated fibers, may contribute to delayed presentation of painful conditions (8).

To provide better perioperative care and minimize the risk factors for postoperative complications, a thoughtful preoperative anesthesiologic evaluation is a landmark and allows detection of the presence and stability of the patient's medical condition, as well as a review of the medication list (9). Other measures may include evaluation of risk factors for postoperative delirium (POD), assessment of preexisting cognitive status, and screening for depression and nutrition status (10). Patients and relatives should be informed about possible complications and treatment perspectives. This proactive approach together with medical team (e.g., surgeon, geriatrician, nurses, and caregivers) cooperation helps to develop an individual and gentle treatment plan for aged patients and may result in fewer cases of neurological complications.

Elderly patients undergoing cardiac and noncardiac surgery go through complex postoperative complications such as longer length of stay, cardiac, pulmonary and gastrointestinal complications, postoperative infections, venous thromboembolism, POD, and POCD. All these conditions are associated with increased costs for postoperative rehabilitations (11).

POCD was originally described in an observational study that enrolled 4250 surgical patients (>65 years old) who received general anesthesia in order to evaluate the possible relationship between anesthesia and development of postoperative cognitive impairment (12). In the presented case series it was often reported that in geriatric practice "the patient has never been the same after operation." It was also reported by relatives and friends of enrolled patients that some of them lost interest in family and in previously enjoyable activities such as book reading, and had difficulties with concentration or doing everyday activities such as driving and shopping. POCD can lead to premature

withdrawal from the labor market, increased social costs, and higher mortality. Since the introduction of open-heart surgery, postoperative alteration of cognitive status has been discussed mainly in regard to brain microembolization after cardiopulmonary bypass (CPB) (13).

However, cognitive complications have been widely recognized even after noncardiac operations and nonsurgical procedures such as coronary angiography or sedation as well. Consequently, the focus of POCD has shifted from type of surgery and anesthesia to the preexisting physical and mental status of the patients.

DEFINITION OF POCD

POCD is a subtle neurological complication associated with cognitive decline in two or more cognitive domains detected by validated neurophysiological tests administered before and after surgery. It has been described in several researches as a transit disorder with a full recovery, but it could boost or enhance ongoing chronic cognitive decline such as AD as well (14).

However, POCD has not been defined by the Diagnostic and Statistical Manual of Mental Disorders, fifth edition (DSM-V), and there is no code in the tenth revision of the International Statistical Classification of Diseases and Health-Related Problems (ICD-10). The spectrum of abilities referred to cognition includes learning, memory, verbal abilities, perception, attention, executive functions, and abstract thinking (10). In the presence of POCD, it is possible to have a decrement in one area without a deficit in another. POCD occurs in all types of surgery, but cardiac patients have the highest incidence (43%), while among noncardiac patients, the orthopedic ones have the highest occurrence (17%). Other incidence rates reported are 12.7% after major noncardiac surgery and 10.4% after major abdominal (15,16).

PATHOPHYSIOLOGY OF POCD

Despite the fact that POCD has been an area of increased interest for anesthesiologists and neurophysiologists, its exact causes remain unknown. Neurostructure modifications presented in patients experiencing POCD are subtle and difficult to visualize or detect despite advances in imaging technology. Therefore, the only instruments to approach neuropsychological assessment on cognitive status are batteries of neurophysiological tests that evaluate changes in the main cognitive domains. This method also has its limitations, as there is no gold standard for the testing batteries used to diagnose POCD, as well at what point the tests should be administered. The possible mechanisms of the pathogenesis of POCD are been reported below (17,18):

1. Neurotransmitter imbalance such as acetylcholine deficiency or dopamine excess
2. Reduced cerebral blood flow and metabolism
3. Dysregulation of stress response and the sleep–wake cycle
4. Neuroinflammation

RISK FACTORS

The potential causes of POCD can be divided into two groups: the first group associated with type of surgery and anesthesia, called modifiable factors, and the second one associated with patient characteristics, called nonmodifiable factors (19).

Major risk factors for POCD

- Age (more than 60 years old)
- Severity of surgery and duration
- History of alcohol abuse
- Medications with anticholinergic properties
- Previous cerebral vascular accident, previous POCD, poor cognition
- Respiratory complications
- Infection complications
- Comorbidities

Modifiable factors

The first studies of POCD were conducted in patients treated for cardiovascular disease.

The mechanisms of PODC development were thought to be strongly related with CPB and microemboli. Over the last 10 years, several studies provided no evidence of CPB as an independent risk factor for POCD. Comparison between incidence of POCD in coronary artery bypass graft (CABG) surgery patients with and without CPB (on-pump vs off-pump) was reported in a large randomized controlled trial (RCT) that included 281 patients (139 on-pump surgery and 142 off-pump surgery). The authors concluded that 29% of on-pump and 21% of off-pump patients had cognitive decline 3

months postoperatively, while there were no differences between two groups at 12 months (20). A meta-analysis further reported that there are no significant neurocognitive benefits when comparing on-pump to off-pump CABG in the early postoperative period (within 3 months) or later (6–12 months) (21).

However, microemboli remains a controversial issue and can occur during cardiac as well as joint replacement surgery. The association between microemboli and POCD was analyzed in a prospective study that enrolled 37 orthopedic patients. Cognitive function was evaluated with a battery of 13 tests at 1 week and at 3 months. POCD was found in 41% and 18%, respectively, but no statistically significant association with microemboli after using transcranial Doppler imaging was reported (22).

The relationship between POCD (at 7 days, 3 months, and 1 year) and aortic atheroma (embolization/microemboli) was assessed in a prospective study that enrolled 311 patients undergoing CABG surgery. The incidence of POCD 7 days postoperatively was higher in patients with larger border of aortic atheroma, but not at 3 months and 1 year postoperatively. According to the outcomes, authors suggested that microemboli and atheroma are not the primary cause of POCD, but are strong indicators for severe vascular disease, which may be a risk factor of POCD (23).

The possible association between incidence of POCD (at 7 days and 3 months postoperatively) and type of surgery (CABG surgery under general anesthesia and total hip joint replacement under general anesthesia) was determined in a prospective study that enrolled 644 patients. The incidence of POCD at day 7 was higher in CABG surgery patients compared to total hip joint replacement (43% vs 17%), while no difference between the groups was reported at 3 months postoperatively (24). In patients with coronary artery disease treated medically, undergoing percutaneous coronary procedures or cardiac surgery, the risk for POCD over 6 years is higher than in patients without coronary artery disease. This review suggests that specific comorbidities, like vascular disease, are more likely to be the reason for cognitive decline than cardiac surgery or general anesthesia (25).

The relationship between possible risk factors and POCD has been further confirmed in a large prospective study that reported data from 1218 elderly patients and 176 healthy volunteers undergoing major noncardiac surgery with general anesthesia. POCD was found in 25.8% at 1 week postoperatively and 9.9% at 3 months after surgery, compared to 3.4% and 2.8%, respectively, in the control group. Increased age, low education level, duration of anesthesia, and postoperative respiratory complication were strongly associated with POCD. On the other hand, type of anesthesia (general vs regional) was not found to be a risk factor for postoperative neurological complication (17,26).

Nonmodifiable factors

AGE

Age has been described by a majority of studies as main risk factor for development of POCD. Therefore, the relationship between age and POCD should not be neglected. A prospective study of 1064 patients showed that the incidence of POCD in patients over 60 years old was 12.7% at 3 months postoperatively, whereas POCD in the younger population (40–60 years) was significantly lower (6% at 3 months) (27). Another prospective study reported that incidence of POCD was higher in elderly patients (>60 years old) than in young or middle-aged patients (<60 years); $p < 0.001$ (18).

GENETIC FACTORS

The literature reports conflicting results for the possible association between the ε4 allele and POCD after cardiac surgery (28,29). The possible relationship between the ε4 allele and POCD at 1 week and 3 months postoperatively after noncardiac surgery was defined in a multicenter study that recruited a total of 976 patients (≥40 years old). The ε4 allele was not found to be a risk factor for POCD at 1 week or 3 months after noncardiac surgery (30). The possible relationship between the ε4 allele and incidence of POCD after carotid endarterectomy was evaluated in a prospective study that enrolled 75 patients. The presence of the ε4 allele increased the risk of POCD at 1 month 62-fold (31). Other genetic factors could be important in the general surgical population—for instance, individual differences in inflammation and drug metabolism, with polymorphism of the drug metabolism system's cytochrome P450 (8). Very slow metabolism of certain drugs could be associated with prolonged recovery, and very fast metabolism could lead to high concentrations of intermediary degradation products (32). Both

situations could result in a disturbance of receptor function, but the relationship with POCD remains to be established.

COMORBIDITIES AND PREEXISTING COGNITIVE IMPAIRMENT

Aging of an organism accompanies a decline in physiological reserve and deficit in the central nervous system. Preoperative mental health is an important factor that could determine higher incidence of POCD, especially in elderly surgery patients (33). This is the reason studies often suggest a cognitive evaluation preoperatively. A statistically significant relationship was found between lower baseline Mini-Mental Status Examination (MMSE) score, depressed basal mood, preexisting cognitive impairment and working memory deficit, and incidence of POCD in cardiac and noncardiac surgery patients at 3 days, 1 week, 3 months and 1 year postoperatively (10,34,35). Preoperative high serum creatinine levels, chronic obstructive pulmonary disease, and poor left ventricular function is associated with higher risk of POCD (36). A systematic review published in 2009 and a prospective study published in 2016 reported that a history of alcohol or drug abuse, diabetes mellitus, Parkinson's disease (PD), and other neurodegenerative diseases increases the incidence and severity of POCD (37,38). Cerebrovascular disease is another significant trigger that could contribute to development of postoperative cognitive complications. Different reports demonstrated that preoperative craniocervical atherosclerosis lesions, stroke, and silent brain ischemia detected by magnetic resonance imaging (MRI), were more likely to have POCD after cardiac and noncardiac surgery (39).

DIAGNOSTIC METHODS

Comprehensive neurophysiological testing is required to diagnose POCD. These batteries of tests should satisfy specific criteria and should not be complex or time consuming.

In 1995, a multidisciplinary expert team developed a Statement of Consensus on assessment of neurobehavioral outcomes after cardiac surgery. It recommended a core battery of neurological tests that could be administered quickly and easily at any time (40).

Incorporating the above recommendations, pioneers of POCD study, the International Study of

Post-Operative Cognitive Dysfunction (ISPOCD) group, used a Z-score to diagnose POCD. A Z-score is nondimensional composite unit that indicates deviation in personal test performance of individuals according to the average test performance of control group. The criteria for POCD is decline of more than two standard deviations (2SD) in two cognitive domains or decline of 2SD in a composite score (Z-score). Neurological test batteries vary in different studies, but all were designed to assess functioning of the main cognitive domains (Table 17.1).

Several factors can influence postoperative cognitive status, including pain, anxiety, nausea, effects of drugs used preoperatively, sleep deprivation, etc. Therefore, baseline cognitive testing is highly important to detect the changes occurring after surgery. Furthermore, neurophysiological follow-up at 1 week, 3 months, and 1 year postoperatively is needed for patients who were diagnosed with any cognitive decline in the early post-surgical period, or high-risk patients (41).

Apart from the patient's health status, staff and time availability have to be considered when choosing a test for routine use, as some tests can take hours to be administer (41,42). Shorter screening tests are preferable for routine use but many of them have a "ceiling effect" (scoring high results without perfect performance on the test's item content) (43,44). One of the most widely used tests is the Mini-Mental State Examination (MMSE), and more recently, the Montreal Cognitive Assessment

(MoCA) has gained popularity. Both of these tools are quick to administer but are not sensitive to subtle cognitive impairment. The neuropsychological tests used are hereby reported:

- *Mini-Mental State Examination* (MMSE) examines orientation in time and space, memory, ability to follow instructions, language (write a sentence, name objects), and attention. It can be administered in 10 minutes and returns a maximum score of 30. Below this, scores can indicate severe (≤ 9 points), moderate (10–18 points), or mild (19–23 points) cognitive impairment. A postoperative low score in comparison with the preoperative performance is a cause of concern and may require further postoperative follow-up with neurologic and neuropsychological consultation (44).
- *Montreal Cognitive Assessment* (MoCA) is a brief cognitive screening tool, widely available, with high sensitivity and specificity for detecting mild cognitive impairment as currently conceptualized in patients performing in the normal range on the MMSE. It evaluates executive and visuospatial abilities, language, memory, attention, abstract reasoning, and orientation (45).
- *Digit Symbol Substitution Test* (DSST) is a sensitive tool to detect changes in psychomotor speed, attention, visuoperceptual (including scanning), writing, and drawing functions. It is a pen-and-paper test where the patient is asked

Table 17.1 Neurological tests and cognitive domain

Cognitive domains	Neuropsychological test
1. Memory and learning	Consortium to Establish a Registry for Alzheimer's Disease (CERAD)
	Digit Span Test (DST)
	Rey Auditory Verbal Learning Test (RAVLT)
	Memory Impairment Screen (MIS)
2. Language	Verbal fluency
	Controlled Oral Word Association Test (COWAT)
	S-words
3. Executive function and attention	Trail Making Test, Part A (TMT-A)
	Trail Making Test, Part B (TMT-B)
	Clock Drawing Test (CDT)
	Stroop Color Word Interference Test (SCWIT)
4. Psychomotor function	Grooved Pegboard Test (GPT)
	Digit Symbol Substitute Test (DSST)

to fill in each square as quickly as possible and to substitute numbers with symbols according to the provided instructions. For example, number 1 equals the @ symbol. The time given to complete as many as possible is 90–120 seconds, and results are evaluated according to the number of correct answers given (46).

- *Trail-Making Test* (TMT) consists of two parts, A and B. In Part A, the subject is asked to connect numbers in order which are distributed on a sheet of a paper from 1 to 25. Part B requires the subject to connect numbers (1–13) and letters alternately (A–L). The patient's performance is timed for both parts, and the maximum time to complete both tasks is 5 minutes. Results for both TMT-A and -B are reported as the number of seconds to complete the task; higher scores reveal greater impairment. Average time to complete Trail A is 29 seconds and for Trail B is 75 seconds. A deficient score is >78 seconds, or for Trail B >273 seconds. The TMT has high sensitivity for detection of cognitive impairment associated with dementia and also evaluates visual attention, executive functioning (TMT-B) and scanning, and visual search (47).

- *Digit Span Test* (DST) is a useful method to detect any changes in working memory. It is a simple and fast test to perform. Patients are given a series of numbers or letters and then are asked to recall them in the correct order. The examiner should start with a short number/letter string, for example 957321, and then increase the number of digits in the string. The digit strings will increase in length with each trial, and the test is continued until the patient makes a mistake (48).

DIFFERENTIAL DIAGNOSIS

POCD is the longer-lasting form of a wide variety of postoperative neurological complications, and sometimes it is difficult to formulate a differential diagnosis based on the patient's symptoms. The pathologic conditions that enter into differential diagnosis are delirium, central anticholinergic syndrome (CAS), dementia, and akinetic crisis (AC). Nowadays, literature reports that POD syndrome is very complex, can be triggered by predisposing and precipitating factors, and is not just a consequence of type of surgery or anesthesia. CAS consists of an absolute or relative reduction in cholinergic activity in the central nervous system induced by drugs that have or not anticholinergic effects. Dementia is an acquired cognitive disorder that interferes with relationships and the patient's quality of life. AC is a complication of PD that can occur as a result of interruption of PD therapy during surgery. Manifestations, diagnostic methods, duration, and prognosis are reported in Table 17.2.

Delirium

Occurrence of POD is a relatively common and sometimes unrecognized postoperative complication. The incidence varies between 25%–60% in the elderly postsurgical population (49). POD is a disturbance of consciousness with a reduced ability to focus, sustain, or shift attention, a change in cognition, or the development of a perceptual disturbance (49). POD can occur soon after surgery, and it can last up to 5 days. It is associated with increased mortality, prolonged hospital stay, functional and cognitive decline, and poor long-term outcome. Development of POD is strongly associated with risk factors (age, preexisting cognitive impairment, frailty, depth of anesthesia, postoperative pain, infection complications, administration of benzodiazepine and anticholinergic drugs, sleep deprivation, and inadequate nutritional status) (19).

The gold standard method to diagnose POD is the Confusion Assessment Method (CAM) Test, or the Confusion Assessment Method Intensive Care Unit (CAM-ICU), for intubated patients (50). Management of POD includes preventive strategies and a multicomponent approach implementing nonpharmacological methods and eliminating any clinical causes that can contribute to the condition.

Central anticholinergic syndrome

CAS is a pathologic condition reported after drugs used in anesthesia and is ICU-associated (51).

Its development cannot be predicted by laboratory findings as there is an individual predisposition for it. Symptoms are identical to the central symptoms of atropine intoxication and consist of agitation, seizures, hallucinations, disorientation, stupor, coma, respiratory depression, etc. Drugs that may induce these disturbances include opiates,

Table 17.2 Differential diagnostics of cognitive impairment

	Manifestations	Diagnostic methods	Timing	Prognosis
POCD	Cognitive deficits postoperatively (impairment of memory, ability to combine tasks, concentration, etc.)	Pre- and postoperative psychometric testing	Several days or weeks after surgery	Reversible in days to months
POD	Impairment of cognitive (attention and memory) and/or spatial/temporal perception	Various delirium scales (e.g., CAM, Nu-DESC, CAM-ICU)	Immediately after surgery (1–3 days postoperatively)	Reversible if the underlying condition is treatable
CAS	Agitated or somnolent/comatose type	Reversal of manifestations on administration of physostigmine	Immediately after surgery	Reversible with medication
Dementia	Impaired memory, impairment of abstract thinking and judgment, aphasia, apraxia, agnosia, executive dysfunction, personality changes	Dementia tests (e.g., MMSE, Short Syndrome Test, Dementia Detection Test)	Develops over months to years	Poor prognosis, no cure available
AC	Worsening of parkinsonism with marked akinesia and inability to verbalize	Interruption of anti-parkinsonian medications during time of surgery	Within hours after surgery	Reversible with antiparkinsonian medication

Abbreviations: AC, akinetic crisis; CAM, Confusion Assessment Method Test; CAM-ICU, Confusion Assessment Method Intensive Care Unit; CAS, central anticholinergic syndrome; MMSE, Mini-Mental Status Examination; Nu-DESC, The Nursing Delirium Screening Scale; POCD, postoperative cognitive dysfunction; POD, postoperative delirium.

benzodiazepines, phenothiazines, ketamine, pro-pofol, halogenated inhalation anesthetics, and H2-blocking agents such as cimetidine.

Dementia

Dementia is considered a family of major neu-rocognitive disorders characterized by memory impairment and/or deficit in other cognitive domains. The worldwide prevalence of dementia was 35.6 million people in 2010 and it is expected to increase to 65.7 million people by 2030 (52). The impairment must be acquired and represent a sig-nificant decline from a previous level of function-ing and interfere with independence in everyday activities. The onset of disease is insidious; the evo-lution is progressive and non-reversible. Dementia can be present in various forms: vascular (multi-infarct) dementia (VaD), AD, PD, dementia with Lewy body (DLB), and frontotemporal dementia (FTD) (53).

Akinetic crisis

AC is a life-threating postoperative complication characterized by an acute severe akinetic-hyper-tonic state, consciousness disturbance, hyperther-mia, and muscle enzyme elevation (54). It can be complicated by infection, pulmonary embolism, renal failure, disseminated intravascular coagula-tion (DIC), and cardiac arrhythmias.

MANAGEMENT OPTIONS AND PREVENTIVE STRATEGIES

There is still no well-defined protocol for treatment of POCD, and a nonpharmacological approach plays the most important role among management options. In order to reduce incidence of POCD, collaboration between surgeon and anesthetist is required to choose the right surgical and anes-thetic technique.

Duration of surgery is important, as shorter and less invasive techniques lead to decreased inflam-matory response (release of proinflammatory cytokines IL-1B, IL-6, TNF) and lower POCD. On the other hand, anesthetics may cause direct toxic effect on neural structures. Low-dose dexa-methasone (0.1 mg/kg) was shown to reduce inci-dence of POCD (10). Mild hypothermia and slow rewarming procedures reduce incidence of POCD

in patients undergoing cardiac surgery. Among nonpharmacological interventions, frequent visits by family and friends, early discharge from hos-pital, nutrition status, sufficient oxygenation and hemodynamic support, regular measurement of vital signs and sleep-wake cycle (adequate room light with variations in light intensity in order to achieve a normal circadian rhythm) should be considered. A clock in a prominent position, a cal-endar, and watching the news on television can help reorientation (55).

OUTCOME

POCD is a very important burden for patients, their families, and society, causing short- and long-term consequences. POCD at both 3 and 12 months postoperatively has been shown to cause higher short-term mortality (between 3 months and 1 year postoperatively), long-term mortality (for a median follow-up of 7.5–8.5 years postop-eratively), while POCD at 1 week after surgery was found to influence mortality. POCD can prolong hospital stay and welfare payments and cause premature withdrawal from the labor market, reduced quality of life, and a less productive work-ing status (10,56).

REFERENCES

1. Hermanides J, Qeva E, Preckel B, Bilotta F. Perioperative hyperglycaemia and neurocog-nitive outcome after surgery: A systematic review. *Minerva Anestesiol.* 2018;84(10): 1178–88.
2. Jungwirth B, Zieglgänsberger W, Kochs E, Rammes G. Anesthesia and postoperative cognitive dysfunction (POCD). *Mini Rev Med Chem.* 2009;9(14):1568–79.
3. Bilotta F, Qeva E, Matot I. Anesthesia and cognitive disorders: A systematic review of the clinical evidence. *Expert Rev Neurother.* 2016;16(11):1311–20.
4. Partridge JS, Collingridge G, Gordon AL, Martin FC, Harari D, Dhesi JK. Where are we in perioperative medicine for older surgical patients? A UK survey of geriatric medicine delivered services in surgery. *Age Ageing.* 2014;43(5):721–4.
5. Marchant NL, Reed BR, DeCarli CS et al. Cerebrovascular disease, β-amyloid, and

cognition in aging. *Neurobiol Aging.* 2012; 33(5):1006, e25–1006.e36.

6. Aubrun F, Gazon M, Schoeffler M, Benyoub K. Evaluation of perioperative risk in elderly patients. *Minerva Anestesiol.* 2012;78(5): 605–18.

7. O'Malley K, Crooks J, Duke E, Stevenson IH. Effect of age and sex on human drug metabolism. *Br Med J.* 1971;3(5775):607–9.

8. Hallingbye T, Martin J, Viscomi C. Acute postoperative pain management in the older patient. *Aging Health.* 2011;7(6): 813–28.

9. Fischer SP. Development and effectiveness of an anesthesia preoperative evaluation clinic in a teaching hospital. *Anesthesiology.* 1996;85(1):196–206.

10. Rundshagen I. Postoperative cognitive dysfunction. *Dtsch Arztebl Int.* 2014;111(8): 119–25.

11. Gelsomino S, Lorusso R, Livi U et al. Cost and cost-effectiveness of cardiac surgery in elderly patients. *J Thorac Cardiovasc Surg.* 2011;142(5):1062–73.

12. Bedford PD. Adverse cerebral effects of anaesthesia on old people. *Lancet.* 1955;269: 259–63.

13. Bokeriia LA, Golukhova EZ, Polunina AG. Postoperative delirium in cardiac operations: Microembolic load is an important factor. *Ann Thorac Surg.* 2009;88(1):349–50.

14. Kat MG, Vreeswijk R, de Jonghe JF et al. Long-term cognitive outcome of delirium in elderly hip surgery patients. A prospective matched controlled study over two and a half years. *Dement Geriatr Cogn Disord.* 2008;26:1–8.

15. Goto T, Maekawa K. Cerebral dysfunction after bypass surgery. *J Anesth.* 2014;28(2): 242–8.

16. Monk TG, Weldon BC, Garvan CW et al. Predictors of cognitive dysfunction after major noncardiac surgery. *Anesthesiology.* 2008;108: 18–30.

17. Krenk L, Rasmussen LS, Kehlet H. New insights into the pathophysiology of postoperative cognitive dysfunction. *Acta Anaesthesiol Scand.* 2010;54(8):951–6.

18. Maclullich AM, Ferguson KJ, Miller T, de Rooij SE, Cunningham C. Unravelling the pathophysiology of delirium: A focus on the role of

aberrant stress responses. *J Psychosom Res.* 2008;65:229–38.

19. Bilotta F, Lauretta MP, Borozdina A, Mizikov VM, Rosa G. Postoperative delirium: Risk factors, diagnosis and perioperative care. *Minerva Anestesiol.* 2013;79(9):1066–76.

20. Van Dijk D, Jansen EW, Hijman R et al. Cognitive outcome after off-pump and on-pump coronary artery bypass graft surgery: A randomized trial. *JAMA.* 2002;287:1405–12.

21. Marasco SF, Sharwood LN, Abramson MJ. No improvement in neurocognitive outcomes after off-pump versus on-pump coronary revascularisation: A meta-analysis. *Eur J Cardiothorac Surg.* 2008;33:961–70.

22. Rodriguez RA, Tellier A, Grabowski J et al. Cognitive dysfunction after total knee arthroplasty. *J Arthroplasty.* 2005;20:763–71.

23. Evered LA, Silbert BS, Scott DA. Postoperative cognitive dysfunction and aortic atheroma. *Ann Thorac Surg.* 2010;89:1091–7.

24. Evered LA, Scott DA, Silbert BS, Maruff P. Postoperative cognitive dysfunction is independent of type of surgery and anaesthetic. *Anesth Analg.* 2011;112:1179–85.

25. Selnes OA, Gottesman RF, Grega MA, Baumgartner WA, Zeger SL, McKhann GM. Cognitive and neurologic outcomes after coronary-artery bypass surgery. *N Engl J Med.* 2012;366:250–7.

26. Rasmussen LS, Johnson T, Kuipers HM et al. Does anaesthesia cause postoperative cognitive dysfunction? A randomised study of regional versus general anaesthesia in 438 elderly patients. *Acta Anaesthesiol Scand.* 2003;47:260–6.

27. Johnson T, Monk T, Rasmussen LS et al. Postoperative cognitive dysfunction in middle-aged patients. *Anesthesiology.* 2002;96(6): 1351–7.

28. Tardiff BE, Newman MF, Saunders AM et al. Preliminary report of a genetic basis for cognitive decline after cardiac operations. *Ann Thorac Surg.* 1997;64:715–20.

29. Steed L, Kong R, Stygall J et al. The role of apolipoprotein E in cognitive decline after cardiac operation. *Ann Thorac Surg.* 2001;71: 823–6.

30. Abildstrom H, Christiansen M, Siersma VD, Rasmussen LS; ISPOCD2 Investigators. Apolipoprotein E genotype and cognitive

dysfunction after noncardiac surgery. *Anesthesiology*. 2004;101:855–61.

31. Heyer EJ, Wilson DA, Sahlein DH et al. APOE-epsilon4 predisposes to cognitive dysfunction following uncomplicated carotid endarterectomy. *Neurology*. 2005;65: 1759–63.

32. Galley HF, Mahdy A, Lowes DA. Pharmacogenetics and anesthesiologists. *Pharmacogenomics*. 2005;6:849–56.

33. Kulason K, Nouchi R, Hoshikawa Y, Noda M, Okada Y, Kawashima R. Indication of cognitive change and associated risk factor after thoracic surgery in the elderly: A pilot study. *Front Aging Neurosci*. 2017;9:396.

34. Radtke FM, Franck M, Herbig TS et al. Incidence and risk factors for cognitive dysfunction in patients with severe systemic disease. *J Int Med Res*. 2012;40(2):612–20.

35. Monk TG, Price CC. Postoperative cognitive disorders. *Curr Opin Crit Care*. 2011;17(4): 376–81.

36. Ghaffary S, Hajhossein Talasaz A, Ghaeli P et al. Association between perioperative parameters and cognitive impairment in post-cardiac surgery patients. *J Tehran Heart Cent*. 2015;10(2):85–92.

37. Hudetz JA, Patterson KM, Byrne AJ et al. A history of alcohol dependence increases the incidence and severity of postoperative cognitive dysfunction in cardiac surgical patients. *Int J Environ Res Public Health*. 2009;6(11):2725–39.

38. Vizcaychipi MP. Post-operative cognitive dysfunction: Pre-operative risk assessment and peri-operative risk minimization: A pragmatic review of the literature. *J Intensive Crit Care*. 2016;2(2):13.

39. Norkienė I, Samalavičius R, Misiūrienė I, Paulauskienė K, Budrys V, Ivaškevičius J. Incidence and risk factors for early postoperative cognitive decline after coronary artery bypass grafting. *Medicina (Kaunas)*. 2010; 46(7):460–4.

40. Murkin JM, Newman SP, Stump DA, Blumenthal JA. Statement of consensus on assessment of neurobehavioral outcomes after cardiac surgery. *Ann Thorac Surg*. 1995;59: 1289–95.

41. Ramaiah R, Lam AM. Postoperative cognitive dysfunction in the elderly. *Anesthesiol Clin*. 2009;27:485–96.

42. Steinmetz J, Christensen KB, Lund T, Lohse N, Rasmussen LS; ISPOCD Group. Long-term consequences of postoperative cognitive dysfunction. *Anesthesiology*. 2009; 110:548–55.

43. Gunther ML, Morandi A, Ely EW. Pathophysiology of delirium in the intensive care unit. *Crit Care Clin*. 2008;24(1): 45–65.

44. Folstein MF, Folstein SE, McHugh PR. "Mini Mental State." A practical method for grading the cognitive state of patients for the clinician. *J Psychiatr Res*. 1975;12(3):189–98.

45. Nasreddine ZS, Phillips NA, Bédirian V et al. The Montreal Cognitive Assessment, MoCA: A brief screening tool for mild cognitive impairment. *J Am Geriatr Soc*. 2005;53(4): 695–9.

46. Rosano C, Perera S, Inzitari M, Newman AB, Longstreth WT, Studenski S. Digit Symbol Substitution test and future clinical and subclinical disorders of cognition, mobility and mood in older adults. *Age Ageing*. 2016;45(5):688–95.

47. Tombaugh TN. Trail Making Test A and B: normative data stratified by age and education. *Arch Clin Neuropsychol*. 2004;19(2): 203–14.

48. Blackburn HL, Benton AL. Revised administration and scoring of the digit span test. *J Consult Psychol*. 1957;21(2):139–43.

49. Steiner LA. Postoperative delirium guidelines: The greater the obstacle, the more glory in overcoming it. *Eur J Anaesthesiol*. 2017;34(4):189–91.

50. Vijayakumar B, Elango P, Ganessan R. Postoperative delirium in elderly patients. *Indian J Anaesth*. 2014;58(3):251–6.

51. Schneck HJ, Rupreht J. Central anticholinergic syndrome (CAS) in anesthesia and intensive care. *Acta Anaesthesiol Belg*. 1989;40(3): 219–28.

52. Ngo J, Holroyd-Leduc JM. Systematic review of recent dementia practice guidelines. *Age Ageing*. 2015;44(1):25–33.

53. Dening T, Sandilyan MB. Dementia: definitions and types. *Nurs Stand.* 2015;29(37):37–42.

54. Capasso M, De Angelis MV, Di Muzio A et al. Critical Illness Neuromyopathy complicating Akinetic crisis in Parkinsonism: Report of 3 cases. *Medicine (Baltimore).* 2015;94(28): e118.

55. Sciard D, Cattano D, Hussain M, Rosenstein A. Perioperative management of proximal hip fractures in the elderly: The surgeon and the anesthesiologist. *Minerva Anestesiol.* 77(7):715–22.

56. Abildstrom H, Rasmussen LS, Rentowl P et al. Cognitive dysfunction 1-2 years after non-cardiac surgery in the elderly. ISPOCD group. International Study of Post-Operative Cognitive Dysfunction. *Acta Anaesthesiol Scand.* 2000;44(10):1246–51.

18

Special considerations: Electroconvulsive therapy

DHRITIMAN CHAKRABARTI AND DEEPTI SRINIVAS

INTRODUCTION

Electroconvulsive therapy (ECT) is a therapeutic modality that uses iatrogenically induced seizures for biological therapy of medically resistant and acute cases of depression, psychosis, and bipolar disorder. The number of patients receiving ECT relative to those on medication for psychiatric disorders is proportionately higher in the geriatric population, mainly due to unresponsiveness to medication, responsiveness to ECT, and also due to intolerance of medication-associated adverse effects. This chapter discusses the relevance and anesthetic considerations of ECT in the geriatric population.

HISTORY OF ECT

The neuropsychiatrist Ladislas Meduna introduced the concept of "biological antagonism between epilepsy and schizophrenia" in 1934 as a case report of dramatic improvement in a patient with catatonic schizophrenia, using a chemically induced seizure. Electrically stimulated seizures were introduced by Ugo Cerletti, again as a single case, in 1938, and these cases have slowly morphed into the modified ECT procedure of today (1). In 1950, a retrospective study published by Slater showed dramatic improvement in the mortality rate among the elderly mentally ill population at his hospital with the introduction of ECT (2). In the 1940s and 1950s, unmodified ECT was being used as the mainstay of biological therapy in severely diseased patients, which led to increased reports of adverse effects, such as fractures, dislocations, and dental injuries (3). During the 1950s, an attempt was made using succinylcholine and barbiturates as muscle relaxants to improve the safety profile of the procedure (4). Today, modified ECT is a standard and relatively safe procedure with well-researched guidelines in place regarding all aspects of this therapeutic modality.

MECHANISM OF ECT

The mechanism of the physiologic effects of ECT have not been fully elucidated to date. Various investigative modalities, including functional Magnetic Resonance Imaging (fMRI), electroencephalogram (EEG), positron emission tomography

(PET), and single photon emission computed tomography (SPECT) have been used to identify various components of the physiologic changes. Postulated theories center around changes in the hypothalamo—pituitary axis (HPA) and the meso-corticolimbic dopaminergic system, and changes in the neuronal networks in the frontal and temporal lobes.

Immediately following the high-amplitude fast activity during the ictal period, a brief period of generalized slowing and diminished amplitude of EEG occurs. This is followed by a gradual increase in power of the delta and theta bands over the frontal and temporal regions in the interictal period, which is found to be correlated with clinical improvement in the patient.

Changes in brain activation pattern measured by PET are found to be in sync with the EEG changes, with reductions noted in anterior cingulate, dorsolateral, and medial frontal regions. The reductions are strongly correlated with improvement in depression scores. Task-based functional MRI reveals a dichotomy of changes, with mild decrease in activation with a working memory task and a large reduction in activation following an emotional picture-viewing task.

ECT also produces a strong short-term activation of the HPA, with abrupt increases of adrenocorticotrophic hormone, cortisol, and arginine vasopressin noted in human subjects up to 1 hour after the procedure. There is also a relative increase in mesocorticolimbic dopamine levels after completion of an ECT course. All these mechanisms prove beneficial in improving multiple features of depression such as recall bias for negative events, ruminative thoughts, misrepresentations of self-worth (frontotemporal slowing), and improvement in mood, concentration, attention, motivation, and anhedonia (dopaminergic and HPA activation) (5).

MENTAL DISEASE BURDEN IN THE ELDERLY

Old age is characterized by deteriorating physical status, lack of functional autonomy, and a high risk of comorbid illnesses, all of which reduce the quality of life. This segment of the population also carries a higher risk of mental disorders that frequently remain undiagnosed and untreated. As such, the elderly have a high yet unmet need for rehabilitation and psychosocial services (6).

Psychopathological syndromes and clinically defined psychiatric disorders have been diagnosed in approximately 70% and 40% of the geriatric population, respectively (7).

The common mental disorders in the elderly are depression, anxiety disorders, dementia, and delirium. Depression, especially in its minor forms such as dysthymia, is frequent and chronic in this age group and is frequently misconstrued as a normal feature of aging. Such disorders are often more challenging in the elderly as they impair functioning and induce somatic complaints. Associated organic comorbid illnesses such as diabetes, stroke, and dementia have been associated with higher risk of depression. Treatment with antidepressants is at least as effective in old age as in younger patients (8).

Anxiety disorders have a prevalence of approximately 10% in the elderly population, with generalized anxiety disorder being the most common (7%) followed by phobic, panic, and compulsive disorders (9). Anxiety is often a prodromal event followed by depressive illness in these patients, and is also associated with benzodiazepine use and chronic somatic diseases (10).

Other disorders that are uncommon but require urgent electroconvulsive therapy are acute mania, catatonia, treatment-refractory psychotic spectrum illness, and organic neurological syndromes (11).

PHYSIOLOGY OF ECT IN THE GERIATRIC POPULATION

Although the mechanism and physiology of ECT in this age group is similar to the younger population, there are a few notable differences. The seizure threshold is higher in the elderly, probably due to greater thickness of the skull and reduced excitability of the brain. Because of the higher threshold, a higher intensity of stimulus is required for eliciting a seizure of adequate duration. Seizure duration is also reduced with shorter slow-wave duration and weaker seizure strength based on electroencephalographic waveform morphology (12).

Electrode placement in ECT is done usually in a bilateral temporal (BT) format or the left unilateral temporal (UT) format, the prior associated with better and faster remission rates and the latter associated with lower cognitive deficits. The question of the better format for electrode placement for the geriatric population has not been studied rigorously, but the overall evidence suggests no difference in efficacy of treatment or in memory function decline between the two. That said, the choice between the two boils down to other adjunctive individual factors such as severity of symptoms, response to ongoing treatment, and systemic comorbidities (13,14).

Stimulus intensity for UT format is at least 2.5 times the seizure threshold, and that for BT is 1.5 times, with upward titration based on duration of seizure and treatment effectiveness. Due to the higher seizure threshold in the elderly, they have requirements for higher stimulus intensity, which theoretically increases the risk for cognitive deficits after the ECT course. The usual protocol for this age group is to start with ultra-brief pulse of UT format stimulation with switchover to BT if response is slow or insufficient. ECT is switched back to UT or discontinued if cognitive deficits are intolerable with BT (15).

ROLE OF ECT

ECT is an important therapeutic tool in the management of depressive illnesses and specific psychotic syndromes, especially in cases requiring urgent intervention such as catatonia, or those with severe suicidal intent. The evidence base is increasing regarding its efficacy in depression, mania, psychosis, and Parkinson's disease. Despite this, there is a general reluctance among physicians to utilize this modality, with fears based on cognitive impairment, which has been demonstrated to be a major adverse effect in the younger age groups. However, recent studies refute the claim of retrograde amnesia resulting from or being aggravated by ECT even in patients with compromised baseline cognition (16,17).

INDICATIONS

1. *Depression*: When refractory to pharmacotherapy, both unipolar and bipolar depression are amenable to remission with ECT, which is the most effective and commonly used modality of treatment in this context. In cases of life-threatening depressive episodes, ECT is the first line of treatment, with response in 63% of the elderly population. Remission rates in the geriatric population for depression were much higher with ECT (63%) than with medication

(33%). The latest evidence in this respect has been provided by the Prolonging Remission in Depressed Elderly (PRIDE) study in which 240 patients age >60 years were treated with UT ECT and venlafaxine. Response rate was 70% with remission in 62%. The response speed and likelihood of response improves with age, with those above 70 years being 1.89 times more likely to respond than those between 60 and 69 years. The reason for this is unclear and probably multifactorial, including earlier referral for ECT and higher rates of medication intolerance (17,18).

2. *Mania*: Although medication is the first-line therapy for mania in the younger population, ECT has its role firmly entrenched in emergent situations requiring rapid correction. Data are scanty in the elderly population, but mixed-age sample studies report better remission rates with ECT than with pharmacotherapy (19,20).

3. *Catatonia*: Catatonia is a physical manifestation of serious mood disorder characterized by disturbed motor activity, and is more commonly observed in the elderly. Benzodiazepines are considered the first-line treatment, with response rate being 60%–70%, but they become less efficacious over time due to development of tolerance. If catatonia is concomitant with severe illness, ECT is the preferred choice for initial treatment (21,22). Although explicit data in the elderly population for this disorder are lacking, case series suggest similar response rates to those of the general population (23).

4. *Psychosis*: Bilateral temporal ECT is effective in treatment of refractory schizophrenia in adults. Data for the older age group come from nonrandomized low-quality studies, which show high variability in success rates but overall concur that BT ECT is safe and effective for this spectrum of disorders (24). ECT is also useful when rapid control is required when schizophrenia is comorbid with catatonia, suicidality, or aggression. ECT is more useful for control of positive symptoms than negative symptoms (25).

5. *Neurological disorders*: ECT is has a long history of being anecdotally useful in a variety of neurological disorders with or without comorbid psychiatric disorder. Parkinson's disease, movement disorders, tardive dyskinesia, dementia with depression, or post-stroke depression are all amenable to treatment.

a. Dementia carries an inherent risk of depression, with up to 50% of patients experiencing it. Although ECT of patients with dementia with depression might carry a theoretical risk of aggravating or hastening cognitive decline, the risk is overstated. A transient cognitive deficit has been demonstrated, but the course of dementia is unaltered. The format of ECT to be used carries considerations similar to other disorders, with UT being used for those at higher risk of cognitive decline and BT being used for those requiring urgent intervention (13,26).

b. ECT in patients with Parkinson's disease benefits both motor and depressive symptoms, with motor symptoms showing a transient improvement, probably due to enhancement in the dopaminergic outflow (27,28). Due to the dual benefit, this treatment modality is an attractive option, albeit with requirement of repeated sessions due to the transience of effect. UT format is preferred to reduce the chance of cognitive decline.

c. Post-stroke depression affects approximately 30% of patients within first 2 years after stroke, with ECT being a useful treatment modality (29).

ADVERSE EFFECTS OF ECT IN THE ELDERLY

Due to the physiological status of patients with old age and comorbid conditions, ECT and anesthesia carry an inherently higher risk in the geriatric population. Side effects common with the younger population include headache, muscle pain, and confusional states/delirium. Mortality is extremely low with this procedure and is estimated to be 2.1 per 100,000 procedures (30). The mortality risk is increased by the presence of cardiac dysfunction, intracranial lesions, respiratory diseases, and American Society of Anesthesiologists class 4/5, while age of patient does not come across as an independent predictor (11). Overall, ECT is deemed a relatively safe procedure in this age group, barring individual concerns stemming from systemic risk factors. Specific adverse effects which increase morbidity of the procedure are:

1. *Cognitive deficits*: This is by far the most common concern among physicians prescribing ECT as a treatment option. The usual timeline of events following a course of ECT includes an acute confusional state which usually lasts approximately 1 hour (prolonged confusional state is a risk factor for amnesia), which is likely to be prolonged in patients with dementia. This is followed by anterograde and/or retrograde amnesia, which is self-limiting and resolves over 1–3 weeks. Physiological factors such as advanced age, organic brain disorders, prolonged acute confusional state, and iatrogenic factors such as BT format of electrode placement, higher stimulus intensity, and frequency predispose to worsening of amnesic state (31). Long-term cognitive changes are unaffected by ECT (17).

2. *Cardiovascular effects*: Cardiovascular (CVS) adverse effects take precedence in this age group because of inherently higher risk due to CVS comorbidities, and should be factored in to the decision for undertaking the procedure. The initial electrical impulse triggers a parasympathetic surge, which is observed as bradycardia and sometimes asystole. This is followed by the seizure activity, which causes an elevation in the sympathetic output and is associated with hypertension and tachycardia. These transient changes are benign in the younger population but may lead to arrhythmias or myocardial ischemia/infarction in those with CVS comorbid diseases. Patients with recent myocardial infarction, heart block, and atrial fibrillation with atrial clot are especially prone to adverse events. Such cases should be identified and medically optimized before taking up ECT, and the implications of these disorders should be explained during informed consent (13).

3. *Cerebral adverse events*: ECT does not cause any direct structural harm to the cortex but does produce neurotrophic changes, as evidenced in neuroimaging studies (13). Hippocampal volume loss in major depressive disorders seems to be reversed as part of the neuroplastic processes induced by ECT (32). The cerebral adverse events due to ECT stem from the systemic hemodynamic changes induced by the procedure, with highest risk being in those with recent stroke and cerebral aneurysms. ECT is usually not performed within the first 2 months of stroke, and

thereafter only after weighing the risk against the benefit, and with careful intraprocedure hemodynamic management (33,34). Intracranial tumors associated with increased intracranial pressure may be considered a relative contraindication; however, patients with stable intracranial masses without edema may be safely administered ECT (35).

4. *Respiratory adverse events*: Respiratory comorbidities such as pulmonary hypertension, asthma, chronic obstructive pulmonary disease, and airway-related problems such as sleep apnea and loose teeth may complicate the anesthetic procedure during ECT administration (36). Taking appropriate precautions such as prior optimization and careful drug selection for respiratory diseases and specially designed bite blocks for tongue and tooth protection greatly reduce the associated risks (13).

5. *Musculoskeletal adverse events*: The geriatric age group is associated with osteoporosis and spinal degenerative changes which could lead to fractures or worsening of disc prolapse. A higher dose of muscle relaxant to ensure immobility can help circumvent iatrogenic morbidity (13).

MANAGEMENT OF PROCEDURE

1. *Pre-ECT evaluation*: Management of ECT in the elderly requires an intensive multidisciplinary approach involving communication between the treating psychiatrist and anesthesiologist, along with involvement of the patient and their relatives. A comprehensive risk-benefit analytic approach should be followed while deciding the need for ECT. Assessments include past and present psychiatric history, substance use, medical comorbidities, and any prior anesthesia experience. Further testing includes baseline cognition assessment, neuropsychiatric tests, and optionally, neuroimaging to rule out organic disorders. Preanesthetic checkup should include medical comorbidities and their optimization, airway and dental examination, electrocardiogram, and standard laboratory testing of biochemistry and hemogram.

2. *Anesthetic protocol*: The choice of anesthetic agents is determined by the patient's physical status and comorbidities as well as the proposed course of ECT in the patient.

   a. *Premedication*: Anticholinergic agents are often administered to counter the initial parasympathetic surge, and glycopyrrolate is the preferred drug in a dose of 0.01 mg/kg administered intravenously immediately before the hypnotic agent injection. In known hypertensive patients or those at risk for myocardial ischemia during the ictal sympathetic surge, esmolol or labetalol may be administered. Other drugs such as alpha-2 receptor agonists or calcium channel blockers may also be considered.

   b. *Preoxygenation*: This is a mandatory step in any anesthetic induction process and its importance in this procedure cannot be overstated due to increase of cerebral oxygen consumption by 200% during the ictal period. In addition, hyperventilation may be used to prolong seizure duration (37).

   c. *Hypnotic agent*: Methohexital (0.75–1 mg/kg) is considered the gold standard due to least effect on seizure threshold and duration compared to other agents. However, due to lack of availability, propofol, ketamine, thiopentone, or etomidate are used more commonly. Individual agent properties regarding CVS depression and seizure suppression should be kept in mind when choosing the agent. Overall, propofol is associated with higher seizure thresholds and shorter seizure durations. However, due to its property of predicable and smooth awakening, propofol is very commonly used in this regard. Etomidate and ketamine are associated with lower threshold and longer seizure duration but are used selectively due to adrenergic suppression by etomidate and propensity to induce psychotic symptoms and longer emergence time with ketamine. The inhalational agent sevoflurane (5%–8% for induction and 2% for maintenance) may be preferred in cases who are uncooperative for intravenous access placement (38). A recent meta-analysis compared efficacy and tolerability of these anesthetic agents and found significantly higher reduction in depression scores and longer seizure durations with methohexital compared to propofol. They concluded that ketamine and methohexital may be preferred over propofol and etomidate in the context of increasing seizure duration and efficacy in improvement of depression scores (39).

   d. *Muscle relaxant*: Short-acting muscle relaxants are preferred, and unless contraindicated, succinylcholine (1–2 mg/kg) is the default choice. If contraindicated in cases of malignant hyperthermia, atypical pseudocholinesterase, hyperkalemia, or recent burn injuries, mivacurium or atracurium may be used.

   e. A bite block must mandatorily be placed between the teeth while pushing the tongue posteriorly before the shock is administered.

3. *Monitoring*: Standard intraoperative monitoring including electrocardiogram, pulse oximetry, noninvasive blood pressure, and end-tidal carbon dioxide should be used in every case. Additional monitoring includes electroencephalography for measuring seizure duration. Although this is optional, it is preferable in cases of modified ECT where motor seizure activity may be attenuated by muscle relaxants. Minimum seizure duration for an effective ECT is 25 seconds for motor seizure and 40 seconds for electroencephalographic seizure (38). Another method used for clinical motor seizure monitoring includes inflating a cuff to above systolic blood pressure on a leg before administration of muscle relaxant and monitoring clinical seizures in the unparalyzed limb.

4. *Electrode placement and stimulus characteristics*: Electrode placement format is dictated by the diagnosis of the patient, the urgency of ECT, and the neurological comorbidities of the patient that may be associated with cognitive decline. The BT format is used when urgency is high and higher efficacy of treatment is required, while the UT format is used when cognitive deficits are a constraining factor. The stimulus is provided as an ultra-brief pulse, with pulse width of 0.5–2 ms, in a constant current format, with the intensity determined by electrode placement, seizure threshold of the patient, and the clinical improvement over the course of ECT (36).

CONCLUSION

ECT is a remarkably efficacious therapeutic modality for treatment of medically refractory mental diseases in the elderly. With careful selection of patients and appropriate precautions, ECT can be used safely to improve the burden of mental health in this age group. Close communication between the psychiatrist and the anesthesiologist is important for a successful outcome.

ACKNOWLEDGEMENT

This chapter could not have been possible without the support of Arpitha Anna Jacob, who was instrumental in reviewing the manuscript and getting it to its final form.

REFERENCES

1. Endler NS. The origins of electroconvulsive therapy (ECT). *Convuls Ther.* 1988;4(1):5–23.
2. Slater ETO. Evaluation of electric convulsion therapy as compared with conservative methods of treatment in depressive states. *J Ment Sci.* 1951;97(408):567–9.
3. Consensus Conference. Electroconvulsive therapy. *JAMA.* 1985;254(15):2103–8.
4. Kral VA. Somatic therapies in older depressed patients. *J Gerontol.* 1976;31(3):311–3.
5. Fosse R, Read J. Electroconvulsive treatment: Hypotheses about mechanisms of action. *Front Psychiatry.* 2013;4:94.
6. Linden M, Horgas AL, Gilberg R, Steinhagen-Thiessen E. Predicting health care utilization in the very old. *J Aging Health.* 1997;9(1):3–27.
7. Wernicke TF, Linden M, Gilberg R, Helmchen H. Ranges of psychiatric morbidity in the old and the very old—Results from the Berlin Aging Study (BASE). *Eur Arch Psychiatry Clin Neurosci.* 2000;250(3):111–9.
8. Katona C. Managing depression and anxiety in the elderly patient. *Eur Neuropsychopharmacol.* 2000;10(Suppl 4):S427–32.
9. Beekman AT, Bremmer MA, Deeg DJ et al. Anxiety disorders in later life: A report from the Longitudinal Aging Study Amsterdam. *Int J Geriatr Psychiatry.* 1998;13(10):717–26.
10. van Balkom AJ, Beekman AT, de Beurs E, Deeg DJ, van Dyck R, van Tilburg W.

Comorbidity of the anxiety disorders in a community-based older population in The Netherlands. *Acta Psychiatr Scand*. 2000; 101(1):37–45.

11. Meyer JP, Swetter SK, Kellner CH. Electroconvulsive therapy in geriatric psychiatry. *Psychiatr Clin North Am*. 2018;41(1):79–93.

12. Sackeim H, Decina P, Prohovnik I, Malitz S. Seizure threshold in electroconvulsive therapy. Effects of sex, age, electrode placement, and number of treatments. *Arch Gen Psychiatry*. 1987;44(4):355–60.

13. Andrade C, Arumugham SS, Thirthalli J. Adverse effects of electroconvulsive therapy. *Psychiatr Clin North Am*. 2016;39(3): 513–30.

14. Fraser RM, Glass IB. Unilateral and bilateral ECT in elderly patients. A comparative study. *Acta Psychiatr Scand*. 1980;62(1):13–31.

15. McLoughlin DM. Response to Kellner and Farber: Addressing crossover of high-dose right unilateral ECT to bitemporal ECT. *Am J Psychiatry*. 2016;173(7):731–2.

16. Verwijk E, Comijs HC, Kok RM et al. Short- and long-term neurocognitive functioning after electroconvulsive therapy in depressed elderly: A prospective naturalistic study. *Int Psychogeriatrics*. 2014;26(2):315–24.

17. Kellner CH, Husain MM, Knapp RG et al. Right unilateral ultrabrief pulse ECT in geriatric depression: Phase 1 of the PRIDE study. *Am J Psychiatry*. 2016;173(11):1101–9.

18. Spaans H-P, Sienaert P, Bouckaert F et al. Speed of remission in elderly patients with depression: Electroconvulsive therapy v. medication. *Br J Psychiatry*. 2015;206(1):67–71.

19. McCabe MS. ECT in the treatment of mania: A controlled study. *Am J Psychiatry*. 1976; 133(6):688–91.

20. Mukherjee S, Sackeim HA, Schnur DB. Electroconvulsive therapy of acute manic episodes: A review of 50 years' experience. *Am J Psychiatry*. 1994;151(2):169–76.

21. Luchini F, Lattanzi L, Bartolommei N et al. Catatonia and neuroleptic malignant syndrome. *J Nerv Ment Dis*. 2013;201(1):36–42.

22. Medda P, Toni C, Luchini F, Giorgi Mariani M, Mauri M, Perugi G. Catatonia in 26 patients with bipolar disorder: Clinical features and response to electroconvulsive therapy. *Bipolar Disord*. 2015;17(8):892–901.

23. Suzuki K, Awata S, Matsuoka H. One-year outcome after response to ECT in middle-aged and elderly patients with intractable catatonic schizophrenia. *J ECT*. 2004;20(2):99–106.

24. Liu AY, Rajji TK, Blumberger DM, Daskalakis ZJ, Mulsant BH. Brain stimulation in the treatment of late-life severe mental illness other than unipolar nonpsychotic depression. *Am J Geriatr Psychiatry*. 2014;22(3):216–40.

25. Pompili M, Lester D, Dominici G et al. Indications for electroconvulsive treatment in schizophrenia: A systematic review. *Schizophr Res*. 2013;146(1–3):1–9.

26. Semkovska M, McLoughlin DM. Objective cognitive performance associated with electroconvulsive therapy for depression: A systematic review and meta-analysis. *Biol Psychiatry*. 2010;68(6):568–77.

27. Borisovskaya A, Bryson WC, Buchholz J, Samii A, Borson S. Electroconvulsive therapy for depression in Parkinson's disease: Systematic review of evidence and recommendations. *Neurodegener Dis Manag*. 2016;6(2):161–76.

28. Rudorfer MV, Risby ED, Hsiao JK, Linnoila M, Potter WZ. ECT alters human monoamines in a different manner from that of antidepressant drugs. *Psychopharmacol Bull*. 1988;24(3): 396–9.

29. Robinson RG, Jorge RE. Post-stroke depression: A review. *Am J Psychiatry*. 2016;173(3): 221–31.

30. Tørring N, Sanghani SN, Petrides G, Kellner CH, Østergaard SD. The mortality rate of electroconvulsive therapy: A systematic review and pooled analysis. *Acta Psychiatr Scand*. 2017;135(5):388–97.

31. Greenberg RM, Kellner CH. Electroconvulsive therapy: A selected review. *Am J Geriatr Psychiatry*. 2005;13(4):268–81.

32. Wilkinson ST, Sanacora G, Bloch MH. Hippocampal volume changes following electroconvulsive therapy: A systematic review and meta-analysis. *Biol Psychiatry Cogn Neurosci Neuroimaging*. 2017;2(4):327–35.

33. Currier MB, Murray GB, Welch CC. Electroconvulsive therapy for post-stroke depressed geriatric patients. *J Neuropsychiatry Clin Neurosci*. 1992;4(2):140–4.

34. Saito S. Anesthesia management for electroconvulsive therapy: Hemodynamic and

respiratory management. *J Anesth*. 2005; 19(2):142–9.

35. Sajedi PI, Mitchell J, Herskovits EH, Raghavan P. Routine cross-sectional head imaging before electroconvulsive therapy: A tertiary center experience. *J Am Coll Radiol*. 2016;13(4):429–34.

36. Kerner N, Prudic J. Current electroconvulsive therapy practice and research in the geriatric population. *Neuropsychiatry (London)*. 2014; 4(1):33–54.

37. Abrams R. Technique of electroconvulsive therapy: Theory. In: Abrams R (ed). *Electroconvulsive Therapy*. 4th ed. Oxford University Press; 2002. pp. 142–71.

38. Kadiyala PK, Kadiyala LD. Anaesthesia for electroconvulsive therapy: An overview with an update on its role in potentiating electroconvulsive therapy. *Indian J Anaesth*. 2017; 61(5):373–80.

39. Fond G, Bennabi D, Haffen E et al. A Bayesian framework systematic review and meta-analysis of anesthetic agents effectiveness/ tolerability profile in electroconvulsive therapy for major depression. *Sci Rep*. 2016;6: 19847.

19

Special considerations: Alzheimer's disease

CHRISTOPHER G. SINON, SONA SHAH ARORA, AMY D. RODRIGUEZ, AND
PAUL S. GARCÍA

ALZHEIMER'S DISEASE: GENERAL INFORMATION AND OVERLAP WITH ANESTHETIC MECHANISMS

Definitions, diagnosis, incidence, and impact

Alzheimer's disease (AD) is a progressive neuro-degenerative disease and the most common cause of dementia worldwide (1–3). One in ten individuals over the age of 65 has dementia that can be attributed to AD. The characteristic symptoms of dementia involve problems in learning, memory, language, and problem-solving that arise from dying or damaged neurons in brain areas important for cognitive function (1). AD pathology is characterized by the formation of extracellular plaques of beta-amyloid peptide and intracellular tangles of hyperphosphorylated tau protein. The accumulation of plaques and tangles in the brains of patients with AD leads to widespread neurodegeneration, causing progressive declines in cognitive ability and eventually leading to death.

Due to its progressive nature, AD often presents in elderly patients. The primary risk factor for AD is age. AD affects nearly 5.7 million people in the United States, with greater than 95% of those affected over the age of 60 (1,2). The illness is diagnosed in patients who present with decline in cognitive function, but a preclinical AD stage may be recognized before an official diagnosis is made. Diagnosis of AD involves cognitive testing and neurological examination of the patient along with family input on behavioral changes. In addition, imaging methods may be used to rule out other potential explanations for cognitive decline (1). Quantifiably, the risk of acquiring an AD diagnosis doubles every 5 years after the age of 65, and 95% of AD cases occur after age 60 (3).

With life expectancy of the general population on the rise, the projected prevalence of AD worldwide is expected to rise to 65 million people by 2030 and 115 million people in 2050 (4–6). Geriatric patients undergoing surgery are more likely to have AD or to be at risk for AD development. With this in mind, it is important for anesthesiologists to consider the effects of anesthesia, surgery, and approaches to perioperative care in patients with AD. We are only beginning to understand how anesthesia affects the development and progression of AD, and currently there are no standards of best practice for the anesthetic management of patients with AD. Research interest is building, however, and researchers have identified commonalities between the pathophysiology of neurodegeneration in AD and the cellular and systematic effects of anesthesia (7). Further, several studies have identified that AD pathogenesis may be affected by anesthesia and perioperative care (8,9). The goal of this chapter is to help the anesthesiologist to better understand (i) the potential for anesthetics and surgery to exacerbate symptoms of AD, and (ii) recommendations for anesthetic practices in patients with mild cognitive impairment (MCI) and AD to avoid perioperative and postoperative complications.

The relation of Alzheimer's disease to perioperative neurocognitive disorders

MECHANISMS AND PATHOGENESIS

Although the definitive etiology remains unknown, two pathological features serve to define AD: amyloid plaques and neurofibrillary tangles. Amyloid plaques are composed of abnormally folded proteins that deposit extracellularly, while neurofibrillary tangles arise from abnormal regulation of intraneuronal cytoskeletal proteins (10). Plaques and tangles result from accumulations of beta-amyloid peptide and hyperphosphorylated tau protein, respectively. Buildup and aggregation of both plaques and neurofibrillary tangles particularly affect the temporal lobe (11–13).

Beta-amyloid is produced following cleavage of the transmembrane protein amyloid precursor protein (APP) by beta-secretase and gamma-secretase (14). It is unclear exactly what role APP or beta-amyloid play in a normally functioning neuron, but an imbalance between the production and clearance of beta-amyloid can lead to pathologic accumulation that may play a causative role in AD (15). Tau protein is an important microtubule-associated protein that helps to stabilize the neuron's cytoskeleton by binding to microtubules (13). In vitro studies suggest that in normal cellular function the activity of tau protein is regulated by phosphorylation. When tau is phosphorylated, there is a reduction in the binding of tau to microtubules which could be an important step for the regulation of neurite outgrowth and axonal transport in the neuron. In AD, as well as all other known diseases involving dysregulated tau, there is rampant phosphorylation of tau proteins resulting in cytoskeletal abnormalities and accumulation of hyperphosphorylated tau. While neurofibrillary tangles formed from hyperphosphorylated tau can generate over decades independent of plaques or the presence of AD (16), both beta-amyloid and hyperphosphorylated tau are necessary for AD pathology.

The presence of plaques and tangles can lead to the damage and death of neurons in many ways, including increased neuroinflammation and oxidative stress as well as disruptions of specific neurotransmitter systems (14,17). Amyloid plaques trigger an immune response via activated microglia. Although microglia serve an important physiologic purpose in neuroprotection and clearance of beta-amyloid via phagocytosis, studies suggest that these macrophages of the brain may also take part in fibril formation (18). In addition, microglia, along with the complement system, also likely facilitate loss of synapses, which correlates with cognitive decline in AD (19). Inflammation also affects tau protein, worsening the severity of its pathology (20,21). Beta-amyloid also impairs normal mitochondrial function by inhibiting important enzymes. The resulting damage to mitochondria causes an increase in the release of reactive oxygen species and oxidative stress in AD (17). Some evidence has shown that certain muscarinic receptors are bound by beta-amyloid disrupting both acetylcholine release and potentiation of synapses. Neurodegeneration of cholinergic pathways is also typical in the progression of AD (14).

The effects of beta-amyloid on multiple disease pathways, including dysregulation of tau phosphorylation, has led to the formation of the amyloid cascade hypothesis for AD pathogenesis (22,23). The amyloid cascade hypothesis posits that the formation of beta-amyloid plaques acts as a trigger, causing the full range of symptoms associated with AD. The hypothesis has been controversial based primarily on two observations. Mouse models of AD expressing mutated genes coding for synthesis of beta-amyloid do not develop tauopathies, and the severity of amyloid plaque deposition does not correlate well with the severity of cognitive symptoms in human AD. More recently, newer rat models of AD that share isoforms of tau with humans have demonstrated the full symptomology of AD following expression of mutated genes in the amyloid precursor protein synthesis pathway (22).

CLINICAL EVIDENCE OF A LINK BETWEEN ANESTHESIA AND AD

Several limits exist to identifying a true association between the risk of developing AD, anesthesia, and surgery. For the most part, surgical processes rarely do not require anesthesia, and anesthesia is rarely administered without surgery; thus, no randomized, double-blind, controlled studies have prospectively and directly tested for the relationship between anesthesia and AD development (24,25). Using a retrospective approach, several larger studies reported that anesthesia and surgery were associated with an increased incidence of AD (8,9). The nature of AD, however, is progressive, suggesting that anesthesia and surgery may play a role in accelerating the underlying disease process more so than serving as the sole "cause" of AD (24). This acceleration of trajectory is illustrated in Figure 19.1. As a normal brain ages, cognitive trajectory decreases exponentially. Similar processes are occurring for a brain on the "AD path," however, the degree of exponential decay is greater. It is important to remember that the pathology and pattern of neurodegeneration seen in AD is fundamentally different than that seen in normal aging. Interactions between surgery with anesthesia and the previously described pathogenic processes occurring in AD may increase the rate of decay in cognitive trajectory for patients with AD.

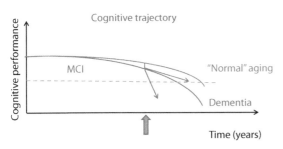

Figure 19.1 Trajectory of average cognitive decline due to normal aging and dementia. The blue arrow represents the timepoint for an intervention or event that accelerates the rate of decay in cognitive performance. While surgery with anesthesia may impact cognitive performance in an individual aging normally, this individual still performs well above threshold for identification of mild cognitive impairment (MCI). Alternatively, an individual with dementia has an accelerated rate of decay in cognitive performance over time and the pathology underlying dementia may make them more susceptible to dramatic declines cognitive performance following surgery.

The content of beta-amyloid, total tau protein, and phosphorylated tau present in cerebrospinal fluid (CSF) is promising as a biomarker for MCI and AD in humans. One study of a cohort of humans between ages 55–90 containing probable MCI and AD volunteers found that the beta-amyloid$_{1-42}$ peptide content in CSF was the most sensitive biomarker for determining which individuals belonged to the "probable AD" group. Also, the ratio of total tau protein to beta-amyloid$_{1-42}$ peptide accurately predicted which volunteers with MCI transitioned into AD within 1 year (26). A similar experiment was performed in patients undergoing aortic valve replacement with propofol anesthesia. CSF samples were collected from each patient the day before and the day after surgery. Following surgery, there was a significant increase in beta-amyloid$_{1-42}$ and neuroinflammatory markers present in CSF (27). CSF samples taken from patients at 0, 6, 24, and 48 hours from the end of a procedure to correct nasal CSF leak displayed a persistent increase in levels of total tau protein and phosphorylated tau over the 48 hours from the end of surgery and an increase in inflammatory markers at 24 hours (28). While these patients showed no difference in beta-amyloid over the course of the study, significant increases in contents of tau in CSF indicate that neurological injury occurred during the peri- or postoperative period. When neurons are damaged or die, tau protein can leak from the injured cells out into the CSF. Lastly, studies support the idea that AD and anesthesia both affect the gross structure of the brain. As discussed previously, structures of the temporal lobe are affected by AD pathology (12,13). Similarly, researchers observed a loss of tissue in the temporal lobe, particularly in the hippocampal region, several months after surgical intervention (29). Although the exact mechanism for how these effects relate to long-term AD progression is unknown, anesthesia and AD have similar effects on shared molecular and structural targets, such as beta-amyloid, tau, and temporal structures.

While these three studies capture transient changes in the central nervous system during surgery, the effects are consistent, with surgery and general anesthesia acting as a stimulus that increases circulating and structural biomarkers of AD and inflammation. It is worth noting that while chronic neuroinflammation may accelerate neurodegeneration in AD, transient increases in neuroinflammation can help to clear beta-amyloid plaques. As we find more accurate biomarkers of MCI and AD, we will be increasingly able to track patients over time to better determine the influence of surgery on neurodegeneration.

PRECLINICAL EVIDENCE OF A LINK BETWEEN ANESTHESIA AND AD

Beyond possibly initiating and contributing to formal AD development, do anesthetics affect AD long term—for instance, increasing cognitive decline? In vitro studies have shown that single exposures to volatile anesthetics can increase the rate of beta-amyloid oligomerization and reduce the concentration of beta-amyloid necessary to form oligomers (30,31). Total tau protein and phosphorylated tau have been shown to increase in CSF following surgery with general anesthesia (28,32). It appears that anesthetics affect both tau and beta-amyloid, thus potentially influencing the pathogenesis of AD.

Why does this association between AD and anesthesia and surgery exist? In order to elucidate this association, multiple studies have aimed to identify the role that anesthesia and surgery may play in accelerating the underlying disease process of AD (24). General anesthesia has been shown to increase beta-amyloid as monomers in mice (33), possibly through inhibition of one of the proteins that degrades beta-amyloid, beta-amyloid—cleaving enzyme (BACE) (34). Experiments in cell culture suggest that some anesthetics may lower the clearance of beta-amyloid (35).

Not only does anesthesia appear to affect some of the same proteins and gross structural components that are impacted in AD, but its effects may act synergistically with AD pathogenesis, contributing to disease progression (24). For example, beta-amyloid accumulation can damage neuronal function by interrupting intracellular calcium homeostasis, leaving neurons susceptible to excitotoxic injury (36). Several anesthetic agents also increase intracellular calcium levels, possibly advancing development of AD (37,38).

Mechanisms underlying inflammation also overlap in AD and anesthesia. Research has found that anesthesia during surgery activates the body's inflammatory response (28,39). This surgery-induced inflammation adds to the already inflamed brain of a patient on an AD path, possibly exacerbating pathology. In an effort to identify options to limit this synergism, studies have identified that some anesthetics may be less inflammation-inducing than others; some agents have even shown anti-inflammatory effects (24).

PHARMACOLOGIC CONSIDERATIONS FOR THOSE WITH OR AT RISK FOR AD

When employing anesthetic in the geriatric population, one must consider the implications that age-related changes have on perioperative anesthetic management. Although most organ systems continue to function at a similar basal level throughout life, a reduction in functional reserve and in ability to compensate for physiologic stress occurs during aging. In general, anesthetic requirements are lower in geriatric patients, but administration of each agent must be tailored to each individual.

Drug dosing due to altered physiology in the elderly

Generally speaking, reduced dosage of any medicine is prudent in elderly patients. Glomerular filtration rate (GFR) progressively declines with age, resulting in an impaired sodium homeostasis and limited response to acid loads. This may result in subclinical hyponatremia, which may be more significant in the setting of a geriatric patient presenting for surgery. Hyponatremia or rapid correction will only worsen cognitive problems in AD patients. Elderly patients overall have a decrease in total body water (typically as much as 20%–30%). As a result, administration of typical drug doses may result in supratherapeutic effects (40).

With advanced age there is also decreased renal tubular function leading to impaired ability to concentrate and dilute urine, increasing the risk of urinary retention and polyuria. During surgical stress, hemodynamic instability may occur if the patient cannot properly respond to volume changes. As a result, particular attention needs to be given to intraoperative fluid and electrolyte management (41).

Further, age-related loss of endoplasmic reticulum results in lowered protein synthesis. Lower levels of proteins, such as albumin, means serum levels of protein-bound drugs increase. There is decreased liver mass and conjugation activity with age. This can lead to changes in the pharmacologic effects of medications due to decreased metabolism and protein binding.

Reduced clearance due to renal or liver dysfunction also leads to increased drug half-lives. In addition, the elderly are more susceptible to the psychoactive effects anesthetic medications, necessitating decreased dosing of anesthetic agents in an effort to reduce perioperative complications (reviewed in [42]).

Although it is common to reduce dosage of opioids and other pain medicine in the elderly and those with or at risk for AD, withholding pain medicine does not avoid complications. Analgesia can be difficult to control in these patients, and frequent assessments (objective and subjective) of the patient's pain should be performed by staff. Pain and heightened sensitivity to the sedating effects of pain medicine make these patients at very high risk of delirium related to pain or treatment of pain.

A decrease in insulin production predisposes to perioperative hyperglycemia even without a diagnosis of diabetes. High glucose levels can lead to swelling of neurons, increased infection risk, impaired wound healing, and altered mental status. Also, dysphagia is known to be common and underdiagnosed in this population (43). Patients with AD may be unreliable in response to recent meals and liquids and may need to be observed for signs of aspiration while advancing their diet postoperatively.

Perioperative considerations for patients receiving drugs to treat Alzheimer's disease

Outpatient drug therapy for alleviating some of the memory problems associated with AD is a new and changing field. Increasingly, patients on either the N-methyl-D-aspartate receptor (NMDA) antagonist, memantine, or one of the three acetylcholinesterase inhibitors, galantamine, rivastigmine, and donepezil, are presenting for surgery. No specific interactions with common anesthetic drugs have been discovered, and a comprehensive review of these drugs in anesthesiology practice has not been undertaken. The acetylcholinesterase inhibitors are associated with signs of increased cholinergic signaling in the periphery: vomiting and nausea. In the case of galantamine, bradycardia is also possible (44). It has been suggested that donepezil be used more routinely in the post-anesthesia care unit (PACU) to aid in recovery as an attempt to remedy a potential anticholinergic cause, either by undiagnosed dementia or as a consequence of

administering drugs known to contribute to anticholinergic situations perioperatively (e.g., diphenhydramine) (45).

CLINICAL APPROACH FOR GERIATRIC PATIENTS WITH OR AT RISK FOR ALZHEIMER'S DISEASE

Preoperative evaluation

In a preoperative setting, anesthesiologists should personalize their care plan to each patient, similar to any other specialty. When a patient has mild cognitive impairment, suggesting they may be on the path to AD development or in the subclinical phase of AD, individualized evaluation may hold even greater significance. Several studies have identified increased risks regarding anesthesia and surgery for patients with mild cognitive impairment: greater sensitivity in general to anesthetic agents, lower bispectral indices (BIS), and greater risk of postoperative complications, such as delirium and cognitive decline (46–49). These variables hold great clinical significance and can affect the quality of care provided if not considered during preoperative evaluation (Figure 19.2).

Research is ongoing regarding ways for anesthesiologists to reduce the risk of AD development during perioperative care. Some labs have shown consistent results suggesting that anesthesia with sevoflurane results in

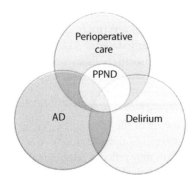

Figure 19.2 Reprinted from Berger et al. 2014 (24). Possible overlapping relationships among perioperative care, delirium, Alzheimer's disease (AD), and persistant postoperative neurocognitive dysfunction (PPND). Each circle represents a group of patients who are undergoing perioperative care and/or who have the given disorder. Circles are not drawn to epidemiologic scale.

more inflammation and increased expression of AD-associated proteins and peptides when compared with propofol anesthesia (31). Propofol has been suggested as preferred anesthetic over sevoflurane for patients with MCI and AD. However, attempts to replicate these findings have been inconsistent, and the mechanism by which propofol would be protective for central nervous system damage is not immediately clear (24).

Intraoperative management and monitoring

The EEG represents the summation of electrical inputs onto dendrites of cortical neurons. EEG recordings are noninvasive and thus can be implemented as a monitor of brain activity before, during, and/or after surgery for most patients. Electrodes are affixed to the skin and will record electrical activity from the brain through the skin and skull. During recording, the higher-frequency activity of brain will be filtered out of the signal by the skull, and the power of the EEG signal recorded will be affected by the number of neurons present in the recording area and the distance between the electrode and the surface of the brain. During normal aging, on average there is a decrease in the mass of white and gray matter present in the brain, which subsequently leads to a decrease in the average EEG power due to age.

While decreases in EEG power are also common for patients with AD, the specific progression of AD pathology leads to EEG characteristics that are well correlated with the severity of AD (summarized in Figure 19.3). In early stages of AD, the spectral power of the EEG increases in the theta range (4–8 Hz) while beta (14–40 Hz) power decreases. With later stages of AD, EEG delta (0.5–4 Hz) power increases as alpha power decreases (50). There is room for speculation that the slowing of the EEG and especially the shift of resting-state EEG alpha band dominance toward a slower rhythm may reflect a "disconnection" of cortical from subcortical networks (51). Recent and preliminary results point to an increased relative theta power in beta-amyloid positive subjects without any symptoms of AD onset (52). While spectral power gives a first impression regarding the changes AD has on the EEG, it does not tell anything regarding functional changes in the EEG (51).

The progression of AD also leads to a change in EEG features that represent connectivity and

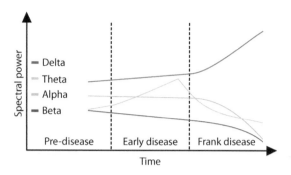

Figure 19.3 Summary of the stereotypical changes in spectral power over the progression of AD. The early disease state is characterized by increases in theta activity and decreasing power in the beta range. Once AD has progressed to the frank disease state, power across all frequencies except for those in the delta range.

synchronization within the brain's neural network. EEG spectral coherence seems to decrease over a wide frequency range in patients diagnosed with AD when compared to healthy patients of same age. The degree of EEG abnormality, specifically lower alpha and delta wave coherences, is often associated with greater severity of AD (53,54). As an example, there is a difference in resting-state alpha coherence between aged healthy, MCI, and AD subjects (51). More sophisticated measures like synchronization likelihood that include nonlinear properties of the EEG showed decreased functional connectivity in alpha and beta frequencies, but not gamma (>40 Hz) (55). This finding may point toward AD disconnecting long range connectivity (beta) while not affecting local patches of neural network activity (gamma) (56). Furthermore, EEG analysis revealed a reduction of frontoparietal synchrony likelihood in AD patients (57). A negative effect on frontoparietal connections is also observable in healthy patients or volunteers transitioning from wakefulness to anesthetic-induced anesthesia and is considered a key mechanism of the anesthetic-induced loss of consciousness (58,59).

Intraoperative "consciousness monitors" can help to simplify the use of EEG recording to guide perioperative anesthetic maintenance for patients with AD. As previously mentioned, anesthetic requirements are generally lower for geriatric patients, and this is especially true for patients with MCI or AD. Titrating anesthetic drugs to remain within the recommended index range for surgical anesthesia can reduce the likelihood of postoperative complications. Burst suppression has been linked to postoperative delirium (POD) and in some studies, persistent perioperative neurocognitive disorders (PPNDs) (see next section). Burst suppression varies in its detection by processed EEG monitors. Many devices simultaneously display the raw EEG waveform and may be of benefit beyond the dimensionless index derived from the EEG. It is reasonable to avoid certain medications associated with paroxysmal nocturnal dyspnea (PND) including benzodiazepines, long-acting narcotics, and known anticholinergics

Postoperative complications: Delirium and other perioperative neurocognitive disorders

The DSM-V defines delirium primarily as a disturbance in cognition (60), which may variably include changes in perception, memory, language, coherent reasoning, and visuospatial processing (Figure 19.4). POD is of particular interest for AD

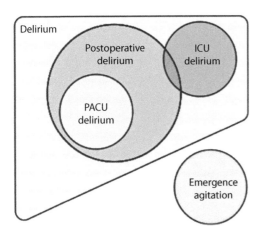

Figure 19.4 Reprinted from Safavynia et al. (2018). Classification of delirium subtypes. Postoperative delirium is a subtype of delirium that occurs between postoperative days 0–5. Post-anesthesia care unit (PACU) delirium is a further subtype of postoperative delirium that occurs in the PACU. Intensive care unit (ICU) delirium is defined by its identification in the ICU; there may be some overlap depending on when patients are admitted to the ICU. Emergence agitation is seen on emergence from anesthesia and has unique etiologies and treatments.

patients, who have an increased risk of developing such cognitive disturbance while in the hospital (48). A diagnosis of delirium is associated with long-term cognitive decline in patients, especially those with preexisting AD.

There are three motoric subtypes of delirium that can present in patients during recovery from anesthesia: a *hyperactive* subtype, marked by agitation, a *hypoactive* subtype, marked by lethargy, and a *mixed* subtype, featuring aspects of both (61). Previous cohort studies have identified hypoactive and mixed subtypes as the most commonly presenting forms of delirium seen in elderly patients during the postoperative period. Unfortunately, delirium is difficult to detect postoperatively without systematic screening tools, especially the hypoactive subtype.

Delirium can be further classified by its clinical setting, such as intensive care unit (ICU) delirium (62) or PACU delirium (63). In contrast, the term *emergence delirium* has been used to describe an agitated state upon emergence from anesthesia (64). This is less likely to occur in patients with AD as opposed to younger patients. Many researchers are beginning to describe this as *emergence agitation*, because consciousness (impaired or unimpaired) was not yet restored before the hyperactivity began. Encouraging the use of assistive devices such as eyeglasses, hearing aids, and dentures would be expected to decrease delirium. No pharmacologic intervention has been proven to be effective in prevention or treatment of PPND, but risk awareness, brain monitoring for titration of anesthetic medications, and post-procedural assessments may decrease the incidence and severity.

The term postoperative cognitive decline (POCD) was previously used to describe abnormal cognition diagnosed or associated with surgery and general anesthesia. In 2018, a change in nomenclature has been recommended. Cognitive decline diagnosed up to 30 days after the procedure is referred to as delayed neurocognitive recovery. Postoperative neurocognitive disorder can persist to 12 months (67) The risk factors are the same as for POD and include dementia diagnosis, increased age, lower initial educational level, long operative time, major or emergency surgery, surgical complications, and previous stroke.

Identification of risk factors for POD/PACU-D prior to surgery can reduce the likelihood of a

Mini-Cog©

Instructions for Administration & Scoring

ID: _____   Date: _____

Step 1: Three Word Registration

Look directly at person and say, "Please listen carefully. I am going to say three words that I want you to repeat back to me now and try to remember. The words are [select a list of words from the versions below]. Please say them for me now." If the person is unable to repeat the words after three attempts, move on to Step 2 (clock drawing).

The following and other word lists have been used in one or more clinical studies.[1-3] For repeated administrations, use of an alternative word list is recommended.

Version 1	Version 2	Version 3	Version 4	Version 5	Version 6
Banana	Leader	Village	River	Captain	Daughter
Sunrise	Season	Kitchen	Nation	Garden	Heaven
Chair	Table	Baby	Finger	Picture	Mountain

Step 2: Clock Drawing

Say: "Next, I want you to draw a clock for me. First, put in all of the numbers where they go." When that is completed, say: "Now, set the hands to 10 past 11."

Use preprinted circle (see next page) for this exercise. Repeat instructions as needed as this is not a memory test. Move to Step 3 if the clock is not complete within three minutes.

Step 3: Three Word Recall

Ask the person to recall the three words you stated in Step 1. Say: "What were the three words I asked you to remember?" Record the word list version number and the person's answers below.

Word List Version: _____   Person's Answers: _____

Scoring

Word Recall: _____ (0-3 points)	1 point for each word spontaneously recalled without cueing.
Clock Draw: _____ (0 or 2 points)	Normal clock = 2 points. A normal clock has all numbers placed in the correct sequence and approximately correct position (e.g., 12, 3, 6 and 9 are in anchor positions) with no missing or duplicate numbers. Hands are pointing to the 11 and 2 (11:10). Hand length is not scored. Inability or refusal to draw a clock (abnormal) = 0 points.
Total Score: _____ (0-5 points)	Total score = Word Recall score + Clock Draw score. A cut point of <3 on the Mini-Cog™ has been validated for dementia screening, but many individuals with clinically meaningful cognitive impairment will score higher. When greater sensitivity is desired, a cut point of <4 is recommended as it may indicate a need for further evaluation of cognitive status.

Figure 19.5 Instructions for completion of the Mini-Cog assessment for cognitive performance. The Mini-Cog assessment can be performed quickly during preparation for surgery. Use of the Mini-Cog with a cut point of <3 has been used with success to identify aged patients with a higher risk for developing postoperative delirium.

missed a diagnosis during recovery (68). Brief cognitive assessments, such as the Mini-Cog (Figure 19.5), can be employed to quickly gauge whether a patient is going into surgery with a preexisting cognitive impairment. Guiding perioperative anesthesia maintenance with EEG, as well as avoiding the use of longer-acting intraoperative opioids, can reduce patient risk for POD. When delirium is present postoperatively, there are recommended steps that can be taken in the PACU to help reduce recovery time, including early mobilization, addressing sensory impairments, and avoiding sleep disturbances. There are currently no pharmacological agents that are effective for the treatment of POD.

PPNDs are characterized by disordered thoughts: changes in memory, visuospatial and language comprehension, and/or attention. AD has been identified to increase susceptibility to or exacerbation of PPNDs, especially after receiving perioperative care (49,65). Other predictors of PPND include hospital-stay delirium and administration of multiple pharmacologic agents, both of which may be common in elderly patients at risk of AD undergoing an anesthetic procedure. The presence of PPNDs alone within the first postoperative year is associated with increased mortality, particularly if the patient experiences a persistent (greater than 3 months) rapid decline in cognitive function (66).

SUMMARY

Alzheimer's disease is increasing in prevalence in our operating rooms. The mechanisms involved in the progression of this neurodegenerative disease overlap with cellular pathways important for our anesthesia drugs. After identifying at-risk patients—such as geriatric patients with or at risk of AD—anesthesiologists can take steps to limit PPNDs. Although further research is necessary, it appears that educating patients about the perioperative experience and introducing a geriatrician to the preoperative care team may be helpful. From a pharmacologic standpoint, limiting the use of drugs such as benzodiazepines and anticholinergics that have an association with delirium already may reduce its incidence. Since polypharmacy is a risk factor for PPNDs, continuous reevaluation of a geriatric patient's overall medication regimen may allow anesthesiologists to eliminate unneeded agents and to have a greater appreciation of possible negative synergistic effects.

REFERENCES

1. Alzheimer's Association. 2018 Alzheimer's Disease Facts and Figures. *Alzheimers Dement.* 2018;14(3):367–429.
2. Hebert LE, Weuve J, Scherr PA, Evans DA. Alzheimer disease in the United States (2010–2050) estimated using the 2010 census. *Neurology.* 2013;80(19):1778–83.
3. Hirtz D, Thurman DJ, Gwinn-Hardy K, Mohamed M, Chaudhuri AR, Zalutsky R. How common are the 'common' neurologic disorders? *Neurology.* 2007;68(5):326–37.
4. Garcia PS, Duggan EW, McCullough IL, Lee SC, Fishman D. Postanesthesia care for the elderly patient. *Clin Ther.* 2015;37(12):2651–65.
5. Prince M, Bryce R, Albanese E, Wimo A, Ribeiro W, Ferri CP. The global prevalence of dementia: A systematic review and metaanalysis. *Alzheimers Dement.* 2013;9(1):63–75.e2.
6. Silbert B, Evered L, Scott DA, Maruff P. Anesthesiology must play a greater role in patients with Alzheimer's disease. *Anesth Analg.* 2011;112(5):1242–5.
7. Arora SS, Gooch JL, Garcia PS. Postoperative cognitive dysfunction, Alzheimer's disease, and anesthesia. *Int J Neurosci.* 2014;124(4):236–42.
8. Chen CW, Lin CC, Chen KB, Kuo YC, Li CY, Chung CJ. Increased risk of dementia in people with previous exposure to general anesthesia: A nationwide population-based case-control study. *Alzheimers Dement.* 2014;10(2):196–204.
9. Chen PL, Yang CW, Tseng YK et al. Risk of dementia after anaesthesia and surgery. *Br J Psychiatry.* 2014;204(3):188–93.
10. Gandy S. The role of cerebral amyloid beta accumulation in common forms of Alzheimer disease. *J Clin Invest.* 2005;115(5):1121–9.
11. Malek N, Baker MR, Mann C, Greene J. Electroencephalographic markers in dementia. *Acta Neurol Scand.* 2017;135(4):388–93.
12. Poorkaj P, Bird TD, Wijsman E et al. Tau is a candidate gene for chromosome 17 frontotemporal dementia. *Ann Neurol.* 1998;43(6):815–25.

13. Ballatore C, Lee VM, Trojanowski JQ. Tau-mediated neurodegeneration in Alzheimer's disease and related disorders. *Nature Rev Neurosci.* 2007;8(9):663–72.

14. Querfurth HW, LaFerla FM. Alzheimer's disease. *N Engl J Med.* 2010;362(4):329–44.

15. Mawuenyega KG, Sigurdson W, Ovod V et al. Decreased clearance of CNS beta-amyloid in Alzheimer's disease. *Science.* 2010; 330(6012):1774.

16. Braak H, Thal Dr, Ghebremedhin E, Ghebremedhin E, Del Tredici K, Del Tredici K. Stages of the pathologic process in Alzheimer disease: age categories from 1 to 100 years. *J Neuropathol Exp Neurol.* 2011 70(11):960–9.

17. Petrasek T, Skurlova M, Maleninska K et al. A rat model of Alzheimer's disease based on Abeta42 and pro-oxidative substances exhibits cognitive deficit and alterations in glutamatergic and cholinergic neurotransmitter systems. *Front Aging Neurosci.* 2016;8:83.

18. Rajendran L, Paolicelli RC. Microglia-mediated synapse loss in Alzheimer's disease. *J Neurosci.* 2018;38(12):2911–9.

19. Hong S, Beja-Glasser VF, Nfonoyim BM et al. Complement and microglia mediate early synapse loss in Alzheimer mouse models. *Science.* 2016;352(6286):712–6.

20. Kitazawa M, Oddo S, Yamasaki TR, Green KN, LaFerla FM. Lipopolysaccharide-induced inflammation exacerbates tau pathology by a cyclin-dependent kinase 5-mediated pathway in a transgenic model of Alzheimer's disease. *J Neurosci.* 2005;25(39):8843–53.

21. Lee DC, Rizer J, Selenica ML et al. LPS-induced inflammation exacerbates phospho-tau pathology in rTg4510 mice. *J Neuroinflammation.* 2010;7:56.

22. Cohen RM, Rezai-Zadeh K, Weitz TM et al. A transgenic Alzheimer rat with plaques, tau pathology, behavioral impairment, oligomeric abeta, and frank neuronal loss. *J Neurosci.* 2013;33(15):6245–56.

23. Hardy J, Allsop D. Amyloid deposition as the central event in the aetiology of Alzheimer's disease. *Trends Pharmacol Sci.* 1991;12(10): 383–8.

24. Berger M, Burke J, Eckenhoff R, Mathew J. Alzheimer's disease, anesthesia, and surgery: A clinically focused review. *J Cardiothoracic Vasc Anesth.* 2014;28(6):1609–23.

25. Hussain M, Berger M, Eckenhoff RG, Seitz DP. General anesthetic and the risk of dementia in elderly patients: Current insights. *Clin Interv Aging.* 2014;9:1619–28.

26. Shaw LM, Vanderstichele H, Knapik-Czajka M et al. Cerebrospinal fluid biomarker signature in Alzheimer's disease neuroimaging initiative subjects. *Ann Neurol.* 2009;65(4):403–13.

27. Reinsfelt B, Westerlind A, Blennow K, Zetterberg H, Ricksten SE. Open-heart surgery increases cerebrospinal fluid levels of Alzheimer-associated amyloid beta. *Acta Anaesthesiol Scand.* 2013;57(1):82–8.

28. Tang JX, Baranov D, Hammond M, Shaw LM, Eckenhoff MF, Eckenhoff RG. Human Alzheimer and inflammation biomarkers after anesthesia and surgery. *Anesthesiology.* 2011;115(4):727–32.

29. Kline RP, Pirraglia E, Cheng H et al. Surgery and brain atrophy in cognitively normal elderly subjects and subjects diagnosed with mild cognitive impairment. *Anesthesiology.* 2012;116(3):603–12.

30. Eckenhoff RG, Johansson JS, Wei H et al. Inhaled anesthetic enhancement of amyloid-beta oligomerization and cytotoxicity. *Anesthesiology.* 2004;101(3):703–9.

31. Carnini A, Lear JD, Eckenhoff RG. Inhaled anesthetic modulation of amyloid beta(1-40) assembly and growth. *Curr Alzheimer Res.* 2007;4(3):233–41.

32. Palotas A, Reis HJ, Bogats G et al. Coronary artery bypass surgery provokes Alzheimer's disease-like changes in the cerebrospinal fluid. *J Alzheimer's Dis.* 2010;21(4):1153–64.

33. Xie Z, Culley DJ, Dong Y et al. The common inhalation anesthetic isoflurane induces caspase activation and increases amyloid beta-protein level in vivo. *Ann Neurol.* 2008; 64(6):618–27.

34. Xie Z, Dong Y, Maeda U et al. The inhalation anesthetic isoflurane induces a vicious cycle of apoptosis and amyloid beta-protein accumulation. *J Neurosci.* 2007;27(6):1247–54.

35. Miller MC, Tavares R, Johanson CE et al. Hippocampal RAGE immunoreactivity in early and advanced Alzheimer's disease. *Brain Res.* 2008;1230:273–80.

36. Mattson MP, Cheng B, Davis D, Bryant K, Lieberburg I, Rydel RE. beta-Amyloid peptides destabilize calcium homeostasis and

render human cortical neurons vulnerable to excitotoxicity. *J Neurosci.* 1992;12(2): 376–89.

37. Hossain MD, Evers AS. Volatile anesthetic-induced efflux of calcium from IP3-gated stores in clonal (GH3) pituitary cells. *Anesthesiology.* 1994;80(6):1379–89; discussion 27A-28A.

38. Xu Z, Dong Y, Wu X et al. The potential dual effects of anesthetic isoflurane on Abeta-induced apoptosis. *Curr Alzheimer Res.* 2011; 8(7):741–52.

39. Marik PE, Flemmer M. The immune response to surgery and trauma: Implications for treatment. *J Trauma Acute Care surg.* 2012;73(4): 801–8.

40. Rana MV, Bonasera LK, Bordelon GJ. Pharmacologic considerations of anesthetic agents in geriatric patients. *Anesthesiology clinics* 2017; 35(2) 259–271.

41. Messina A, Longhini F, Coppo C et al. Use of the fluid challenge in critically ill adult patients: a systematic review. *Anesthesia & Analgesia.* 2017 Nov 1;125(5):1532–43.

42. Deiner S, Silverstein JH. Anesthesia for geriatric patients. *Minerva anestesiologica.* 2011 Feb;77(2):180–9.

43. Stark DC. Aspiration in the surgical patient. *International anesthesiology clinics.* 1977 Apr 1;15(1):13–48.

44. Fisher AA-O, Carney G, Bassett K, Dormuth CR. Tolerability of cholinesterase inhibitors: a population-based study of persistence, adherence, and switching. *Drugs & aging.* 2017 Mar 1;34(3):221–31.

45. Mellios G. Donepezil: It is time to replace physostigmine in anesthesiology. *Medical hypotheses.* 2016;100(94):23–4.

46. Erdogan MA, Demirbilek S, Erdil F et al. The effects of cognitive impairment on anaesthetic requirement in the elderly. *Eur J Anaesthesiol.* 2012;29(7):326–31.

47. Renna M, Handy J, Shah A. Low baseline Bispectral Index of the electroencephalogram in patients with dementia. *Anesth Analg.* 2003;96(5):1380–5, table of contents.

48. Gross AL, Jones RN, Habtemariam DA et al. Delirium and long-term cognitive trajectory among persons with dementia. *Arch Intern Med.* 2012;172(17):1324–31.

49. Steinmetz J, Siersma V, Kessing LV, Rasmussen LS. Is postoperative cognitive dysfunction a risk factor for dementia? A cohort follow-up study. *Br J Anaesth.* 2013;110 Suppl 1:i92–7.

50. Jeong J. EEG dynamics in patients with Alzheimer's disease. *Clin Neurophysiol.* 2004;115(7):1490–505.

51. Babiloni C, Lizio R, Marzano N et al. Brain neural synchronization and functional coupling in Alzheimer's disease as revealed by resting state EEG rhythms. *Int J Psychophysiol.* 2016;103:88–102.

52. Gouw AA, Alsema AM, Tijms BM, Scheltens P, Stam CJ, van der Flier WM. The relation between eeg spectral analysis and clinical progression in non-demented, amyloid-positive subjects. *Alzheimers Dement.* 2015; 11(7):P255–P6.

53. Miyauchi T, Hagimoto H, Ishii M et al. Quantitative EEG in patients with presenile and senile dementia of the Alzheimer type. *Acta Neurol Scand.* 1994;89(1):56–64.

54. Brunovsky M, Matousek M, Edman A, Cervena K, Krajca V. Objective assessment of the degree of dementia by means of EEG. *Neuropsychobiology.* 2003;48(1):19–26.

55. Pijnenburg Y, Vd Made Y, Van Walsum AVC, Knol D, Scheltens P, Stam C. EEG synchronization likelihood in mild cognitive impairment and Alzheimer's disease during a working memory task. *Clin Neurophysiol.* 2004;115(6):1332–9.

56. Von Stein A, Sarnthein J. Different frequencies for different scales of cortical integration: From local gamma to long range alpha/theta synchronization. *Int J Psychophysiol.* 2000;38(3):301–13.

57. Babiloni C, Ferri R, Binetti G et al. Fronto-parietal coupling of brain rhythms in mild cognitive impairment: A multicentric EEG study. *Brain Res Bull.* 2006;69(1):63–73.

58. Jordan D, Ilg R, Riedl V et al. Simultaneous Electroencephalographic and Functional Magnetic Resonance Imaging Indicate Impaired Cortical Top–Down Processing in Association with Anesthetic-induced Unconsciousness. *Anesthesiology.* 2013; 119(5):1031–42.

59. Lee U, Ku S, Noh G, Baek S, Choi B, Mashour GA. Disruption of Frontal–Parietal Communication by Ketamine, Propofol, and Sevoflurane. *Anesthesiology.* 2013;118(6): 1264–75.

60. *Diagnostic and statistical manual of mental disorders: DSM-5. American Psychiatric A, American Psychiatric Association DSMTF.* Arlington, VA: American Psychiatric Association; 2013.

61. Peterson JF, Pun BT, Dittus RS et al. Delirium and its motoric subtypes: A study of 614 critically ill patients. *J Am Geriatr Soc.* 2006; 54(3):479–84.

62. Miller RR 3rd, Ely EW. Delirium and cognitive dysfunction in the intensive care unit. (1069–3424 (Print)).

63. Hernandez BA, Lindroth H, Rowley P et al. Post-anaesthesia care unit delirium: Incidence, risk factors and associated adverse outcomes. *Br J Anaesth.* 2017;119(2):288–90.

64. Eckenhoff JE, Kneale DH, Dripps RD. The incidence and etiology of postanesthetic excitment. A clinical survey. *Anesthesiology.* 1961;22:667–73.

65. Xie Z, McAuliffe S, Swain CA et al. Cerebrospinal fluid abeta to tau ratio and postoperative cognitive change. *Ann Surg.* 2013;258(2):364–9.

66. Monk TG, Weldon BC, Garvan CW et al. Predictors of cognitive dysfunction after major noncardiac surgery. *Anesthesiology.* 2008;108(1):18–30.

67. Evered L, Silbert B, Knopman DS et al. The Nomenclature Consensus Working Group. Recommendations for the nomenclature of cognitive change associated with anaesthesia and surgery—2018. *Br J Anaesth.* 2018; 121(5):1005–12.

68. Safavynia SA, Arora S, Pryor KO et al. An update on postoperative delirium: Clinical features, neuropathogenesis, and perioperative management. *Curr Anesthesiol Rep.* 2018;8(3):252–62.

20

Special considerations: Parkinson's disease

ADRIANA MARTIN AND SHOBANA RAJAN

INTRODUCTION

Parkinson's disease (PD) is a disorder of the central nervous system (CNS) clinically characterized by tremor, bradykinesia, and rigidity. It is caused by loss of dopaminergic neurons in the substantia nigra of the basal ganglia. This neuronal degeneration leads to reduced facilitation of voluntary movements. The incidence of PD varies between 12–19 per 100,000 person-years and it is estimated to affect 1% of the population above 60 years old (1,2). PD is the most common movement disorder and the second most common neurodegenerative disease worldwide (2). Given the fact that our population is getting older and life expectancy is rising, it is expected that the prevalence of the disease will increase. For this reason, these patients are being seen in the operating room more often and anesthesiologists must be aware of the nuances related to their management. This chapter provides an overview of the disease and its perioperative management.

The cause of PD remains unknown for most of the cases. Genetic and environmental risk factors have been identified (3). Increasing age is the greatest risk factor for PD. Gender is another established risk factor, with the male-to-female ratio being approximately 3:2 (4). Environmental risk factors include pesticide exposure, prior head injury, rural living, and beta-blocker use. Some environmental factors are associated with decreased risk of developing PD, and include tobacco smoking, coffee drinking, nonsteroidal antiinflammatory drug (NSAID) use, calcium channel blocker use, and alcohol consumption.

Neuropathologically, the disease is characterized by the presence of intracytoplasmic inclusion bodies containing alpha-synuclein. These inclusion bodies are called Lewy bodies, and are mainly present in the substantia nigra (5). The presence of Lewy bodies helps in the postmortem diagnosis during autopsies and is considered the gold standard for diagnosis. Neuroinflammation is another feature of PD pathology and is displayed by increase in the number as well as in the activation state of astrocytes and microglia (3).

CLINICAL MANIFESTATIONS

The disease is clinically manifested by three cardinal symptoms: tremor, rigidity, and bradykinesia. The tremor consists of a resting tremor that decreases with purposeful movement. It usually starts unilaterally in the hand and is described as a "pill-rolling" tremor. It is initially intermittent, but as the disease progresses it becomes more frequent and evident. Rigidity is characterized by increased resistance to passive movement. It also usually starts unilaterally, and usually in the same side affected by the tremor. Cogwheel rigidity is an example, and

Table 20.1 Summary of motor symptoms of PD

Resting tremor	Dysphagia
Bradykinesia	Blurred vision and other visual disturbances
Rigidity	Dystonia
Postural instability	Micrographia
Masked facial expression	Myoclonus
Speech disturbances	Shuffling, short-stepped gait

is characterized by a ratchety pattern of resistance and relaxation during a range-of-motion maneuver. Bradykinesia is a generalized slowness of movement and is the most common symptom. Patients may describe it as weakness, feeling unsteady, tiredness, or difficulty performing simple tasks with the hand, such as buttoning clothes.

Another common motor symptom is postural instability. It is the feeling of imbalance caused by impairment of centrally-mediated postural reflexes. Usually it does not appear until later in the course of the disease, and it is typically a feature of more advanced disease. Other motor symptoms are summarized in Table 20.1.

Nonmotor symptoms are also of major importance, although they are usually seen later in the course of the disease. Nearly all patients have at least one nonmotor symptom (6). These symptoms have significant impact on quality of life and contribute to institutionalization at advanced stages of the disease (6). The most frequent nonmotor symptoms are fatigue, psychiatric symptoms such as anxiety and cognitive decline, gastrointestinal symptoms, and sleep disorders like insomnia. They also commonly have symptoms from autonomic dysfunction like constipation, impaired bladder emptying, sexual dysfunction, seborrhea, and sialorrhea.

DIAGNOSIS

The diagnosis of PD is clinical and based on the presence of the three cardinal symptoms (3). Most frequently, patients will have bradykinesia and one of the other symptoms. There are no physiologic tests or blood tests to confirm the clinical diagnosis of PD, and neuroimaging is usually unrevealing. Although the gold standard for diagnosis is the pathologic examination, this is not needed for diagnosis.

The diagnostic criteria by the Movement Disorder Society states that motor parkinsonism

is the core symptom and defines it by bradykinesia plus resting tremor or rigidity (7). The patient should not have any red flag symptoms that would favor other diagnoses. Another supportive feature to establish a diagnose of PD is response to dopaminergic therapy. This response is generally reduced in patients with parkinsonism due to parkinsonian syndromes, and is used to clarify the differential diagnosis.

TREATMENT OF PARKINSON'S DISEASE

There is a wide array of treatment modalities for PD. Unfortunately, until now there has been no established disease-modifying or neuroprotective therapy. The decision to initiate therapy and which one to use is individualized and takes into consideration the patient's symptoms, age, stage of disease, degree of functional disability, and level of physical activity. Treatment can be divided into pharmacological and surgical modalities. Since there is no disease-modifying treatment, therapy should be started and guided by the patient's discomfort and impairment in quality of life.

Medical management

There are six main classes of drugs used to treat PD. Table 20.2 lists those classes and their common side effects. Drugs that increase dopamine concentration or stimulate dopamine receptors remain the mainstay in the treatment of motor symptoms (3,8).

LEVODOPA

Levodopa is the most effective drug in the treatment of motor symptoms (9). It is usually initiated for those with more severe impairment of activities of daily living. Levodopa acts by being converted to dopamine in the CNS. It is generally combined

Table 20.2 Classes of drugs for treatment of Parkinson's disease and adverse effects of treatment

Medication class	Adverse effects
Levodopa-carbidopa	Nausea, headache, orthostatic hypotension, dyskinesia, hallucinations, psychosis, and neuroleptic malignant syndrome
Dopamine agonists	Same as levodopa-carbidopa; also, edema
MAO-B inhibitors	Stimulant effect, dizziness, headache, confusion, and serotonin syndrome
Anticholinergics	Hallucinations, delirium, cognitive impairment, nausea, dry mouth, blurred vision, urinary retention, and constipation
COMT inhibitors	Dark-colored urine and exacerbation of levodopa adverse effects
Amantadine	Hallucinations, confusion, blurred vision, ankle edema, livedo reticular, nausea, dry mouth, and constipation

with carbidopa, a peripheral decarboxylase inhibitor that inhibits the conversion of levodopa to dopamine in the systemic circulation. Dosage varies from patient to patient and it is usually clinically titrated to the lowest dose with an effective response. Levodopa is usually given three times a day but can be divided into more doses.

Some common side effects of levodopa include nausea, orthostatic hypotension, somnolence, dizziness, and headache. Side effects are decreased by the use of peripheral decarboxylase inhibitors. Elderly patients are susceptible to more serious adverse reactions like confusion, hallucinations, and agitation. Wearing-off phenomenon is a complication that starts within years of treatment and is characterized by involuntary movements like dyskinesia and others. The effect of levodopa can begin to wear off approximately 2 hours after a dose.

Levodopa, as well as dopamine agonists, should not be stopped abruptly, because sudden withdrawal has been associated with parkinsonism-hyperpyrexia syndrome. This potentially fatal condition presents similar to neuroleptic malignant syndrome, with mental status change, muscular rigidity, hyperthermia, and autonomic instability.

DOPAMINE AGONISTS

Dopamine agonists (DA) are medications that directly stimulate the dopamine receptors in the brain. The most commonly used ones are bromocriptine, pramipexole, and ropinirole. Apomorphine and rotigotine are DA available for subcutaneous and transdermal use, respectively. An advantage of DA over levodopa is that it does not require metabolic conversion and does not depend upon neuronal uptake and release. DAs

are effective as monotherapy in patients with early and advanced disease, but they are less effective than levodopa (1). Dosage varies between agents, but they are usually given at least three times a day. They cause similar adverse effects as levodopa. Patients who abruptly stop taking DA are at risk for withdrawal syndrome. Withdrawal syndrome from DA presents with anxiety, nausea, sweating, fatigue, and dizziness.

MONOAMINE OXIDASE (MAO) INHIBITORS

Monoamine oxidase type B (MAO-B) inhibitors act by inhibition of the enzyme responsible for the breakdown of dopamine at the synaptic cleft. MAO-B inhibitors include selegiline, rasagiline, and safinamide. They are modestly effective as symptomatic treatment, and recent studies have suggested that they may have some neuroprotective properties (9). Common side effects are headache, nausea, insomnia, and confusion. Although these drugs selectively inhibit MAO type B and not MAO type A, which is the enzyme involved in the breakdown of serotonin, it is recommended to not use them concomitantly with tricyclic antidepressants or selective serotonin reuptake inhibitors due to a low risk of causing serotonin syndrome, especially when using them at higher doses. Serotonin syndrome would manifest by altered mental status, muscular rigidity, hyperreflexia, hyperpyrexia, and autonomic hyperactivity with tachycardia and hypertension. As discussed later in this chapter, opioids with serotoninergic properties should also avoided in patients on MAO-B inhibitors. Because this class of drugs selectively inhibits MAO type B, they do not precipitate hypertensive crisis in patients who ingest tyramine-containing food.

ANTICHOLINERGIC

The dopamine depletion that occurs in the substantia nigra in PD causes an imbalance between the dopaminergic and cholinergic neurological pathways. Anticholinergic drugs antagonize this cholinergic sensitivity and have been proven to improve Parkinson's symptoms, especially tremor. They were the first drugs used to treat PD and were proven to be effective in controlling motor symptoms (9). The most commonly used anticholinergics to treat PD are trihexyphenidyl and benztropine. The limitations to their use are the significant side effects. They can cause memory impairment, confusion, hallucinations, urinary retention, blurred vision, constipation, and tachycardia. For this reason, they are avoided in elderly patients. Abrupt discontinuation can cause withdrawal manifested by acute exacerbation of parkinsonism. They should be avoided in patients with prostatic hypertrophy and acute-angle glaucoma.

AMANTADINE

Amantadine is an antiviral agent that has mild antiparkinsonian activity. It increases dopamine release, stimulates dopamine receptors, and decreases dopamine reuptake (10). Adverse effects include lived reticularis, peripheral edema, confusion, and hallucinations.

CATECHOL-O-METHYLTRANSFERASE INHIBITORS

Catechol-O-methyltransferase (COMT) inhibitors inhibit the metabolism of levodopa. The most common used COMT inhibitors are tolcapone and entacapone. They are always given in combination with levodopa and have been found to have a small benefit. They are infective if given as monotherapy.

Surgical management

Functional neurosurgery is another treatment modality for PD. It is an option especially for patients who respond to levodopa but are suffering from disabling dyskinesia and motor fluctuations.

Deep brain stimulation (DBS) is the most frequent surgical intervention performed in PD patients. Stimulation of the subthalamic nucleus and globus pallidus internus are the most studied targets. DBS is effective in treating motor and non-motor symptoms of patients with moderate to advanced PD, and it has been shown to decrease the need for

medications (3). It is reversible and can be adjusted as the disease progresses. Preoperative levodopa responsiveness is a predictor of good response to DBS (11). The procedure consists of implantation of a DBS lead in the target nucleus and implantation of a pulse generator in the chest. Disadvantages of DBS include the requirement for stereotactic brain surgery for electrode placement, the introduction of hardware with risk of infection, and the need for periodic reprogramming.

ANESTHETIC IMPLICATIONS

With the aging of our population, geriatric patients, and consequently patients with PD, are more frequently seen in the surgical setting. Patients with PD are at increased risk of postoperative morbidity and mortality. It is extremely important for the anesthesiologist and all providers involved in the care of these patients to be aware of the complications related to this condition and the specific requirements in its management.

Aspiration pneumonia is the leading cause of death in patients with PD (12). It is related to the impairment of pharyngeal muscles and swallowing. Reduced swallowing causes secondary sialorrhea. Drugs used to treat parkinsonism have little effect on dysphagia. These patients are also known to have decreased gastric emptying, another factor that can contribute to increase aspiration risk in the perioperative period (13). Difficulty with swallowing also contributes to a poor nutritional status preoperatively, and higher risk of postoperative complications. Patients may also have gastrointestinal side effects like nausea and vomiting from antiparkinsonian medications.

Reduced respiratory function is another important contributor to morbidity by predisposing patients to respiratory infections, atelectasis, and postoperative respiratory failure (14). Respiratory dysfunction is due to a combination of factors including restrictive lung changes, decreased muscle strength, and upper airway obstruction (15). Patients with PD are also at greater risk of primary and postoperative laryngospasm due to dysfunction of the laryngeal muscles (16).

Orthostatic hypotension due to cardiovascular autonomic dysfunction is a predominant symptom and is associated with postoperative hypotension (17). Patients with PD have special sensitivity to drugs that may cause hypotension. Orthostatic hypotension may be even more exacerbated in patients taking dopaminergic medications or antidepressants to treat non-motor symptoms. Associated with autonomic dysfunction, patients may have defective temperature regulation, constipation, urinary retention, and dehydration from profuse sweating (18). Cardiac arrhythmias, hypertension, and hypovolemia are additional cardiac risk factors in these patients (19).

Surgical patients with PD have an increased morbidity risk (20). They also have a higher in-hospital mortality (21). After total hip arthroplasty, patients with PD had 50% higher chances of postoperative complications (22). These patients are at increased risk for postoperative delirium, bacterial infection, altered mental status, and urinary tract infection (21). They are also at greater risk for postoperative fall, increased length of stay, and increased ICU stay (20). Thus optimal perioperative management and anticipation of issues related to the disease can promote a reduction in complication rates and improve outcomes in this population.

ANESTHETIC MANAGEMENT

Patients with PD most often present for orthopedic, urological, gynecological, and incidental general surgery procedures. They are also seen in the surgical unit for procedures related to the disease. Approaches to functional neurosurgery and DBS are discussed in Chapter 11. Awareness of potential complications to which these patients are susceptible allows anticipation of possible adverse events. Effective management can reduce morbidity by decreasing complications from the disease, the anesthesia, and the surgery. Table 20.3 summarizes important factors involved in the perioperative management of PD.

PREOPERATIVE

A detailed history of the disease course with a complete medication list, including dosage, time of administration, and time of last dose is important to prevent complications associated with the disease. Apart from routine history and physical examination, patients with PD may require additional assessment and testing (18). Pulmonary function tests, arterial blood gas, and chest X-ray may be needed if pulmonary reserve is in doubt. If malnourished, patients ideally should have their nutritional status optimized as this may improve surgical outcomes. Scheduling these patients as the earliest surgery in the day allows greater predictability over time of fasting and surgery (23).

Table 20.3 An overview of recommendations for perioperative management of patients with PD

Preoperative	• History and physical
	• Detailed medication history (drugs, dosages, timing)
	• Discontinue MAO-B inhibitors 1–2 weeks prior to surgery
	• Assess duration of disease and presence of "wearing-off" effect
	• Pulmonary function tests if questionable pulmonary reserve
	• Schedule as first surgery of the day
	• Continue medication regimen until just prior to induction
	• Assess risk of aspiration (history of dysphagia, sialorrhea, gastroparesis, comorbidities) and need for intubation
Intraoperative	• Avoid dopamine antagonists (droperidol, haloperidol, promethazine, prochlorperazine and metoclopramide)
	• Avoid fentanyl and alfentanil
	• Avoid serotoninergic opioids if patient on MAO-B inhibitors
	• If long surgery, place gastric tube for antiparkinson drug administration or consider alternative medications
	• Ensure adequate ventilation prior to extubation
Postoperative	• Resume patients antiparkinson drug regimen as soon as possible
	• Multimodal analgesia
	• Communicate and reorient patients to avoid delirium; if postoperative delirium, avoid antipsychotics
	• Early mobilization and physical therapy
	• Incentive spirometry

The actual medication regimen should be continued until just prior to induction of anesthesia. Trying to reproduce patient's exact drug regimen is very important. Levodopa has a short half-life of 1–2 hours, and its interruption has been associated with a "wearing off" effect, delayed recovery, and reports of severe rigidity upon emergence of anesthesia (24). Sudden abrupt discontinuation of levodopa is also associated with parkinsonism-hyperpyrexia syndrome. The use of gastric tubes has been suggested to continue antiparkinson medications, especially during prolonged surgeries. Because levodopa is absorbed in the proximal small bowel and these patients can have gastroparesis related to the disease, a duodenal feeding tube may be more effective. Some studies have investigated switching patients from their usual treatment to medications available in the parenteral form, and they have been successful in avoiding side effects from dopamine withdrawal (23). Patients with significant ileus may benefit from apomorphine or rotigotine since enteric absorption may be significantly compromised. Apomorphine is a potent dopamine agonist that can be used subcutaneously. However, it can cause significant nausea and vomiting, and premedication with antiemetics should be concomitantly administered. Rotigotine is a newer dopamine agonist available as a transdermal patch. It aims to maintain a steady concentration over 24 hours and is usually well tolerated, but it is not as potent as apomorphine (25).

If the patient is being treated for PD with MAO-B inhibitors, it is recommended to discontinue it 1–2 weeks before surgery to minimize drug interactions (26). These medications may contribute to labile blood pressure and increase the risk for serotonin syndrome. If they are continued in the preoperative period, avoid medications that interact with them and watch for signs and symptoms of serotonin syndrome.

TYPE OF ANESTHESIA

The choice of anesthesia should take into consideration many factors, such as the procedure scheduled, preferences of the patient, and risk factors for complications. When appropriate, regional anesthesia has advantages over general anesthesia as it avoids the side effects of general anesthetics and muscle relaxants. Regional anesthesia also allows monitoring of Parkinson's symptoms

during surgery and dosing of antiparkinson agents if needed. Lastly, regional anesthesia avoids postoperative nausea and vomiting (PONV), which is particularly beneficial in this group of patients since they have contraindications to multiple antiemetic drugs. At the same time, tremor will not be eliminated with regional anesthesia, and it can make surgery and electrocardiographic monitoring difficult. PD is associated with impaired swallowing and excessive salivation. Sialorrhea may worsen with sedation and can result in aspiration. Anesthesiologists should assess the risk of aspiration, particularly if there is significant dysphagia and sialorrhea, and should proceed with intubation when safer. Glycopyrrolate by mouth and ipratropium spray have been found to be effective for short-term treatment of sialorrhea (26).

If it is decided to proceed with general anesthesia, halothane should be avoided in patients taking levodopa because it can increase cardiac sensitivity to catecholamines and increase the risk of arrhythmias (26). Propofol can have antiparkinsonian effects but can also induce dyskinesia, a common side effect of levodopa (27). Propofol is still commonly used to induce anesthesia in these patients, but the risk of dyskinetic effects should be considered. Isoflurane, sevoflurane, and enflurane have been recommended as safe alternatives (19). There are no reported cases of neuromuscular blocking agents that worsen PD symptoms (28). Non-depolarizing blocking agents should be fully reversed at the end of the surgery to avoid further compromising their ventilatory function. Adequacy of ventilation and capacity to secure the airway should be carefully assessed prior to extubation. Drugs that are used for PONV treatment that have dopamine antagonist actions are contraindicated in PD. Examples of these drugs are butyrophenones (droperidol, haloperidol, benperidol), phenothiazines (promethazine, perphenazine, prochlorperazine), and metoclopramide. Ondansetron may be used safely without exacerbating parkinsonism (19).

FLUCTUATIONS IN BLOOD PRESSURE

Patients with PD can have autonomic failure with autonomic instability and special sensitivity to hypotensive drugs, including antiparkinson drugs. Autonomic failure impairs the patient's ability to respond to hypovolemia and to the vasodilation associated with anesthetic agents. Levodopa has a hypotensive effect through central mechanisms that are more pronounced in patients with a high baseline blood pressure (29). Dopamine agonists are associated with even more severe hypotension than levodopa as they also cause peripheral vasodilation. Maintaining adequate hydration is important, as this can exacerbate hypotension.

ANALGESIA

Opioid-induced muscle rigidity results from presynaptic inhibition of dopamine release (28). Fentanyl has been associated with muscle rigidity and severe bradykinesia in patients with PD. There are also reports of acute dystonia after alfentanil (30). Phenylpiperidine opioids such as meperidine, methadone, pethidine, tramadol, and fentanyl should be avoided in patients on MAO-B inhibitors. These are serotoninergic opioids that can precipitate agitation, rigidity, and serotonin syndrome in patients taking MAO-B inhibitors, especially when on higher doses of MAO-B inhibitors. Overactivation of serotonin receptors can manifest by altered mental status, rigidity, hyperreflexia, and autonomic hyperactivity. Oxycodone, hydromorphone, oxymorphone, and buprenorphine are not serotonin uptake inhibitors, but they may increase intrasynaptic serotonin levels and have also been reported in serotonin syndrome (31). More attention to avoid these opioids should be paid in patients who are taking selective serotonin reuptake inhibitor (SSRIs) and tricyclic antidepressants (TCAs) in addition to MAO-B inhibitors. MAO inhibitors also inhibit the metabolism of narcotics in the liver, so the dose of any opioids should be decreased. In order to minimize opioids, multimodal analgesia techniques should be favored. It is recommended that MAO-B inhibitor be stopped 1–2 weeks prior to surgery to avoid these complications, but this is not always feasible, especially in cases of emergent surgery.

PATIENTS WITH DEEP BRAIN STIMULATION

Patients with DBS presenting for incidental surgery require particular considerations. They may need to have the stimulator turned off during certain procedures. It is recommended to consult a movement disorder specialist for more specific recommendations. Electrocautery may damage the leads and should be used with caution. If necessary, bipolar cautery is preferred and the stimulator should be turned off.

POSTOPERATIVE CARE

Postoperative care of patients with PD should emphasize airway protection, incentive spirometry, and early mobilization. Longer times without antiparkinsonian drugs may lead to worsening in motor symptoms and delayed recovery. It is essential to ensure that patients are medicated appropriately, as this can reduce their perioperative morbidity. Physical therapy is a key component in the recovery phase as it can facilitate overall recovery.

As discussed earlier, these patients are more prone to postoperative delirium, confusion, and hallucinations. This risk is particularly increased in patients with preoperative dementia. Most typical and atypical antipsychotics can worsen parkinsonism and must be avoided. Clozapine is the preferred antipsychotic medication for patients with PD. Patients with PD seem to be more sensitive to benzodiazepines, and it is recommended to use them with caution (26). Shivering is common after anesthesia and should be distinguished from parkinsonian symptoms and managed appropriately.

REFERENCES

1. Tysnes OB, Storstein A. Epidemiology of Parkinson's disease. *J Neural Transm.* 2017;124(8):901–5.
2. Timothy RM, James TB, Hamill RW et al. Parkinson's disease. *Subcell Biochem.* 2012;65:389–455.
3. Kalia LV, Lang AE. Parkinson's disease. *Lancet.* 2015;386(9996):896–912.
4. De Lau LM, Breteler MM. Epidemiology of Parkinson's disease. *Lancet Neuro.* 2006;5:525–35.
5. Kenji K. Lewy body disease and dementia with Lewy bodies. *Proc Jpn Acad Ser B Phys Biol.* 2014;90(8):301–6.
6. Hussl A, Seppi K, Poewe W et al. Nonmotor symptoms in Parkinson's disease. *Expert Rev Neurother.* 2013;13:581.
7. Postuma RB, Berg D. MDS clinical diagnostic criteria for Parkinson's disease. *Mov Disord.* 2015;30(12):1591–601.
8. Connolly BS, Lang AE. Pharmacological treatment of Parkinson disease: A review. *JAMA.* 2014;311(16):1670–83.

9. Ferreira J, Katzenschlager R, Bloem BR et al. Summary of the recommendations of the EFNS/MDS-ES review on therapeutic management of Parkinson's disease. *Eur J Neurol.* 2012;20(1):5–15.

10. Amantadine and other antiglutamate agents: Management of Parkinson's disease. *Mov Disord.* 2002;17(S4):S13–22.

11. Kleiner-Fisman G, Fisman D, Sime E et al. Long-term follow up of bilateral deep brain stimulation of the subthalamic nucleus in patients with advanced Parkinson disease. *J Neurosurg.* 2003;99(3):489–95.

12. Mu L, Sobotka S, Chen J et al. Altered pharyngeal muscles in Parkinson disease. *J Neuropathol Exp Neurol.* 2012;71(6):520–30.

13. Byrne K, Pfeiffer R, Quigley EMM et al. Gastrointestinal dysfunction in Parkinson disease. *J Clin Gastroenterol.* 1994;19(1):11–6.

14. Easdown L, Tessler M, Minuk J et al. Upper airway involvement in Parkinson's disease resulting in postoperative respiratory failure. *Can J Anaesth.* 1995;42(4):344–7.

15. Torsney K, Forsyth D. Respiratory dysfunction in Parkinson's disease. *J R Coll Physicians Edinb.* 2017;47(1):35–9.

16. Gdynia H, Kassubek J, Sperfeld A-D et al. Laryngospasm in neurological diseases. *Neurocritical Care.* 2006;4(2):163–7.

17. Kim J, Lee S, Oh Y-S et al. Arterial stiffness and cardiovascular autonomic dysfunction in patients with Parkinson's disease. *Neurodegener Dis.* 2017;17(2-3):89–96.

18. Nicholson G, Pereira A, Hall GM et al. Parkinson's disease and anaesthesia. *Br J Anaesth.* 2002;89(6):904–16.

19. Robert D, Lewis S. Considerations for general anaesthesia in Parkinson's disease. *J Clin Neurosci.* 2018;48:34–41.

20. Mueller M, Jüptner U, Wuellner U et al. Parkinson's disease influences the perioperative risk profile in surgery. *Langenbecks Arch Surg.* 2008;394(3):511–5.

21. Pepper P, Goldstein M. Postoperative complications in Parkinson's disease. *J Am Geriatr Soc.* 1999;47(8):967–72.

22. Newman JM, Sodhi N, Dalton SE et al. Does Parkinson's disease increase the risk of perioperative complications after total hip arthroplasty? A nationwide database study. *J Arthroplasty.* 2018;33(7S):S162–6.

23. Brennan K, Genever R. Managing Parkinson's disease during surgery. *BMJ.* 2010;341:c5718.

24. Stagg P, Grice T. Nasogastric medication for perioperative Parkinson's rigidity during anaesthesia emergence. *Anaesth Intensive Care.* 2011;39(6):1128–30.

25. Wullner U, Kassubek J, Odin P et al. Transdermal rotigotine for the perioperative management of Parkinson's disease. *J Neural Transm.* 2010;117(7):855–9.

26. Katus L, Shtilbans A. Perioperative management of patients with Parkinson's disease. *Am J Med.* 2014;127(4):275–80.

27. Krauss J, Akeyson KE, Giam P, Jankovic J. Propofol-induced dyskinesias in Parkinson's disease. *Anesth Analg.* 1996;83(2):420–2.

28. Rudra A, Rudra P, Chatterjee S et al. Parkinson's disease and anaesthesia. *Indian J Anaesth.* 2007;51:382–8.

29. Irwin RP, Nutt JG, Woodward WR et al. Pharmacodynamics of the hypotensive effect of levodopa in Parkinsonian patients. *Clin Neuropharmacol.* 1992;15(5):365–74.

30. Mets B. Acute dystonia after alfentanil in untreated Parkinson's disease. *Anesth Analg.* 1991;72(4):557–8.

31. Rastogi R, Swarm R, Patel TA et al. Case scenario: opioid association with serotonin syndrome: Implications to the practitioners. *Anesthesiology.* 2011;115(6):1291–8.

21

Fluids and electrolyte management

INDU KAPOOR AND ROBERT G. HAHN

INTRODUCTION

Water is an essential part of life and is required to maintain normal body function. As a rule of thumb, water occupies 60% of the body weight in adult males and 50% in women. The total body water (TBW) content decreases with age mainly due to a reduced intracellular fluid volume. The National Confidential Enquiry into Patient Outcome and Death (NCEPOD) estimated that 20% of elderly patients have poorly documented fluid balance or have fluid imbalance that is unrecognized or untreated (1). Fluid and electrolyte impairment and age-related changes in the elderly body can lead to substantial variation in daily fluid requirements between patients (2). Elderly patients are more prone to water and electrolyte imbalance because of age-related physiological changes like reduced thirst sensation, impaired ability of kidney to conserve water, and disease-related factors like diabetes. For these reasons, fluid therapy in the elderly is challenging and should be considered with precise indication, contraindication, and adverse effects.

BODY WATER DISTRIBUTION AND COMPOSITION

Total body water makes up a significant fraction of the human body, by both weight and volume. There is considerable variation in body water percentage based on factors like age, gender, health, weight, etc. In a large study of adults of all ages and both sexes, the adult human body averaged ~65% water. The figure for water fraction by weight in this sample was found to be $58 \pm 8\%$ water for males and $48 \pm 6\%$ for females (3,4). Some obese people have as little as 45% water by weight. Most of the body fluid is contained in the intracellular and extracellular compartments, but water is also contained inside various body organs like gastrointestinal, cerebrospinal, peritoneal, and ocular fluids. Muscle tissue and fat also contain 75% and 10% of water, respectively. Two-thirds of the body water is contained within cells, i.e. intracellular fluid, whereas one-third is contained in areas outside of cells, i.e. extracellular fluid. The extracellular compartment is further divided in plasma, interstitial fluid, and transcellular fluid. Plasma

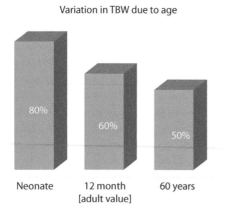

Variation in TBW due to age

Neonate   12 month [adult value]   60 years

Figure 21.1 Variation in total body water (TBW) content due to aging.

constitutes one-fifth of extracellular fluid, interstitial fluid (IF) constitutes four-fifths of extracellular fluid, and transcellular fluid (or "third space") is mostly ignored but is contained inside the body organs. Blood plasma has high concentrations of sodium, chloride, bicarbonate, and protein. The IF has high concentrations of sodium, chloride, and bicarbonate, but a relatively lower concentration of protein. In contrast, the intracellular fluid (ICF) has elevated amounts of potassium, phosphate, magnesium, and protein. Cell membranes are freely permeable to water and the fluid compartments are therefore in osmotic equilibrium. The same osmolarity (290–300 mOsm/L) is ensured in the extracellular fluid (ECF) by sodium salts and in the ICF by potassium salts. Several studies have demonstrated that TBW (Figure 21.1) and ICF decrease with age due to fat-free mass loss and an increase in ECF and ECF/TBW ratio (4–10). These physiological fluid changes make it necessary to investigate normal hydration and fluid retention in the elderly with a view to distinguishing fluid imbalance from normality (11).

PHYSIOLOGY AND PATHOPHYSIOLOGY IN GERIATRICS

The minimum fluid requirement in an adult human is 1 mL/kg/hour, half of which is lost by evaporation, mainly from the airways, while the other half is needed to maintain minimum urinary excretion. The excretion of water through the kidneys is regulated through numerous hormonal axes. The kidney can change the osmolarity of urine from 50 to 1200 mOsmol/L, which helps in keeping plasma values within range despite variations in input or output. However, the ability to concentrate the urine becomes impaired with age, and it is rare to see an elderly person with a urine osmolality reaching 900 mOsmol/kg.

There are three key hormones that play roles in regulating fluid and electrolyte balance.

1. *Antidiuretic hormone* (ADH), released from the posterior pituitary; the most important hormone, regulating the renal excretion of free water. A small increase in plasma osmolarity of only 1 mOsmol/L triggers an increase in ADH secretion (12). ADH secretion may also change in response to many other factors such as pain, stress, nausea, and various drugs. ADH binds to two major receptors, V1 and V2. While V1 receptors are responsible for the vasoconstricting effect of ADH, V2 receptors mediate its water-retaining function.

2. *Aldosterone*, secreted from the adrenal cortex; primarily involved in the regulation of plasma potassium concentration and the effective circulating volume. Aldosterone increases potassium excretion, at the level of the distal nephron, in response to a rise in its plasma concentration, and mainly acts in the distal nephron by increasing sodium and chloride reabsorption and potassium excretion. Consequently, water will be reabsorbed along with the primary extracellular solutes. The stress hormone cortisol also has water-retaining properties, albeit weaker than for aldosterone.

3. *Atrial natriuretic peptide* (ANP), produced by the heart in response to atrial wall stretch, i.e., in cases of volume expansion. ANP increases renal sodium and water excretion by means of a reduced sodium reabsorption at the level of the collecting tubules and through an increased glomerular filtration rate. ANP has also direct vasodilating effects, determining a reduction in blood pressure (13).

Elderly adults are susceptible to dehydration and electrolyte abnormalities, with causes including impaired thirst sensation, mental disability, and physical disability restricting access to fluid intake, and iatrogenic causes including polypharmacy and unmonitored diuretic usage. They are also predisposed to water retention and related electrolyte abnormalities, exacerbated at times of physiological stress. Positive fluid balance has been shown to be an independent risk factor for morbidity and mortality in critically ill patients with acute kidney injury (14). Age-related physiological changes, including renal senescence, also increase the susceptibility of the older adult population to dehydration. Dehydration of as little as 2% of TBW can result in a significant impairment in physical, visuomotor, psychomotor, and cognitive performances (15). One study reported a 30-day mortality of 17% in elderly adults with the principal diagnosis of dehydration as per the International Statistical Classification of Diseases and Related Health Problems (ICD) classification, with the 1-year mortality being close to 50% (16). In a study of patients admitted to acute geriatric care, the 30-day mortality was 21% in those with dehydration, which should be compared to 8% in the others (17).

The elderly also have weakened autonomic responses, which makes it more difficult for them to cope with hemodynamic changes and cooling. Hence, goal-directed fluid therapy is more useful in them than in younger subjects. In the elderly, preload becomes very important to hemodynamic stability. Moreover, the reactions to both inotropic and chronotrophic impulses are impaired. Hence higher concentrations of vasoactive drugs are required to exert desired effects.

ELECTROLYTE ABNORMALITIES IN GERIATRICS

Dehydration is classified as *isotonic, hypotonic,* or *hypertonic* (Figure 21.2).

- *Isotonic* dehydration can occur following equal loss of water and sodium. Therefore, the serum sodium concentration is normal. This type of dehydration may occur as a result of diarrhea, where there is loss of both water and salt in equal amounts.
- *Hypotonic* dehydration occurs when the sodium loss is greater than the water loss, resulting in increased intracellular fluid volume, reduced thirst, and renal conservation of water. Late signs include hyponatremia and loss of extracellular fluid volume, which may proceed to circulatory shock. This may happen when a patient is vomiting or is treated by diuretics.
- *Hypertonic* dehydration occurs when water loss exceeds the losses of sodium, which leads to hypernatremia. This may occur as a result of fever, or more commonly, thirst impairment, as a part of age-related physiological changes in elderly patients. Hypernatremia in particular is associated with higher mortality rate of up to 70% in severe cases (19,20).

Electrolyte abnormalities, specifically sodium imbalance, in elderly patients is very common and occurs following dehydration (18). Hyponatremia, however, is much more common than hypernatremia and is a risk factor for bone fracture in elderly patients (21,22). Other electrolyte abnormalities found to be associated with age-specific physiological changes are hyperkalemia because of impaired ability to secrete potassium, and blunting of renin

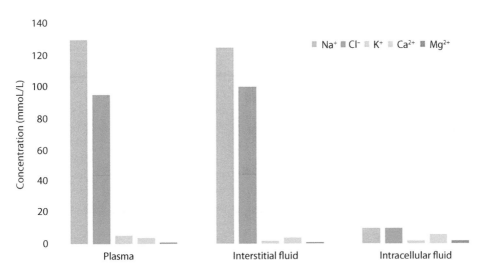

Figure 21.2 Distribution of electrolytes between the body's three major fluid compartments.

angiotensin response to a sudden rise in serum potassium levels (23,24). Decrease in serum magnesium levels has also been reported to be associated with increasing age, mostly related to decrease in dietary intake. Hypomagnesemia along with hypocalcemia can exacerbate osteoporosis and can cause arrhythmias, myocardial infarction, and even death (25).

TYPE OF FLUID IN GERIATRICS

Stress in response to surgery is associated with release of ADH from posterior pituitary resulting in increased water retention. Increased sympathetic activity further leads to an increase in aldosterone concentration resulting in further water and sodium absorption. These changes make elderly patients more prone to water and sodium retention (26). The UK NCEPOD found that at the extremes of age errors in fluid management, usually fluid excess, were the most common cause of avoidable postoperative morbidity and mortality, further highlighting the importance of accurate fluid prescription in older adults (27).

Perioperatively, 0.9% normal saline is the most commonly used intravenous crystalloid worldwide (28). Studies have shown that sodium balance remains abnormal for 2 days following infusion of 0.9% normal saline (29). The mild hyperchloremic acidosis that always follows saline infusion was also found to be associated with prolonged postoperative recovery through reduced gastric blood flow and intramucosal pH in elderly adult patients (30). In contrast, balanced crystalloid solutions that provide a smaller sodium and chloride load do not induce hyperchloremic acidosis (31,32). Moreover, there is a difference in the rate of excretion of these fluids. Also in the elderly, balanced fluid is more readily excreted than saline (48).

The type of fluid and volume regimen given intraoperatively can both impact patient outcome after major surgery. There is a current trend to use more crystalloid fluid, although a recent randomized controlled, double-blind, bi-center superiority study showed fewer postoperative complications with a colloid-based goal-directed fluid therapy than with a crystalloid one. This beneficial effect may be related to a less positive intraoperative fluid balance when a balanced colloid was used (33).

Neuroanesthetists may prefer saline during neurotrauma and neurosurgery because of its

believed hypertonic nature (308 mOsmol/kg), while balanced crystalloids are usually slightly hypotonic (270–285 mOsmol/kg). However, there is no strong evidence of a benefit from using saline, which causes metabolic acidosis in these patients just as it does in others (49). Moreover, saline becomes isotonic (295 mOsmol/kg) when infused to the blood owing to dilution by plasma proteins. Sodium still needs to be added to the fluid if the anesthetist wants to effectively reduce the intracerebral pressure.

Both crystalloids and colloids are used in the care of patients as volume expanders for numerous clinical conditions. The choice of intravenous crystalloid versus colloid solutions depends on the patient's needs and should be based on scientific evidence, not on tradition. Studies have indicated that crystalloids and colloids can be beneficial but also detrimental to patients if used incorrectly. Fluid resuscitation with either crystalloids or colloids must be individualized, and in the future, more preventive supplements may be used with these fluids to improve patient outcomes (34). Current literature is lacking on studies comparing crystalloids with colloids in elderly patients.

PLANNING THE FLUID THERAPY

Patients should be allowed to drink clear fluid up to 2 hours before surgery and should be encouraged to begin taking oral fluid as soon as possible after its completion.

There are three approaches when planning the fluid therapy during a surgical procedure.

1. *Fluid balance method*: Perceived and measured losses of fluid are replaced with infusion fluids so that their volume effect matches 1:1. This is the oldest and still most widely used approach.
2. *Outcome-based fluid therapy*: Fluid is infused in accordance with studies in which different fluid programs have been compared and one has been shown to be superior to others. Such studies show that 3–5 mL/kg/hour is the optimal infusion rate of crystalloids for a group undergoing abdominal surgery. Less volume increases the risk of nausea, and more fluid increases the risk of other complications (37). During the past 15 years, the results of outcome-oriented studies have promoted a more restrictive fluid administration during surgery.

In contrast, a restrictive crystalloid fluid program in the postoperative period does not seem to limit the number of complications (38).

3. *Goal-directed fluid therapy*: Fluid is infused with the aim of reaching a predetermined physiological target. The most common approach is to give a bolus of fluid, usually 250–500 mL of a colloid and examine the resulting change in stroke volume. If the increase exceeds 10% the patient is said to be fluid responsive, and more fluid can be given. A less time-consuming approach is to maintain the stroke volume index at 35–40 mL/m²/beat around which the optimized values seem to cluster (39). Goal-directed fluid therapy requires measurements of central hemodynamics and time to perform the bolus testing, but has been found to be beneficial in the sickest patients. Unselected use in a surgical population is questioned.

VOLUME EFFECTS

The therapeutic effect of infusing fluid is usually to expand the plasma volume. Therefore, the effectiveness by which this is achieved is a key feature of the therapy. There are two components of this effect: an immediate volume expansion and an intravascular half-life. For crystalloids, there is also a third component, distribution.

The colloid fluids used today include albumin 5%, hydroxyethyl starch (HES), dextran 70, and gelatin. Albumin 5% expands the plasma volume by 80% (40), HES by 100% (41), and dextran 70 by slightly more than 100% of the infused amount. There are scarce data on gelatin, but the expansion is probably close to that of HES. The half-life for the intravascular persistence of these colloids is 110 min for albumin and HES, and 175 min for dextran 70 (42). There are no data on the intravascular persistence of colloid fluids during surgery, but a shorter half-life is implicated in inflammatory disease due to increased capillary leakage of macromolecules.

Crystalloid electrolyte-based fluids expand the plasma volume by almost half the infused amount at the end of an infusion lasting 20–30 min (Figure 21.3). The plasma volume expansion decreases over a period of 30 min owing to distribution to the interstitial fluid space. The plasma volume expansion finally reached is 30% provided that

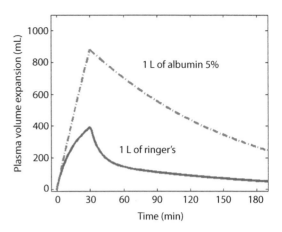

Figure 21.3 Expected plasma volume expansion when 1 liter of albumin 5% and 1 liter of Ringer's solution is infused in a healthy male adult over 30 min. Simulation-based typical kinetic data from volunteers.

no elimination occurs. From there, further reductions of the plasma volume expansion are governed primarily by urinary excretion, which occurs more slowly during surgery due to the anesthesia-induced decrease in arterial pressure (43). Further reduction of the rate of elimination occurs in old age (Figure 21.4). There are abundant data on the kinetics of crystalloid fluids during surgery.

The most clear-cut indications for colloid fluid are hemorrhage and goal-directed fluid therapy. The indication for electrolyte-based crystalloid fluid is expansion of extracellular fluid space,

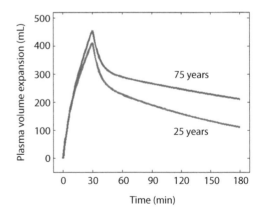

Figure 21.4 Expected plasma volume expansion over time when 1 liter of Ringer's solution is infused in a young male aged 25 years and an older man aged 75 years. Simulation-based kinetic data from Hahn (43) including both volunteers and surgical patients.

which is needed during surgery due to the anesthesia-induced blunting of the adrenergic system. There are also some crystalloid fluids that should be reserved for special indications and require special caution when administered. These include hypertonic saline, mannitol, and glucose solutions.

Hypertonic saline 3%–7.5% and mannitol 15% are crystalloid fluids that should be reserved for therapeutic intervention when the intracerebral pressure rises. They dehydrate the intracellular space by virtue of osmosis, and in consequence, expand the plasma volume. The risk of fluid overload is greater with saline because the mannitol also has a diuretic effect. However, the diuresis is of the osmotic kind, which implies that large amounts of extracellular solutes are lost with the urine. This loss later acts to re-fill the intracellular fluid space ("rebound effect") perhaps in excess of the starting point. Additional sodium administration might help to resolve this problem.

Glucose solutions should be given with caution during neuroanesthesia and neurotrauma, if at all, due to a negative influence of hyperglycemia on brain function if cardiac arrest develops (44). Monitoring of plasma glucose is recommended. In other situations, in patients who are conscious but cannot eat or drink, 25–30 mL/kg of glucose 5% per 24 hours is indicated. Sodium and potassium 1 mmoL/kg per 24 hours should be added. A safe infusion time is 4 hours, which should be extended to 6 hours in debilitated patients. Even slower infusions may be required during surgery due to the hyperglycemic effect of trauma (45).

COMPLICATIONS

Intravenous fluid administration might be associated with adverse effects. Isotonic or nearly isotonic crystalloid fluids are harmless up to a volume of 2 liters. Excessive fluid administration might cause acute hemodynamic overload and a fall in body temperature. Other problems are usually related to their preferential distribution to specific interstitial areas, such as the subcutis, the gastrointestinal tract, and the lungs. The first sign of overload is a prolongation of the gastrointestinal recovery time. Further administration of isotonic fluid causes tissue edema, with all related consequences, including indirect worsening of cellular function (35).

Crystalloid fluid load to 6–7 liters in colon surgery increases the risk of wound infection, suture insufficiency, bleeding, pulmonary edema, and pulmonary infection (46). Providing even more fluid might promote pulmonary edema (47). Old age and low arterial pressure restrict the elimination of fluid during the actual surgical procedure, thereby promoting fluid overload (43).

Adverse effects of colloid fluids include anaphylactic reactions, which occur in about 0.3% of the patients. They span from mild chills and fever to hemodynamic shock. All the colloid fluids increase the surgical blood loss, at least in a major surgery where the bleeding cannot be completely controlled surgically. HES might impair kidney function in septic patients.

CURRENT PRACTICE

In spite of the current understanding and knowledge of age-related changes in the renal and cardiovascular systems, an accurate fluid management strategy remains weakly understood in elderly patients. Goal-directed fluid therapy using minimally invasive cardiac output monitor has been found to be beneficial in this patient population (36).

CONCLUSION

The number of elderly patients has increased in recent times because of improved medical facilities worldwide. The rapid increase in this patient population has imposed multiple challenges to medical professionals because of age-related physiological changes in all organ systems, polypharmacy, and significant fluid and electrolyte abnormalities. Awareness among medical personnel and the patient is a key factor for improved outcome.

REFERENCES

1. Callum KG, Gray AJG, Martin IC, Sherry KM. Extremes of age: The elderly. *NCEPOD Report*. 1999:55–102.
2. Shafiee MAS, Bohn D, Hoorn EJ, Halperin ML. How to select optimal maintenance intravenous fluid therapy. *Q J Med*. 2003;96:601–10.
3. Watson PE, Watson ID, Batt RD. Total body water volumes for adult males and females estimated from simple anthropometric measurements. *Am J Clin Nutr*. 1980;33:27–39.

4. Guyton AC. *Textbook of Medical Physiology.* 5th ed. Philadelphia: WB Saunders; 1976. p. 284, 424.

5. Hansen JT, Koeppen BM. *Netter's Atlas of Human Physiology.* Teterboro, NJ: Icon Learning Systems; 2002.

6. Mazariegos M, Wang Z, Gallagher D, Baumgartner RN, Allison DB, Wang J, Pierson RN JR, Heymsfield SB. Differences between young and old females in the five levels of body composition and their relevance to the two-compartment chemical model. *J Gerontol.* 1994;49:M201–208.

7. Aloia JF, Vaswani A, Flaster E, Ma R. Relationship of body water compartments to age, race, and fat-free mass. *J Lab Clin Med.* 1998;132:483–90.

8. Ritz P. Body water spaces and cellular hydration during healthy aging. *Ann N Y Acad Sci.* 2000;904:474–83.

9. Schoeller DA. Changes in total body water with age. *Am J Clin Nutr.* 1989;50:1176–81.

10. Steen B. Body composition and aging. *Nutr Rev.* 1988;46:45–51.

11. Giuseppe S, Lucia L, Stefania V et al. Body fluid distribution in elderly subjects with congestive heart failure. *Ann Clin Lab Sci.* 2004;34.

12. Verbalis JG. Disorders of body water homeostasis. *Best Pract Res Clin Endocrinol Metab.* 2003;17:471–503.

13. Rose B. *Clinical Physiology of Acid-Base and Electrolyte Disorders.* McGraw-Hill Education/Medical; 2017.

14. El-Sharkawy AM, Lobo DN. The pathophysiology of fluid and electrolyte balance in the older adult surgical patient. *Clin Nutr.* 2014;33:6–13.

15. Grandjean AC, Grandjean NR. Dehydration and cognitive performance. *J Am Coll Nutr.* 2007;26:549S–54S.

16. Warren JL, Bacon WE, Harris T, McBean AM, Foley DJ, Phillips C. The burden and outcomes associated with dehydration among US elderly, 1991. *Am J Public Health.* 1994;84:1265–9.

17. Johnson P, Waldreus N, Hahn RG, Stenström H, Sjöstrand F. Fluid retention index predicts the 30-day mortality in geriatric care. *Scand J Clin Lab Invest.* 2015;75:444–51.

18. Hawkins RC. Age and gender as risk factors for hyponatremia and hypernatremia. *Clin Chim Acta.* 2003;337:169–72.

19. Alshayeb HM, Showkat A, Babar F, Mangold T, Wall BM. Severe hypernatremia correction rate and mortality in hospitalized patients. *Am J Med Sci.* 2011;341:356–60.

20. Snyder NA, Feigal DW, Arieff AI. Hypernatremia in elderly patients. A heterogeneous, morbid, and iatrogenic entity. *Ann Intern Med.* 1987;107:309–19.

21. Gankam Kengne F, Andres C, Sattar L, Melot C, Decaux G. Mild hyponatremia and risk of fracture in the ambulatory elderly. *QJM.* 2008;101:583–8.

22. Kinsella S, Moran S, Sullivan MO, Molloy MG, Eustace JA. Hyponatremia independent of osteoporosis is associated with fracture occurrence. *Clin J Am Soc Nephrol.* 2010;5:275–80.

23. Musso C, Liakopoulos V, De Miguel R, Imperiali N, Algranati L. Transtubular potassium concentration gradient: Comparison between healthy old people and chronic renal failure patients. *Int Urol Nephrol.* 2006;38:387–90.

24. Clark BA, Brown RS, Epstein FH. Effect of atrial natriuretic peptide on potassium-stimulated aldosterone secretion: Potential relevance to hypoaldosteronism in man. *J Clin Endocrinol Metab.* 1992;75:399–403.

25. Safavi M, Honarmand A. Admission hypomagnesemia impact on mortality or morbidity in critically ill patients. *Middle East J Anesthesiol.* 2007;19:645–60.

26. Desborough JP. The stress response to trauma and surgery. *Br J Anaesth.* 2000;85:109–17.

27. Callum KG, Gray AJ, Hoile RW et al. *Extremes of Age: The 1999 Report of the National Confidential Enquiry Into Perioperative Deaths.* London: National Confidential Enquiry into Perioperative Deaths; 1999.

28. Awad S, Allison SP, Lobo DN. The history of 0.9% saline. *Clin Nutr.* 2008;27:179–88.

29. Drummer C, Gerzer R, Heer M et al. Effects of an acute saline infusion on fluid and electrolyte metabolism in humans. *Am J Physiol.* 1992;262:F744–54.

30. Wilkes NJ, Woolf R, Mutch M et al. The effects of balanced versus saline-based hetastarch and crystalloid solutions on acid-base and electrolyte status and gastric mucosal perfusion in elderly surgical patients. *Anesth Analg.* 2001;93:811–6.

31. Reid F, Lobo DN, Williams RN, Rowlands BJ, Allison SP. (Ab)normal saline and physiological Hartmann's solution: A randomized double-blind crossover study. *Clin Sci (Lond).* 2003;104:17–24.

32. Williams EL, Hildebrand KL, McCormick SA, Bedel MJ. The effect of intravenous lactated Ringer's solution versus 0.9% sodium chloride solution on serum osmolality in human volunteers. *Anesth Analg.* 1999;88:999–1003.

33. Joosten A, Delaporte A, Ickx B et al. Crystalloid versus colloid for intraoperative goal-directed fluid therapy using a closed-loop system: A randomized, double-blinded, controlled trial in major abdominal surgery. *Anesthesiology.* 2018;128:55–66.

34. Pierce JD, Shen, Q, Thimmesch A et al. The ongoing controversy: Crystalloids versus colloids. *J Infus Nurs.* 2016;39:40–4.

35. Marik PE. Iatrogenic salt water drowning and the hazards of a high central venous pressure. *Ann Intensive Care.* 2014;4:21.

36. Pearse RM, Harrison DA, MacDonald N et al. Effect of a perioperative, cardiac output-guided hemodynamic therapy algorithm on outcomes following major gastrointestinal surgery: A randomized clinical trial and systematic review. *JAMA.* 2014;311:2181–90.

37. Hahn RG. Adverse effects of crystalloid and colloid fluids. *Anaesthesiol Intensive Ther.* 2017;49:303–8.

38. Vermeulen H, Hofland J, Legemate DA, Ubbink DT. Intravenous fluid restriction after major abdominal surgery: A randomized blinded clinical trial. *Trials.* 2009;10:50.

39. Li Y, He R, Ying X, Hahn RG. Dehydration, hemodynamics and fluid volume optimization after induction of general anesthesia. *Clinics.* 2014;69:809–81.

40. Hedin A, Hahn RG. Volume expansion and plasma protein clearance during intravenous infusion of 5% albumin and autologous plasma. *Clin Sci.* 2005;106:217–24.

41. Hahn RG, Bergek C, Gebäck T, Zdolsek J. Interactions between the volume effects of hydroxyethyl starch 130/0.4 and Ringer's acetate. *Crit Care.* 2013;17:R104.

42. Hahn RG, Lyons G. The half-life of infusion fluids: An educational review. *Eur J Anaesthesiol.* 2016;33:475–82.

43. Hahn RG. Arterial pressure and the elimination of crystalloid fluid: A population-based study. *Anesth Analg.* 2017;124:1824–33.

44. Siemkowicz E. The effect of glucose upon restitution after transient cerebral ischemia: A summary. *Acta Neurol Scand.* 1985;71:417–27.

45. Hahn RG. How fast can glucose be infused in the perioperative setting? *Perioper Med.* 2016;5:1.

46. Brandstrup B, Tonnesen H, Beier-Holgersen R et al. Effects of intravenous fluid restriction on postoperative complications: Comparison of two perioperative fluid regimens. A randomized assessor-blinded multicenter trial. *Ann Surg.* 2003;238:641–8.

47. Arieff AI. Fatal postoperative pulmonary edema. Pathogenesis and literature review. *Chest.* 1999;115:1371–7.

48. Hahn RG, Nyberg Isacson M, Fagerström T, Rosvall J, Nyman CR. Isotonic saline in elderly men: An open-labelled controlled infusion study of electrolyte balance, urine flow and kidney function. *Anaesthesia* 2016;71:155–62.

49. Hahn RG. In response: Fluids in neurosurgery. *Acta Anaesthesiol Scand.* 2018;62:140–1.

22

Palliative care in geriatric patients with neurological diseases

SEEMA MISHRA AND NISHKARSH GUPTA

INTRODUCTION

Neurological diseases are commonly present in older adults and may affect up to 55% of geriatric patients (1,2). These neurological diseases may be associated with high risk of adverse health outcomes, including disability, falls, frequent admissions to the hospital, and death. There is a global trend toward an increasing elderly population due to economic wellbeing, better healthcare system, improved medicines, etc. This increase in the geriatric population may lead to a growing number of elderly patients with neurological diseases (3). In the near future, the rising numbers of elderly patients may be a challenge for the healthcare system.

Neurodegenerative and cerebrovascular diseases are frequent in the elderly and their prevalence increases from age 55–65 years to age 90 years. The most common neurological diseases in the elderly include dementia (Alzheimer's type, vascular) (1%–40%), Parkinson's disease (PD) (0.5%–10.2%) and stroke (1%–10%). Other common diseases include amyotrophic lateral sclerosis (ALS) and multiple sclerosis (MS) (4). The symptom burden in patients living with neurologic disease is often more than for patients with malignancy, and includes cognitive impairment, emotional and psychological distress, speech and communication disorders, disability, and restricted respiration and swallowing. In addition, there may be large impacts on social, family, and work life. Unpredictable disease trajectory, increased symptom burden, cognitive impairments, and associated decreased quality of life in patients with life-limiting neurologic disease suggest that there is a need for comprehensive palliative care (PC) services for these patients (5). The clinical course of neurological diseases is often unpredictable, and prognosis is uncertain. Therefore, PC in geriatric patients with neurological diseases may be more complex, and one needs to assess the specific needs of geriatric patients suffering from neurological diseases.

Unlike cancer patients, these patients receive inadequate symptom control throughout the illness trajectory and do not plan their end of life (EOL) well (6,7). Common reasons include the patient's inability to express the requirements, and inability of the caregivers and physicians to recognize their needs (8).

Due to these difficulties, the PC approach to providing care for these individuals is catching up in the recent development of guidelines (9). PC often challenges traditional care for neurology and places more emphasis on the relief of suffering than the preservation of function and prolongation of life. PC assesses and treats medical, psychosocial, and spiritual issues. It also helps the patient to accept decline in function and death as an expected natural outcome rather than failure of medical treatment (10). In addition, it addresses the need to offer support services to the caregivers and family (11). We briefly discuss the PC needs of common neurological disorders, common symptoms and their management to improve quality of life, and advance care planning in geriatric patients.

APPROACH TO PALLIATIVE CARE FOR NEUROLOGICAL PATIENTS

The care of geriatric people with progressive neurological disease is challenging due to age-related physiological decline and the unique complexities of neurological diseases such as variable rate of progression, increased symptom burden, and limited prognostication markers. This need for PC in neurological diseases increases as the disease progress.

Neurological diseases differ considerably from cancer and initiation of PC is often challenging. The main differences are as follows:

1. It is often difficult to diagnose neurological conditions and many times the diagnosis may be delayed and lead to advanced disease.
2. The progression is variable and difficult to predict. These diseases do not have appropriate biomarkers or indices to predict progression. The neurological disease may have an acute onset leading to death, as in stroke, or a rapid decline over a few years as in ALS, or a prolonged deterioration over several years as in PD. Because of the unpredictable disease progression, it may be difficult to recognize the need for PC and EOL care.
3. Patients have both cognitive and physical disabilities, which may be exaggerated in geriatric patients and result in considerable management challenges.
4. These are complex diseases; in some the diagnosis may be difficult and delayed because of

an inability to biopsy and no clear biomarkers.
5. The disease process is unpredictable, and patients often have waxing and waning of disease progression with repeated attacks of acute exacerbation. The patient's symptoms are partly controlled with treatment, but their psychological suffering and disease severity progress with every acute exacerbation. Prognosis of the disease has been taken as a benchmark for allocating PC services worldwide and may be difficult in geriatric patients with neurological diseases. There is a role for episodic involvement of PC physicians during the progression of the disease at times of acute distressing symptoms or when psychosocial issues arise, such as at the time of diagnosis, assessing need for ventilator support, or at the EOL in these patients. Good communication among the various professionals is required. PC physicians are experienced in communicating about the diagnosis, management, and treatment options and advance planning. They play an important role in management of these patients.

COMMON SYMPTOMS IN GERIATRIC PATIENTS WITH NEUROLOGICAL DISEASE

1. *Respiratory insufficiency*: It is common in elderly patients with neurological diseases to have respiratory symptoms like dyspnea. Opioids are mainstay of dyspnea and can be given via oral, nasal, subcutaneous, transdermal, and inhalation route. In addition, benzodiazepines like lorazepam and midazolam may be required to reduce anxiety. Respiratory insufficiency is also common and may be due to progression of neurological disease as in ALS, or secondary to pulmonary infections or debility (12). The patient's preferences for prolonged invasive ventilation and tracheostomy should be asked for and documented. All efforts should be made to prevent respiratory infections by vaccination (influenza vaccinations or polyvalent pneumococcal vaccines). If feasible, noninvasive positive pressure ventilation (NIPPV) should be preferred. It may often be difficult to wean these patients from NIPPV and this needs to be carefully discussed beforehand (13).

2. *Cognitive decline*: Many people with neurological disease have altered autonomy due to changes in mood, cognitive abilities, communication, dysphasia, or dysarthria. These affect EOL care planning, and can cause distress to patients, families, and professional caregivers. It is necessary for PC physicians to discuss the EOL care plan earlier in the disease progression, when they have the capacity to do so.

3. *Dysphagia*: This is common in the elderly with neurodegenerative disorders due to lack of coordination of the muscles of swallowing, especially at the end-of-life phase (14). The need to plan for feeding is an appropriate approach, especially in very advanced stages of the disease. One needs to ensure appropriate posture, oral care, and food consistency to provide food to very ill and frail patients. In some severe cases like ALS placement of a percutaneous endoscopic gastrostomy (PEG) may be needed to prevent aspiration pneumonia and improve the patient's quality of life (15).

4. *Malnutrition*: Generally, malnutrition occurs due to decreased availability (insufficient food intake or malabsorption of nutrients) or increased requirement of nutrients. In geriatric patients, age-related physiological changes lead to loss of appetite and/or decreased food intake (16). In addition, patients with neurological diseases have additional risk factors for malnutrition including cognitive decline, dementia, poor appetite, poor oral health and dental hygiene, dysphagia, impaired motor and sensory skills, etc. Management depends on the etiology, and a multidisciplinary approach is required to correct various contributing factors. All medical causes (such as tooth loss or dysphagia) have to be specifically addressed. Oral supplementation is preferred, and parenteral nutrition is generally reserved for patients when oral/enteral supplementation is not feasible (17).

5. *Insomnia and sleep disorders*: These patients commonly have insomnia, sleep disturbances, and depression. Treatment of the primary neurological disease may restore normal sleep pattern, but in patients with depression antidepressants (amitriptyline) and hypnotics (zolpidem) may be required (13).

6. *Pain*: Pain is an important symptom and needs to be managed. Pain is common in patients with ALS, PD, and dementia (18,19). Many patients suffer from more than one pain but are less likely to receive adequate painkillers compared with cancer patients (20). Causes of pain in geriatric patients with neurological disease include:

a. Direct damage of the nerves, by demyelization/nerve compression/deafferentation, presenting as neuropathic pain.

b. Disease progression, leading to altered muscle tone, cramps, and spasticity.

c. Secondary to other issues like bed sores, incidental pain from constipation, urinary tract infection, and age-related degenerative changes in the joints such as osteoarthritis of the knee, lumbar disc prolapse, etc. are often present. The American Geriatrics Society found that 25%–50% of older people living in the community have major pain problems, and 45%–80% of nursing home residents have substantial pain that is undertreated (21).

d. The pain assessment may be difficult in patients with communication impairment or cognitive decline. Recent consensus recommendations suggest use of the Pain Assessment in Advanced Dementia (PAINAD) and the Pain Assessment Checklist for Seniors with Limited Ability to Communicate (PACSLAC) for assessing pain in these patients (22). The treatment of pain depends on the assessed or probable cause. Physiotherapy and occupational therapy can help in managing muscular stiffness and maintaining joint elasticity. The choice of analgesia should be planned as per the World Health Organization ladder (23). Considering the decreased metabolism of drugs in the elderly, drugs should be titrated slowly to reduce side effects. In addition, these patients might have swallowing problems, and alternative routes of administration like transdermal buprenorphine or fentanyl may be preferred.

7. *Urinary and bowel problems*: Urinary incontinence or retention is a common problem and may be due to direct neurological damage or as a consequence of a general physical decline of the patient. The patient may require urinary catheterization, which makes them prone to urinary tract infections. Constipation is also a common distressing symptom in these patients

and can occur in all neurological conditions. It may be worsened by the use of symptomatic drugs like opioids, anticholinergics, and disease-specific treatments. The patient should be encouraged to take adequate fluids, increase mobility, and use appropriate laxatives.

8. *Psychosis and psychiatric illness*: People with a neurological disease often have psychological and emotional distress. They may present atypically in patients with neurological disease. This may be further aggravated in an elderly person, who may have additional problems due to other comorbidities. They are particularly faced with fears of increasing disability, loss of cognition and ability to communicate, being a burden on family, and a distressing death (24). These factors may increase the risk of depression or anxiety and make them prone to suicidal tendencies or a request for physician-hastened death (25). However, appropriate symptom control and preemptive assessments to maintain a maximum of autonomy may prevent the patient from such measures. Treatment includes management of the potential causes, various non-pharmacological interventions (music therapy, massage, and physical activity) and drug therapy to reduce the symptoms (26).

COMMON NEUROLOGICAL DISORDERS IN GERIATRIC PATIENTS

Dementia

Dementia is a clinical syndrome with insidious onset and slow progression of at least two cognitive domains, such as short-term memory, language, executive function (reasoning and judgment), personality, and social cognition (27). This cognitive dysfunction interferes with the individual's activities of daily living (ADLs) (28). In advanced cases, the patient may have a complete loss of verbal abilities, mobility, and complete dependence in ADLs (29). Worldwide, 47.5 million individuals were estimated to have dementia, and this number is expected to increase to 135 million as the age of the individuals increases (27).

DIAGNOSIS AND ASSESSMENT

The clinical diagnosis of dementia may be missed in early stages, so it is important for PC physicians to screen for dementia in older individuals

and older adults. Various scales such as the Mini-Mental Sate Examination (MMSE), the Montreal Cognitive Assessment (MoCA), and the Mini-Cog have been used to identify dementia. The MMSE may not detect early stages of dementia. The MoCA has high sensitivity and can be used to detect mild cognitive decline. The Mini-Cog combines a three-item recall with clock-drawing test. It can be done in 3 minutes and a patient unable to recall all three items or able to recall less than three items with abnormal clock draw is considered to have a positive test (27). However, these scales may not be able to stage the severity of cognitive decline. Global severity scales are needed, like the functional assessment stage (FAST) scale and the global deterioration scale (GDS) to categorize dementia on the basis of severity (30,31). In GDS, the scores range from 1–7, and patients in stage 7 have advanced dementia, profound memory deficit, limited speech (less than five words), total functional dependence, and immobility. Similarly, FAST consists of seven major stages and stage 7 suggests advanced dementia. The various causes of dementia are summarized in Table 22.1.

Parkinsonism

PD is a common neurodegenerative disease. Patients experience a wide variety of symptoms including immobility, tremors, postural instability, pain, fatigue, dementia, and cognitive decline (33). PD cannot be cured, but treatment can be given to provide symptomatic relief. It may be difficult to manage PD in advanced stages, and patients may be confined to nursing homes for management without considering the quality of life (34). Many non-motor manifestations may be present in patients with PD such as sleep disturbance, fatigue, autonomic disturbance, pain, sensory abnormalities, etc. Treatment options for these symptoms are limited, and PC plays an important role in their management. In addition to PD, these patients may suffer from atypical parkinsonism-like disorders that do not respond to levodopa. (Table 22.2) The progression of symptoms and disability in patients with PD can be assessed using the Hoehn and Yahr (HY) scale. It divides progression of PD into five stages, and a higher stage signifies motor impairment and worsened quality of life (35).

Table 22.1 Causes of dementia

Cause	Pathophysiology	Clinical features
Alzheimer's disease	Accumulation of extracellular amyloid plaques, intracellular neurofibrillary tangles, and loss of neurons due to abnormal metabolism of amyloid-β 40 and amyloid-β 42	Slowly progressive impairment in memory
Vascular dementia	Multiple lacunar infarcts due to ischemic or hemorrhagic cerebrovascular disease	Sudden onset of cognitive deficits followed by periods where deficits stabilize
Dementia with Lewy bodies	Alpha-synuclein clump (Lewy bodies) deposition	Associated with parkinsonism; very sensitive to neuroleptic medicines
Frontotemporal dementia	Focal degeneration of the frontal and/or temporal lobes	Personality change hallmark; memory and visuospatial functions may be spared in initial stage

Source: Laurila JV et al. Gen Hosp Psychiatry. 2004;26(1):31–5. (32).

Table 22.2 Atypical parkinsonism-like disorders

Disorder	Characteristics
Dementia with Lewy bodies (DLB)	Visual hallucinations, fluctuating cognition, and parkinsonism
Progressive supranuclear palsy (PSP)	Supranuclear vertical ophthalmoparesis or ophthalmoplegia is the hallmark of PSP
	The PSP parkinsonism phenotype is characterized by asymmetric onset of limb symptoms, tremor, and a moderate initial therapeutic response to levodopa
Multiple system atrophy (MSA)	Commonly presents with parkinsonism with varying degrees of dysautonomia, cerebellar involvement, and pyramidal signs
	These patients respond poorly to levodopa
	The cortical involvement is less, and cognitive function is relatively well preserved
Corticobasal degeneration (CBD)	A progressive asymmetric, often unilateral (at onset) movement disorder with cognitive impairment
	May be associated with akinesia, extreme rigidity, dystonia, focal myoclonus, and alien limb phenomenon

Amyotrophic lateral sclerosis

ALS is a common neurological disease that affects primary or secondary motor neurons. It is more common in females, with incidence of approximately 2/100,000 per year and life expectancy of 2–4 years after onset of disease. It has two variants, the spinal variant (asymmetric tetra paresis with cranial nerve deficit in late stages) and the bulbar variant (progressive muscle weakness with speech and swallowing defect). Additional symptoms may include apathy, disinhibition, decreased mobility, progressive dyspnea, dysphagia, muscle cramps, dysarthrophonia, and sleep disturbance (36). It may lead to progressive disability and death, so life-prolonging treatments need to be instituted after considering the patient's preferences, the impact on quality of life, and family burden. Efforts should be made to preserve their mobility to improve overall quality of life (37).

Stroke

Stroke is common in elderly patients and leads to considerable morbidity and mortality. Developments in the management of stroke have reduced the overall mortality related to it, but the disability and associated physiological and psychological symptom burden remains to be addressed. An introduction to PC may benefit patients with stroke by improving symptom control, ensuring good communication, and discontinuing inappropriate medications (38). However, there is limited information for identification and management of the PC needs of these patients. Stroke patients are often referred late for PC to manage EOL decisions.

END-OF-LIFE CARE IN PATIENTS WITH NEUROLOGICAL DISEASES

As disease progress, one needs to prepare the patients and their families for EOL. It is often difficult to recognize the stage at which this should be initiated. Recognition of this stage may be complex; however, certain conditions such as swallowing problems, recurrent infections, marked decrease in functional status, aspiration pneumonia, and severe cognitive impairment should prompt PC physicians to start EOL care planning (39).

This allows the families and carers to be better prepared for the death and to make appropriate preparations to ensure that the person's wishes such as place of death, execution of the will, the funeral arrangements, etc. at the EOL are honored (40). These communications should be made early, as there may be cognitive decline and a reduced ability to communicate as the disease progresses.

Many patients with neurological disease may receive complex treatments to treat primary disease, such as cytotoxic drugs and monoclonal antibodies in MS, or invasive therapies like deep brain stimulation in PD, or ventilator support in ALS. These interventions may pose complex ethical issues. As the disease progresses, treatments may no longer be appropriate and the need to withdraw treatment should also be discussed. The PC physician should work with the primary neuro physician to decide when these complex therapies are medically futile and need to be stopped (41,42).

The planning for EOL is complex and should be executed in an appropriate manner. A six-step approach suggested by the Indian Association of Palliative Care includes Identify, Assess, Plan, Provide, Reassess, and Reflect (43). It is important to identify the need for EOL planning and assess the symptoms and disease severity. Then the EOL care needs to be planned, depending upon the patient's and carers' needs. The existing protocols need to be reviewed, unnecessary medications should be stopped, unnecessary investigations should be avoided, and maximum relief for EOL symptoms such as pain, dyspnea, delirium, respiratory secretions, etc. should be ensured. Moreover, the family and the patient should be communicated with and counseled throughout the process regarding the expected life and symptom burdens and their management. The patient's preferences regarding resuscitation and advance care planning should be documented. The EOL care process should be reviewed for any gaps in communication and acceptance, and any concerns regarding the care process should be addressed. Any improvements in the EOL care process should be initiated depending upon the feedback of the caregivers.

VARIOUS MODELS OF INVOLVEMENT OF PALLIATIVE CARE IN NEUROLOGICAL DISEASES

1. *Traditional model of involvement of specialist PC*: Active curative neurology care is provided to the patient until the end of life, and PC is provided only at the end of life (44).
2. *Model of early and increasing involvement of specialist PC*: Early involvement of specialist PC and their role increases as the disease progresses.
3. *Model of dynamic involvement of PC services based on trigger points*: Specialist PC is provided at the trigger points. The trigger points are points when symptom burden increases and needs to be addressed to improve quality of life. These may occur at any time point of the disease and need to be addressed.

SUPPORT FOR CARERS

It is important to support the family members and other carers who support these patients. They are often worried about the impending death and may be more fearful of the dying process than the death itself. All the caregivers need to adjust to the eventuality and need to be given appropriate information to alleviate their concerns and fears (42). Carers should be educated about and prepared for a gradually worsening neurological condition and should be counseled to adjust to the situation. Carers are prone to develop psychiatric illness and may develop suicidal tendencies. The family and carers should be counseled and their needs and queries regarding supporting the geriatric patients at home should be addressed. A clear plan for EOL should be made in consultation with the patient and their carers so that all are aware of the plan if difficulty arises.

SUMMARY

PC should be considered early in managing geriatric patients with neurological disease. Assessment and care of these patients requires a multidisciplinary team approach, and primary neurologists should be involved in planning PC services. Communication with patients and families is important and should be started before cognitive deterioration occurs due to disease progression. A thorough assessment of physical and psychosocial issues should be done and managed to improve quality of life. Considering the possibility of cognitive decline in patients over time, discussion regarding advance care planning and EOL should be initiated well in time. PC principles should be discussed with treating neurologists so that they can explain these issues to the patients and manage them better.

REFERENCES

1. Hofman A, Murad SD, Van Duijn CM, Franco OH, Goedegebure A, Arfan Ikram M. The Rotterdam Study: 2014 objectives and design update. *Eur J Epidemiol*. 2013;28:889–926.
2. Murray CJ, Vos T, Lozano R et al. Disability-adjusted life years (DALYs) for 291 diseases and injuries in 21 regions, 1990–2010: A systematic analysis for the Global Burden of Disease Study 2010. *Lancet*. 2012;380: 2197–223.
3. Neurology in the elderly: More trials urgently needed. *Lancet Neurol* 2009, 8(11):969.
4. de Rijk MC, Launer LJ, Berger K et al. Prevalence of Parkinson's disease in Europe: A collaborative study of population-based cohorts. *Neurologic Diseases in the Elderly Research Group. Neurology*. 2000;54(11 Suppl 5):S21–3.
5. Boersma I, Miyasaki J, Kutner K, Kluger B. Palliative care and neurology: Time for a paradigm shift. *Neurology*. 2014;83:561–7.
6. Birch D, Draper J. A critical literature review exploring the challenges of delivering effective palliative care to older people with dementia. *J Clin Nurs*. 2008;17(9):1144–63.
7. Hely MA, Morris JG, Traficante R et al. The Sydney Multicentre Study of Parkinson's disease: Progression and mortality at 10 years. *J Neurol Neurosurg Psychiatry*. 1999;67:300–7.
8. Veronese S, Gallo G, Valle A et al. Specialist palliative care improves the quality of life in advanced neurodegenerative disorders: NE-PAL, a pilot randomised controlled study. *BMJ Support Palliat Care*. 2015;7:164–72.
9. Durepos P, Wickson-Griffiths A, Hazzan AA et al. Assessing palliative care content in dementia care guidelines: A systematic review. *J Pain Symptom Manage*. 2017;53(4):804–13.
10. Lanoix M. Palliative care and Parkinson's disease: Managing the chronic-palliative interface. *Chronic Illn*. 2009;5:46–55.
11. Hudson PL, Aranda S, Kristjanson LJ. Meeting the supportive needs of family caregivers in palliative care: Challenges for health professionals. *J Palliat Med*. 2004;7:19–25.
12. Bourke SC, Tomlinson M, Williams TL, Bullock RE, Shaw PJ, Gibson GJ. Effects of non-invasive ventilation on survival and quality of life in patients with amyotrophic lateral sclerosis: A randomised controlled trial. *Lancet Neurol*. 2006;5(2):140–7.
13. Andersen PM, Abrahams S, Borasio GD et al. EFNS guidelines on the clinical management of amyotrophic lateral sclerosis (MALS)—revised report of an EFNS task force. *Eur J Neurol*. 2012;19(3):360–75.
14. Muller J, Wenning GK, Verny M et al. Progression of dysarthria and dysphagia in postmortem–confirmed Parkinsonian disorders. *Arch Neurol*. 2001;58(2):259–64.
15. National Institute for Health and Care Excellence. Motor neurone disease: Noninvasive ventilation. NICE Clinical Guideline (CG105). NICE. 2010.
16. Landi F, Calvani R, Tosato M et al. Anorexia of aging: Risk factors, consequences, and potential treatments. *Nutrients*. 2016;8:69.

17. Volkert D, Berner YN, Berry E et al. ESPEN guidelines on enteral nutrition: Geriatrics. Clin Nutr. 2006;25:330–60.

18. Chio A, Canosa A, Gallo S et al. Pain in amyotrophic lateral sclerosis: A population-based controlled study. Eur J Neurol. 2012;19(4): 551–5.

19. Sampson EL, White N, Lord K et al. Pain, agitation, and behavioural problems in people with dementia admitted to general hospital wards: A longitudinal cohort study. Pain. 2015; 156(4):675–83.

20. Calvert M, Pall H, Hoppitt T, Eaton B, Savill E, Sackley C. Health-related quality of life and supportive care in patients with rare long-term neurological conditions. Qual Life Res. 2013; 22(6):1231–8.

21. AGS Panel. The management of persistent pain in older persons. J Am Geriatr Soc. 2002; 50(6 Suppl):S205–24.

22. Herr K, Bursch H, Ersek M, Miller LL, Swafford K. Use of pain-behavioral assessment tools in the nursing home: Expert consensus recommendations for practice. J Gerontol Nurs. 2010;36(3):18–29.

23. World Health Organization. Cancer pain relief and palliative care. Report of a WHO Expert Committee. World Health Organ Tech Rep Ser. 1990:1–75.

24. Oliver D. Opioid medication in the palliative care of motor neurone disease. Palliat Med. 1998;12(2):113–5.

25. Bascom PB, Tolle SW. Responding to requests for physician assisted suicide: "These are uncharted waters for both of us…" JAMA 2002;288(1):91–8.

26. Aarsland D, Larsen JP, Karlsen K, Lim NG, Tandberg E. Mental symptoms in Parkinson's disease are important contributors to caregiver distress. Int J Geriatr Psychiatry. 1999; 14:866–74.

27. World Health Organization. Dementia. 2016. http://www.who.int/mediacentre/factsheets/fs362/en/. Updated 2017. Accessed August 16, 2017.

28. American Psychiatry Association. Diagnostic and Statistical Manual of Mental Disorders: DSM-5. 5th ed. Washington, DC: American Psychiatric Association; 2013.

29. Reisberg B, Ferris SH, de Ledon MJ, Crook T. The Global Deterioration Scale for assessment of primary degenerative dementia. Am J Psychiatry. 1982;139(9):1136–9.

30. Reisberg B. Functional assessment staging (FAST). Psychopharmacol Bull. 1988;24:653.

31. Reisberg B, Ferris SH, de Leon MJ, Crook T. The Global Deterioration Scale for assessment of primary degenerative dementia. Am J Psychiatry. 1982;139:1136.

32. Laurila JV, Pitkala KH, Strandberg TE, Tilvis RS. Detection and documentation of dementia and delirium in acute geriatric wards. Gen Hosp Psychiatry. 2004;26(1):31–5.

33. Tanner CM, Goldman SM. Epidemiology of Parkinson's disease. Neurol Clin. 1996; 14(2):317–35.

34. Lee MA, Prentice WM, Hildreth AJ, Walker RW. Measuring symptom load in idiopathic Parkinson's disease. Parkinsonism Relat Disord. 2007;13(5):284–9.

35. Goetz CG, Poewe W, Rascol O, Sampaio C, Stebbins GT et al. Movement Disorder Society Task Force report on the Hoehn and Yahr staging scale: Status and recommendations. Mov Disord 2004;19:1020.

36. Voltz R, Lorenzl S, and Nübling GS. Neurological disorders other than dementia. Oxford Textbook of Palliative Medicine. 5th ed. Oxford University Press; 2017. pp. 997–1003.

37. Karam CY, Paganoni S, Joyce N, Carter GT, Bedlack R. Palliative care issues in amyotrophic lateral sclerosis: An evidenced-based review. Am J Hosp Palliat Care. 2016;33(1):84–92.

38. Mead GE, Cowey E, Murray SA. Life after stroke—is palliative care relevant? A better understanding of illness trajectories after stroke may help clinicians identify patients for a palliative approach to care. Int J Stroke. 2013;8:447–8.

39. The National Council for Palliative Care. End of life care in long term neurological conditions: A framework for implementation. NHS National End of Life Care Programme. 2010.

40. Hussain J, Adams D, Allgar V, Campbell C. Triggers in advanced neurological conditions: Prediction and management of the terminal phase. BMJ Supp Palliat Care. 2014;4:30–7.

41. Oliver DJ, Turner MR. Some difficult decisions in ALS/MND. ALS. 2010;11:339–43.

42. Smith S, Wasner M. Psychosocial care. In: Oliver D, Borasio GD, Johnston W (eds). *Palliative Care in Amyotrophic Lateral Sclerosis – from Diagnosis to Bereavement.* 3rd ed. Oxford: Oxford University Press; 2014.

43. Macaden SC, Salins N, Muckaden M et al. End of life care policy for the dying: Consensus position statement of Indian association of palliative care. *Indian J Palliat Care.* 2014; 20(3):171–81.

44. Bede P, Hardiman O, O'Brannagain D. An integrated framework of early intervention palliative care in motor neurone disease as a model to progressive neurodegenerative diseases. *Poster at European ALS Congress, Turin.* 2009.

23

Brain death and ethical issues: Death by neurological criteria

BRITTANY BOLDUC AND DAVID M. GREER

WHAT IS BRAIN DEATH?

Brain death is a medically, legally, and ethically accepted definition of human death within the United States and most other countries. The term "brain death" is misleading, as it suggests that only the brain has died, and not the entire human organism. Rather, the term "death by neurological criteria" better embodies the concept that brain death is as much a form of death as cardiopulmonary arrest (1). Death by neurological criteria requires that clinical functions of the entire brain, including the brainstem, have suffered irreversible damage and have ceased to function completely.

In adults, the most common causes of brain death include massive head trauma, hypoxic ischemic neuronal damage such as cardiopulmonary arrest, and massive intracranial hemorrhage (2). The pathogenesis of brain death occurs in three phases. The initial phase includes the primary brain insult. This leads to edema and increased intracranial pressure. When the intracranial pressure surpasses mean arterial blood pressure, intracranial blood flow ceases and cerebral herniation occurs. In the second phase, remaining cerebral, cerebellar, and brainstem neurons that survived the initial phase are killed due to the lack of intracranial blood flow. The third phase consists of a drop in intracranial pressure and possible reperfusion of infarcted brain (3).

The concept of brain death has been muddled with ethical, legal, and religious challenges throughout the years, and these continue to arise in today's society. As a result, it has been necessary for the scientific world to establish clear, discrete diagnostic criteria and protocols for the determination of death by neurological criteria. The formal, accepted criteria require (4,5):

1. The presence of a catastrophic structural brain lesion sufficient to produce the clinical findings of brain death
2. Irreversible coma with a known etiology
3. Absence of reversible causes, including metabolic and toxic abnormalities
4. Absence of all brainstem reflexes and cranial nerves
5. Apnea

It is important to note that current US guidelines for the diagnosis of death by neurological criteria do not require that a physician be of any certain subspecialty. That is to say, any physician can medically and legally diagnose a patient as brain dead. The clear gravity of this diagnosis for both patients and families leaves no room for error. Thus, it is critical that any physician determining brain death use a strict algorithm and be appropriately trained in the clinical examination and interpretation of diagnostic and ancillary testing. Such criteria have been published by the American Academy of Neurology (AAN) and accepted by the medical community. These published criteria are the foundation of this chapter.

HISTORY

To fully understand the definition and concept of brain death, it is helpful to understand the long history that has led to today's accepted standards and protocols. Prior to the era of modern critical care medicine, the concept of death focused on the human heart as the epicenter of life, and cardiopulmonary arrest was the only accepted form of human death (6).

The first reference of brain death dates back to the twelfth century, when Rabbi Moses Maimonides argued that spasmodic jerking observed in decapitated humans did not represent evidence of life because the movements clearly did not originate from the brain (7). Despite these early observations, the overarching concept that loss of total brain function could represent death did not come to light until the advent of positive pressure ventilation in 1952. In 1959, Pierre Mollaret and Maurice Goulon published their article "Le coma depassé," which was first to describe "irretrievable coma." (8) This groundbreaking article was the first to call into question whether patients with "coma depassé" were alive or dead and whether continued ventilation and medical care in these patients was appropriate. This forced the medical community to reevaluate the definition of death in the new technological era of critical care medicine.

It wasn't until 1968 that the first criteria for the determination of brain death were published by the Harvard Committee. This committee, consisting of physicians, a theologian, a lawyer, and a historian of science, examined irreversible coma as a criterion for death and described four clinical features required for diagnosis of brain death: (i) unreceptivity and unresponsiveness; (ii) absent movements or breathing; (ii) absent reflexes; (iv)

isoelectric electroencephalography (EEG) (9). Prerequisites included correction of hypothermia ($<32.2°C$) and absence of central nervous system (CNS) depressants, and a second confirmatory examination at least 24 hours after the initial evaluation was required. The publication of a formal definition of brain death by the scientific community led to the necessity for a legal recognition of brain death. The Harvard Committee criteria were used to develop the Uniform Determination of Death Act (UDDA), which states: "An individual who has sustained either (1) irreversible cessation of circulatory and respiratory functions, or (2) irreversible cessation of all functions of the entire brain, including the brain stem, is dead. A determination of death must be made in accordance with accepted medical standards." (10)

The Harvard Committee criteria were considered the "accepted medical standard" in determination of brain death until the AAN published an evidence-based guideline in 1995. This protocol provided a methodical approach to the clinical diagnosis of death by neurological criteria and required (i) loss of consciousness, (ii) absent motor response to painful stimuli, (iii) absent brainstem reflexes, and (iv) apnea (11). Like the Harvard criteria, prerequisites of catastrophic CNS injury and exclusion of confounding variables were required. These guidelines have been widely accepted by medical societies and legal bodies and have since been updated by the AAN in 2010. The 2010 update also addressed the potential for misdiagnosis or brain death mimics, appropriate observation times, and the potential use of ancillary tests (4). The 2010 guidelines are the foundation for determination of death by neurological criteria today, and when used correctly, the diagnosis of brain death can be made without error.

Despite the publication and scientific and legal acceptance of stepwise guidelines, studies have shown disturbing variability in brain death determination protocols between major medical centers (12). In particular, institutions varied in who could perform testing, number of examinations required for diagnosis, prerequisites for diagnosis, techniques in testing brainstem function, apnea testing, and ancillary test use. From the legal perspective, despite the existence of the UDDA and recognized AAN protocols, each state has its own legal regulations and each hospital is left to establish its own criteria (5). This has led to much confusion in the public eye and leaves unacceptable room for error. It is critically important to note that in a systematic review, no diagnosis of brain death has ever resulted in neurological recovery when diagnosed strictly by AAN guidelines (4).

Prerequisites

As referenced in the definition of death by neurological criteria, it is first necessary to identify the presence of a catastrophic structural brain lesion leading to the absence of all cerebrally-mediated responses to the environment. If no lesion can be identified, a provider must consider alternative diagnoses (13). The etiology of coma must be identified, and coma must be determined to be irreversible. Per recent AAN guidelines, there is insufficient evidence to dictate a strict period of time that must pass before an injury is determined irreversible (4). Irreversibility is typically identified by neuroimaging (computed tomography [CT] and/or magnetic resonance imaging [MRI]) demonstrating catastrophic diffuse structural damage and by ruling out reversible etiologies. This includes exclusion of a CNS-depressant drug effect or neuromuscular blockade. If confounding pharmaceuticals are identified by history, or serum or urine testing, it is standard to wait at least five drug half-lives before proceeding with brain death determination. It is also important to note that hypothermia may slow drug clearance, and patients who suffered or were treated with hypothermia may require longer than five drug half-lives for full clearance (14). There should be no significant electrolyte or acid-base disturbances, which may be a reversible cause of CNS depression.

A patient must be at or near normal body temperature for brain death declaration. This is defined as body temperature >36°C (15). In patients treated with therapeutic hypothermia post-cardiac arrest, it is standard to wait 72 hours post-rewarming before performing a brain death examination. In those post-cardiac arrest patients not treated with hypothermia, it is recommended that examination be performed no sooner than 24 hours after the initial insult (16).

It is also necessary to achieve normal systolic blood pressure prior to proceeding with diagnosis. This is defined as a systolic blood pressure >100 mmHg. Vasopressors are frequently required (4).

PREREQUISITE CHECKLIST

Prerequisite	Complete
Presence of irreversible coma	
Etiology of coma identified (consider neuroimaging)	
Confounding pharmaceuticals ruled out (obtain urine and serum toxicology, patient history)	
If pharmaceuticals present, wait at least five half-lives (assuming normal hepatic and renal function)	
Normothermia present (>36°C); if hypothermic, wait at least 72 hours after rewarming to proceed	
Blood pressure >100 mmHg (vasopressors may be necessary)	
Correction of major electrolyte/ acid-base disturbances	
Ensure absence of paralysis, if paralytics given	

Clinical examination

When all prerequisites are met, the clinician can proceed with the physical examination. Coma must first be established. Coma is defined as complete unresponsiveness to the environment. There must be no eye opening or eye movement to noxious stimuli and no purposeful motor movement to noxious stimulation. It is important that spinally mediated movements not be mistaken for purposeful movements. These spinal reflexes will be discussed later.

After confirming a comatose state, the physician can move on to cranial nerve testing. All cranial nerve reflexes must be absent for the diagnosis of brain death. Pupillary response to a bright light must be absent in both eyes. The pupils are typically fixed in mid-position (4–9 mm) due to sympathetic and parasympathetic denervation (4). Pinpoint pupils should alert the provider to possible drug effect. A magnifying glass or pupilometer may be used to detect small changes in pupil size. In a patient with proper spinal integrity, oculocephalic reflexes should be tested by rapidly turning the patient's head from side to side and vertically with the eyes held open. There should be no eye movement in the brain-dead patient. Vestibuloocular reflexes should be tested using maximal ice water caloric stimulation. First, otoscopic examination is performed to ensure that tympanic membrane is intact and external auditory canals are patent. The head of the bed should be at 30°. Fifty mL of ice water is infused into one ear through a flexible, dull-ended tube, such as a butterfly catheter with the needle removed. The infusion occurs over 1 minute, while an assistant holds open the patient's eyes. A patient who is brain dead will display no response to this test, including no grimace, eye movements, or motor response. An interval of 5 minutes should exist before testing the other ear (17). The corneal reflex should be tested with a cotton swab applicator pressed carefully on the cornea bilaterally. Facial muscle response to noxious stimuli should be assessed by applying deep pressure to the temporomandibular joint and the supraorbital ridge. No grimace should be seen. Gag and cough reflexes can be tested by suctioning the patient's endotracheal tube or by stimulating the posterior pharynx with a tongue depressor. A jaw jerk reflex should be absent. Again, all cranial nerve reflexes must be absent bilaterally in order to diagnose brain death and to proceed with further testing.

CRANIAL NERVE TESTING CHECKLIST

Cranial nerve	Completed
Pupillary responses to bright light with magnifying glass and/or pupilometer (CN II, III)	
Oculocephalic reflex horizontally and vertically (CN III, IV, VI)	
Cold caloric testing (CN III, VI, VIII)	
Corneal reflex (CN V, VII)	
Jaw jerk reflex (CN V)	
Facial response to noxious stimulus (CN V, VII)	
Cough and gag reflexes (CN IX, X)	

Abbreviation: CN: cranial nerve.

Apnea testing

After confirming the presence of irreversible coma and absent brainstem reflexes, the provider can move on to apnea testing. Apnea is defined as the absence of respiratory drive despite CO_2 challenge. Acidemia from rising pCO_2 provides the stimulus

for an intact medulla to breathe. Thus, apnea testing requires a rise in CO_2 while preserving oxygenation. Prerequisites for apnea testing include normotension (systolic blood pressure [SBP] >100 mmHg), normothermia, euvolemia, eucapnia ($PaCO_2$ 40–45 mmHg), absence of hypoxia, and no prior evidence of CO_2 retention. In some patients, the apnea test is not safe or reliable, such as those with underlying acute or chronic pulmonary disease (18). In those cases, ancillary testing (discussed later) will be necessary. In those who meet criteria, patients should be pre-oxygenated with 100% oxygen to a PaO_2 >200 mmHg. Ventilator frequency should be reduced to 10 breaths per minute. Positive end-expiratory pressure (PEEP) should be reduced to 5 cm H_2O. Patient must remain clinically stable and maintain oxygen saturation >95% at these minimal ventilator settings to proceed with apnea testing (4). Desaturation or hemodynamic instability suggests that apnea testing may not be safe and should be performed with great caution, if at all.

If a patient is deemed appropriate to continue, a baseline blood gas should be obtained, including PaO_2, $PaCO_2$, and pH. The patient should then be disconnected from the ventilator. It is critical that the ventilator be completely disconnected, as ventilator auto-cycling may confound results (19,20). Oxygenation is preserved during testing by placing an insufflation catheter through the endotracheal tube to the level of the carina and administering 100% oxygen passively at 4–6 liters per minute for the duration of the test. A higher flow rate may wash out CO_2 and confound the test. The chest and abdomen should be bared, and the patient is observed for 10 minutes for any signs of respiratory movements including abdominal or chest excursions or gasping. If respiratory effort is observed, the test should be aborted, and the patient is not brain dead. If no respiratory drive is observed, a repeat blood gas should be obtained at approximately 10 minutes if the patient is stable. PCO_2 greater than 60 mmHg or an increase of greater than 20 mmHg from an elevated baseline (for known CO_2 retainers) is consistent with a positive apnea test and supports the diagnosis of brain death (21). PCO_2 rises at a rate of approximately 3 mmHg per minute, which means an adequate amount of time must be allowed for a proper CO_2 challenge (22). If the arterial blood gas (ABG) results are inconclusive but the patient is hemodynamically stable, the test can be repeated for a longer duration of 10–15 minutes, after repeat preoxygenation and once again establishing normocapnia.

Apnea testing should be immediately aborted if the patient's systolic blood pressure drops below 90 mmHg or oxygen saturation drops below 85% for more than 30 seconds (23). The most common complications of apnea testing include hypotension, cardiac arrhythmia, acidosis, and hypoxemia. These are more likely to occur in the setting of inadequate preoxygenation (24,25).

APNEA TESTING CHECKLIST

Sequence of steps	Complete
Normotension (SBP >100 mmHg)	
Normothermia (temp >36°C)	
Eucapnia (pCO$_2$ 40–45)	
Preoxygenate to PaO$_2$ 200 mmHg	
Ventilator frequency 10 breaths per minute	
PEEP 5	
— Is patient stable with above settings? —	
Obtain baseline blood gas	
Uncover patient's abdomen and chest for observation	
Completely disconnect ventilator	
Insert insufflation catheter through endotracheal tube to carina at 4–6 L per minute	
Observe for respiratory effort	
Repeat blood gas at 10 minutes	
Reconnect to ventilator, briefly hyperventilate to remove CO$_2$, and correct acidosis	

ANCILLARY TESTING

When and why

Under current AAN guidelines, ancillary testing is not required for the determination of death by neurological criteria. When a complete clinical neurological examination and apnea test can be properly and safely conducted, this is sufficient for diagnosis and ancillary tests should not be performed (2,4). It is recommended that ancillary testing be used sparingly and only in appropriate cases. Appropriate cases include situations in which a complete neurological examination cannot be completed, such as severe facial trauma preventing complete brainstem testing, preexisting pupillary abnormalities, or tympanic membrane damage. Ancillary testing is also necessary if apnea testing cannot be completed, as in cases of severe acute or chronic pulmonary disease or hemodynamic instability. Lastly, when concurrent metabolic or toxic abnormalities exist which may confound the clinical neurological evaluation and cannot be corrected, ancillary testing should be used. Overall, ancillary tests should never supersede the clinical exam, but they should be used in any case in which there is uncertainty surrounding the clinical diagnosis. The current validated ancillary tests included in the 2010 AAN brain death guidelines include EEG, cerebral angiography, nuclear scan (Single-photon emission computed tomography [SPECT]), and transcranial Doppler ultrasonography (TCD) (4). These tests, as well as other proposed ancillary tests, are discussed in detail in the following section, "Available ancillary tests."

Available ancillary tests

Available ancillary testing can be divided into two categories: those that test electrical activity of the brain and those that test cerebral blood flow. Individual institutions tend to dictate their own protocols for ancillary testing based on testing most readily available.

BIOELECTRICAL STUDIES

EEG

The most commonly used electrophysiologic ancillary study is EEG. A minimum of eight scalp electrodes should be used and interelectrode impedance should be 100–10,000 Ohms. Electrodes should be spaced at least 10 cm from each other. EEG must show absence of electrical activity (isoelectric recording) at a sensitivity of 2 microvolts for 30 minutes for the determination of brain death. There should be no reactivity to external stimuli (4,26). There are significant limitations to this test, causing it to fall out of favor. EEG is very susceptible to false positives. EEG can be affected by medications or sedation, hypothermia, toxic or metabolic derangements, and external artifacts or interference. In addition, large case series have shown that up to 3.5% of patients who are clinically brain dead can maintain rudimentary EEG activity for several hours after clinical diagnosis has been made (27). Finally, EEG does not assess brainstem function, and thus, if used, should only be used in combination with evoked potentials (see the following section, "Somatosensory evoked potentials").

Somatosensory evoked potentials

Somatosensory evoked potentials (SSEP) is an assessment of the function of the posterior columns, medial lemniscus, thalamus, and sensorimotor cortex. Brain death is indicated by absence of the N20-P22 response to median nerve stimulation bilaterally. The 2010 AAN guidelines reviewed the literature regarding SSEP in brain death determination. Two studies examined the use of nasopharyngeal electrode recording of SSEPs and showed disappearance of the P14 wave (presumably representing medial lemniscus and cuneate nucleus) in all clinically brain-dead patients. The P14 was not absent in the control group of comatose patients who were not brain dead (28,29). There was not adequate statistical precision or investigation to approve this as a recommended ancillary test by the AAN guidelines (4). It is also important to note that SSEP can be normal early in the course of brain death due to some residual functioning neurons, and is presumed to disappear over time (30). Lesions of the upper cervical cord and medulla can also confound results (31).

Brainstem auditory evoked responses

Brainstem auditory evoked response (BAER) testing has the appeal of being noninvasive, inexpensive, and feasible in the setting of sedation or hypothermia. However, it does require expertise in performance and interpretation, which is not widely available in all medical institutions. BAER is not a currently recommended ancillary test by the AAN brain death determination guidelines (4). However, studies have shown 100% sensitivity and 73.7% specificity in brain death determination. This is an area that continues to require further investigation (32,33).

CEREBROVASCULAR STUDIES

CT and MRI

Head CT and brain MRI are frequently used early in the assessment of brain death in the context of establishing etiology and diffuse catastrophic cerebral injury. This imaging has been deemed insufficiently specific for use as ancillary testing in the diagnosis of brain death (4). Studies have investigated the use of computed tomographic angiography (CTA) or magnetic resonance angiogram (MRA) for the determination of cessation of cerebral blood flow (34). As of yet, research is deemed insufficient to support the use of CTA or MRA as ancillary brain death testing, and their use cannot be condoned.

Cerebral angiography

Conventional cerebral angiography is considered the gold standard for cerebral blood flow testing in brain death. The proposed pathophysiology exploits the hypothesis that increased intracranial blood pressure due to diffuse cerebral edema leads to complete cessation of blood flow to the brain, thus leading to brain death. The catheter tip should be advanced to the aortic arch and contrast injected under pressure into each of the four arteries supplying blood to the brain. Each artery should be injected individually, and the test should consist of two injections 20 minutes apart. Angiography must show absence of filling of all four arteries as their course becomes intracranial (2).

Disadvantages to angiography include the time-consuming nature, expense of the procedure, invasiveness of the procedure, and possibility for renal damage or allergic reaction with contrast injection (2).

Single-photon emission computed tomography

SPECT imaging uses the radionuclide tracer Tc-99m-HMPAO to confirm absence of cerebral blood flow. The isotope should be injected within 30 minutes of reconstitution. Images of the head are then obtained in the anterior, posterior, and lateral planes at time intervals of 30–60 minutes after injection and 2 hours after injection. There should be no radionuclide uptake in the brain parenchyma, leaving the so-called "hollow skull" appearance (35,36). The nasal area should show uptake, as this is vascularized from the external carotid vasculature. There should be no tracer in the superior sagittal sinus.

SPECT has been validated in the literature for use in brain death determination and is a recommended ancillary study by AAN guidelines. Literature has shown that SPECT confirmed brain death in 95% of patients on initial evaluation and

100% at 48 hours, therefore suggesting that there may be a false negative rate early in the brain death process. Studies have identified no false positive results (37).

Transcranial Doppler ultrasonography

TCD can be useful in the determination of brain death given that as intracranial pressure rises there are subsequent changes in flow patterns through the intracranial arteries. Brain death can be supported by one of two findings on TCD: (i) absence of systolic peaks due to intracranial pressure exceeding systolic blood pressure, and (ii) "reverberating" blood flow with slight anterograde flow during systole and equal reversal of flow during diastole when intracranial pressure exceeds diastolic blood pressure (38,39). These patterns represent no effective forward blood flow. Complete testing requires findings consistent with absent effective forward flow bilaterally in both the anterior and posterior circulation demonstrated by two examinations at least 30 minutes apart.

Sensitivity of TCD in brain death determination has been estimated at 90% and specificity at 98% (40) TCD is a noninvasive bedside study and can be especially useful in patients deemed too unstable to leave the ICU for angiography or SPECT. However, TCD is only useful if reliable signal can be obtained. Transtemporal, suboccipital, or transorbital approaches can be used. It is important to note that complete absence of signal cannot be equated with absence of intracranial circulation. Lack of signal is encountered in 5%–10% of patients, and these studies should be deemed nondiagnostic (41). False negative findings have been reported in females and with sympathomimetic drug use (42). TCD can also be confounded by marked changes in $PaCO_2$, hematocrit, and cardiac output, including in patients with an intra-aortic balloon pump (43).

PITFALLS IN BRAIN DEATH DETERMINATION

As previously stated, there has been no documented recovery of brain function after the diagnosis of brain death since the institution of the 1995 AAN guidelines if the protocol was followed correctly

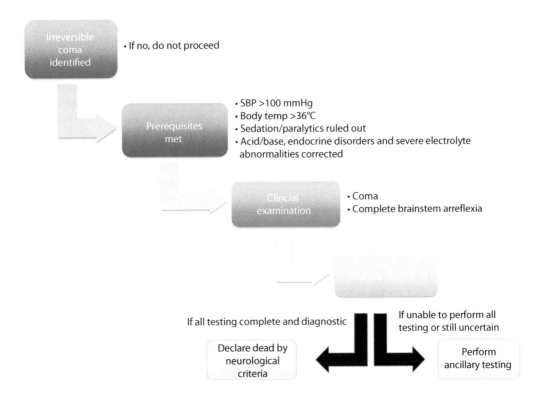

Brain death algorithmic approach.

(4). That said, there are cited cases of brain death mimics, including high cervical cord injury, fulminant Guillain-Barré syndrome (44,45), organophosphate intoxication (46), baclofen overdose (47), barbiturate overdose (48), and delayed vecuronium clearance (49). In all of these cited cases there was at least one deviation from the AAN brain death guideline. There are also a number of "red flags" which should caution providers against proceeding with brain death testing, and many of these are components of the brain death declaration prerequisites previously discussed. These include normal neuroimaging, unsupported blood pressure, hypothermia, metabolic acidosis, or positive urine or serum toxicology (15).

Clinical examination pitfalls

It is a common misconception that a patient who is brain dead is by definition motionless. Rather, many studies have described reflexive, spinally-mediated movements that are consistent with brain death.

Within the cranial nerve distribution, these movements may present as facial myokymias, transient eyelid opening, ocular microtremor, or cyclic pupillary constriction and dilation (50). It has been postulated that some of these movements, such as facial myokymias and tremor, may be the result of denervation or deafferentation (51).

There is also a series of axial and appendicular movements that are spinally mediated and consistent with brain death. These movements have no cerebral origin. They can be categorized as muscle stretch reflexes, cutaneomuscular reflexes, or polysegmental spinal automatisms (50). Most of these movements appear within the first 24 hours of brain death and rarely present after 72 hours (52). Movements recognized by the AAN that do not preclude the diagnosis of brain death include spontaneous movements of the limbs, deep tendon reflexes, superficial abdominal reflexes, triple flexion response, and the Babinski sign (4). The etiology of these complex motor responses is not well understood, but they are thought to be old motor patterns that are released when brainstem and neocortical function ceases (51). It can be difficult for clinicians to differentiate between these reflexive movements from purposeful or voluntary movements. A recent publication describes five clinical aspects that may assist in differentiating spinal versus voluntary movements (53):

1. Spinal responses are characterized by synchronous decorticate or decerebrate (flexion or extension) responses.
2. Spinal responses are typically slow and short in duration with a constant pattern of latency.
3. The most common spinal responses are triple flexion (flexion of the hip, knee, and foot). There are common variations including undulating toe sign or Babinski sign.
4. Most movements are provoked by an external stimulus and not spontaneous.
5. Spinal responses can sometimes be elicited by forceful neck flexion and noxious stimuli below the cervicomedullary junction. They are not stimulated by supraorbital or temporomandibular pressure.

These movements are stereotyped and are never purposeful. Perhaps the most dramatic spinal reflex that can be seen is the Lazarus sign, in which brain-dead patients have been described as elevating both arms and slowly adducting them across the chest (54). For the experienced provider, spinally-mediated movements can even serve as clinical confirmation that brain death has occurred, as these reflexes only emerge after a phase of spinal shock in brain-dead patients (55).

Confounders

Two of the most common confounding factors in brain death determination are drug intoxication and hypothermia. Sedating medications must not be present, and it is standard to wait at least five half-lives before proceeding with brain death evaluation when renal function and hepatic function are normal (14). If a patient has ingested an unknown, unquantifiable amount of a substance, one should wait at least 48 hours before brain death examination (56). It is also important to note that mechanical ventilation may decrease hepatic and renal blood flow and thus decrease clearance of drugs (55).

DOCUMENTATION

Once death by neurological criteria has been determined, the time of death should be recorded in the patient's medical record. The time of death is the official time at which laboratory result of arterial pCO_2 reached the target value during apnea testing (4). If apnea testing could not be performed, time of death is the time at which confirmatory ancillary testing is officially interpreted. Death by neurologic criteria documentation should always include prerequisites for brain death examination, and details of the clinical examination including all cranial nerve reflexes, apnea testing, and ancillary testing results (56). The use of a checklist is recommended to ensure that no component of the clinical examination has been omitted and that the diagnosis of brain death is properly documented and justified. Such a checklist is provided in the 2010 AAN brain death guidelines and in the following table (4).

Brain death determination	Completed
Prerequisites met	
Irreversible coma established	
Etiology of coma established	
Systolic blood pressure >100 mmHg	
Body temperature >36°C	
Sedatives/paralytics ruled out	
Electrolytes/acid-base disturbances corrected, no severe endocrine disorder	
Complete cranial nerve examination	
Pupillary reflex	
Oculocephalic reflex horizontal and vertical	
Oculovestibular testing bilaterally	
Corneal reflex bilaterally	
Jaw jerk reflex	
Facial response to noxious stimulus	
Cough and gag reflexes	
Apnea test performed; use checklist, detail exam	
Ancillary testing as needed, results reported	

AFTER BRAIN DEATH DECLARATION

The family discussion

Delivering bad news in a clear, yet compassionate and comforting, manner is a skill that takes time, experience, and practice to develop. It is preferable that a relationship has been built with the family before brain death testing and discussions, so that they are aware of the steps being taken and understand the management plan. Delivering the news that a family member has been declared brain dead should be a discussion centered on explaining to the family that their loved one has died and is being supported entirely by artificial means. As one can imagine, this is devastating news that can be met with a host of different emotional responses. It is not unusual for families to require time to grieve and compose themselves before proceeding with further discussions. The concept of brain death will likely be met with many questions, and it is best to explain as clearly as possible that their family member is medically and legally dead (56). A randomized controlled trial has even suggested that family members benefit from witnessing the evaluation of brain death and that this may improve the rate of organ donation (57,58). It may require more than one formal meeting to completely explain the process of brain death.

Organ donation

Federal and state law require that the physician contact an organ procurement organization (OPO) following declaration of brain death (4). It is important that the clinician recognize viable candidates early. Criteria for donation include (i) standard criteria: donors younger than 50 years who suffered brain death, and (ii) expanded criteria: donors over the age of 60 or 50–59 years plus having two of the following: stroke or cardiac disease as cause of death, hypertension, or terminal serum creatinine level of >1.5 mg/dL (56,59). The clinician should never bring up the topic of organ donation without coordination with the OPO. A representative from the OPO will approach the family after the diagnosis of death by neurological criteria. The separation of the clinical team from the concept of organ donation has been shown to increase family trust in the clinical providers and diagnosis of brain death and improve the rates of organ donation (60).

A host of pathophysiologic changes occur following brain death, and the intensive care physician should be prepared to manage these pending possible organ donation. Due to deprivation of blood flow to the hypothalamus, loss of temperature regulation is common (59). Hemodynamic instability is also encountered, and typically occurs in three phases. First, there is a sympathetic surge preceding medullary damage due to herniation, resulting in hypertension, left ventricular dysfunction, neurogenic pulmonary edema, and cardiac arrhythmias. Next, spinal cord infarction following herniation results in a loss of sympathetic tone, leading to hypotension. Lastly, lack of cerebral perfusion leads to pituitary dysfunction and diabetes insipidus, causing hypovolemia and further hypotension (61). These pathophysiologic changes should be aggressively managed by an intensive care physician and targeted at optimizing the viability of organs for transplantation.

THE FUTURE OF DEATH BY NEUROLOGICAL CRITERIA

Multiple recent studies have brought to light the unacceptable amount of variability amongst major medical institution protocols for the determination of death by neurological criteria (12). This widespread attention has led to the development of strategies to standardize protocols and improve compliance with AAN guidelines. There has also been a movement toward improved physician training in the clinical diagnosis of brain death, including simulation exercises and a proposal for certification in brain death declaration similar to that of advanced cardiac life support (ACLS) (55).

The advancement of modern medicine has brought to light several potential new ancillary tests for the diagnosis of brain death. These include the use of brain tissue oxygenation, which may be used to determine the moment of brain death (62). One series found 96.6% sensitivity and 99.3% specificity for the ratio of jugular to central venous oxygenation saturation in the determination of brain death (63). As referenced previously, the use of MRA in the determination of brain death continues to be explored (34). Laboratory studies such as protein S-100b are also being investigated. Protein S-100b is a calcium-binding protein found in the cytosol of astroglial and Schwann cells and has been found to be highly specific for CNS lesions (64).

CONCLUSION

Death by neurological criteria is a diagnosis that can currently be determined medically and legally by a physician of any clinical specialty. Any physician evaluating a patient for brain death should be properly trained and confident in the clinical skills necessary. It is critical that all prerequisites be met and that all components of the clinical evaluation be carefully performed, including apnea testing, to avoid misdiagnosis. When the clinical evaluation cannot be completed due to patient safety or pre-existing conditions, ancillary testing can be used to support the diagnosis of brain death. The use of an algorithmic checklist can be helpful to ensure a complete and accurate exam for the diagnosis. When done appropriately according to the AAN guidelines, the physician can be confident in the clinical diagnosis of death by neurologic criteria.

REFERENCES

1. Bernat JL. Death by neurologic criteria 1968–2014: Changing interpretations. Forward. *J Crit Care.* 2014;29(4):671–2.
2. Wijdicks EF. Determining brain death. *Continuum (Minneap Minn).* 2015;21(5 Neurocritical Care):1411–24.
3. Schroder R. Later changes in brain death. Signs of partial recirculation. *Acta Neuropathol.* 1983;62(1–2):15–23.
4. Wijdicks EF, Varelas PN, Gronseth GS, Greer DM. Evidence-based guideline update: Determining brain death in adults: Report of the Quality Standards Subcommittee of the American Academy of Neurology. *Neurology.* 2010;74(23):1911–8.
5. Guidelines for the determination of death: Report of the medical consultants on the diagnosis of death to the President's Commission for the Study of Ethical Problems in Medicine and Biomedical and Behavioral Research. *JAMA.* 1981;246(19): 2184–6.
6. Lizza JP. Defining death for persons and human organisms. *Theor Med Bioeth.* 1999;20(5):439–53.
7. Bernat JL. The concept and practice of brain death. *Prog Brain Res.* 2005;150:369–79.
8. Mollaret P GM. Le coma Depasse (memoire preliminaire). *Rev Neurol.* 1959(101):3–15.
9. A definition of irreversible coma: Report of the Ad Hoc committee of the Harvard Medical School to examine the definition of brain death. *JAMA.* 1968;205(6):337–40.
10. Uniform Determination of Death Act (UDDA). 12 uniform laws annotated 589. 1993.

11. Practice parameters for determining brain death in adults (summary statement). The Quality Standards Subcommittee of the American Academy of Neurology. *Neurology*. 1995;45(5):1012–4.

12. Greer DM, Varelas PN, Haque S, Wijdicks EF. Variability of brain death determination guidelines in leading US neurologic institutions. *Neurology*. 2008;70(4):284–9.

13. Williams MA, Suarez JI. Brain death determination in adults: More than meets the eye. *Crit Care Med*. 1997;25(11):1787–8.

14. Neavyn MJ, Stolbach A, Greer DM et al. ACMT position statement: Determining brain death in adults after drug overdose. *J Med Toxicol*. 2017;13(3):271–3.

15. Hwang DY, Gilmore EJ, Greer DM. Assessment of brain death in the neurocritical care unit. *Neurosurg Clin N Am*. 2013;24(3):469–82.

16. Dhakal LP, Sen A, Stanko CM et al. Early absent pupillary light reflexes after cardiac arrest in patients treated with therapeutic hypothermia. *Ther Hypothermia Temp Manag*. 2016;6(3):116–21.

17. Hicks RG, Torda TA. The vestibulo-ocular (caloric) reflex in the diagnosis of cerebral death. *Anaesth Intensive Care*. 1979;7(2):169–73.

18. Yee AH, Mandrekar J, Rabinstein AA, Wijdicks EF. Predictors of apnea test failure during brain death determination. *Neurocrit Care*. 2010;12(3):352–5.

19. Dodd-Sullivan R, Quirin J, Newhart J. Ventilator autotriggering: A caution in brain death diagnosis. *Prog Transplant*. 2011;21(2):152–5.

20. McGee WT, Mailloux P. Ventilator autocycling and delayed recognition of brain death. *Neurocrit Care*. 2011;14(2):267–71.

21. Wijdicks EF, Rabinstein AA, Manno EM, Atkinson JD. Pronouncing brain death: Contemporary practice and safety of the apnea test. *Neurology*. 2008;71(16):1240–4.

22. Schafer JA, Caronna JJ. Duration of apnea needed to confirm brain death. *Neurology*. 1978;28(7):661–6.

23. Baron L, Shemie SD, Teitelbaum J, Doig CJ. Brief review: History, concept and controversies in the neurological determination of death. *Can J Anaest*. 2006;53(6):602–8.

24. Goudreau JL, Wijdicks EF, Emery SF. Complications during apnea testing in the determination of brain death: Predisposing factors. *Neurology*. 2000;55(7):1045–8.

25. Jeret JS, Benjamin JL. Risk of hypotension during apnea testing. *Arch Neurol*. 1994;51(6):595–9.

26. Szurhaj W, Lamblin MD, Kaminska A, Sediri H. EEG guidelines in the diagnosis of brain death. *Neurophysiol Clin*. 2015;45(1):97–104.

27. Buchner H, Schuchardt V. Reliability of electroencephalogram in the diagnosis of brain death. *Eur Neurol*. 1990;30(3):138–41.

28. Belsh JM, Chokroverty S. Short-latency somatosensory evoked potentials in brain-dead patients. *Electroencephalogr Clin Neurophysiol*. 1987;68(1):75–8.

29. Wagner W. Scalp, earlobe and nasopharyngeal recordings of the median nerve somatosensory evoked P14 potential in coma and brain death. Detailed latency and amplitude analysis in 181 patients. *Brain*. 1996;119(Pt 5):1507–21.

30. Rothstein TL. Recovery from near death following cerebral anoxia: A case report demonstrating superiority of median somatosensory evoked potentials over EEG in predicting a favorable outcome after cardiopulmonary resuscitation. *Adv Exp Med Biol*. 2004;550:189–96.

31. Mauguiere F, Ibanez V. The dissociation of early SEP components in lesions of the cervico-medullary junction: A cue for routine interpretation of abnormal cervical responses to median nerve stimulation. *Electroencephalogr Clin Neurophysiol*. 1985;62(6):406–20.

32. Goldie WD, Chiappa KH, Young RR, Brooks EB. Brainstem auditory and short-latency somatosensory evoked responses in brain death. *Neurology*. 1981;31(3):248–56.

33. Waters CE, French G, Burt M. Difficulty in brainstem death testing in the presence of high spinal cord injury. *Br J Anaesth*. 2004;92(5):760–4.

34. Ishii K, Onuma T, Kinoshita T, Shiina G, Kameyama M, Shimosegawa Y. Brain death: MR and MR angiography. *AJNR Am J Neuroradiol*. 1996;17(4):731–5.

35. Donohoe KJ, Frey KA, Gerbaudo VH, Mariani G, Nagel JS, Shulkin B. Procedure guideline

for brain death scintigraphy. *J Nucl Med.* 2003; 44(5):846–51.

36. Zuckier LS. Radionuclide evaluation of brain death in the post-McMath era. *J Nucl Med.* 2016;57(10):1560–8.

37. Munari M, Zucchetta P, Carollo C et al. Confirmatory tests in the diagnosis of brain death: Comparison between SPECT and contrast angiography. *Crit Care Med.* 2005;33(9): 2068–73.

38. Petty GW, Mohr JP, Pedley TA et al. The role of transcranial Doppler in confirming brain death: Sensitivity, specificity, and suggestions for performance and interpretation. *Neurology.* 1990;40(2):300–3.

39. Ducrocq X, Hassler W, Moritake K et al. Consensus opinion on diagnosis of cerebral circulatory arrest using Doppler-sonography: Task Force Group on cerebral death of the Neurosonology Research Group of the World Federation of Neurology. *J Neurol Sci.* 1998; 159(2):145–50.

40. Chang JJ, Tsivgoulis G, Katsanos AH, Malkoff MD, Alexandrov AV. Diagnostic accuracy of transcranial Doppler for brain death confirmation: Systematic review and meta-analysis. *AJNR Am J Neuroradiol.* 2016;37(3):408–14.

41. Ducrocq X, Braun M, Debouverie M, Junges C, Hummer M, Vespignani H. Brain death and transcranial Doppler: Experience in 130 cases of brain dead patients. *J Neurol Sci.* 1998; 160(1):41–6.

42. de Freitas GR, Andre C. Sensitivity of transcranial Doppler for confirming brain death: A prospective study of 270 cases. *Acta Neurol Scand.* 2006;113(6):426–32.

43. Avlonitis VS, Wigfield CH, Kirby JA, Dark JH. The hemodynamic mechanisms of lung injury and systemic inflammatory response following brain death in the transplant donor. *Am J Transplant.* 2005;5(4 Pt 1):684–93.

44. Rivas S, Douds GL, Ostdahl RH, Harbaugh KS. Fulminant Guillain-Barre syndrome after closed head injury: A potentially reversible cause of an ominous examination. Case report. *J Neurosurg.* 2008;108(3):595–600.

45. Stojkovic T, Verdin M, Hurtevent JF, Laureau E, Krivosic-Horber R, Vermersch P. Guillain-Barre syndrome resembling brainstem death in a patient with brain injury. *J Neurol.* 2001; 248(5):430–2.

46. Peter JV, Prabhakar AT, Pichamuthu K. In-laws, insecticide--and a mimic of brain death. *Lancet.* 2008;371(9612):622.

47. Ostermann ME, Young B, Sibbald WJ, Nicolle MW. Coma mimicking brain death following baclofen overdose. *Intensive Care Med.* 2000;26(8):1144–6.

48. Kirshbaum RJ, Carollo VJ. Reversible iso-electric EEG in barbiturate coma. *JAMA.* 1970;212(7):1215.

49. Kainuma M, Miyake T, Kanno T. Extremely prolonged vecuronium clearance in a brain death case. *Anesthesiology.* 2001;95(4):1023–4.

50. Jain S, DeGeorgia M. Brain death-associated reflexes and automatisms. *Neurocrit Care.* 2005;3(2):122–6.

51. Saposnik G, Basile VS, Young GB. Movements in brain death: A systematic review. *Can J Neurol Sci.* 2009;36(2):154–60.

52. Dosemeci L, Cengiz M, Yilmaz M, Ramazanoglu A. Frequency of spinal reflex movements in brain-dead patients. *Transplant Proc.* 2004;36(1):17–9.

53. Mittal MK, Arteaga GM, Wijdicks EF. Thumbs up sign in brain death. *Neurocrit Care.* 2012; 17(2):265–7.

54. Heytens L, Verlooy J, Gheuens J, Bossaert L. Lazarus sign and extensor posturing in a brain-dead patient. Case report. *J Neurosurg.* 1989;71(3):449–51.

55. Busl KM, Greer DM. Pitfalls in the diagnosis of brain death. *Neurocrit Care.* 2009;11(2): 276–87.

56. Youn TS, Greer DM. Brain death and management of a potential organ donor in the intensive care unit. *Crit Care Clin.* 2014; 30(4):813–31.

57. Curtis JR, Patrick DL, Shannon SE, Treece PD, Engelberg RA, Rubenfeld GD. The family conference as a focus to improve communication about end-of-life care in the intensive care unit: Opportunities for improvement. *Crit Care Med.* 2001;29(2 Suppl):N26–33.

58. Tawil I, Brown LH, Comfort D et al. Family presence during brain death evaluation: A randomized controlled trial*. *Crit Care Med.* 2014;42(4):934–42.

59. Dare AJ, Bartlett AS, Fraser JF. Critical care of the potential organ donor. *Curr Neurol Neurosci Rep.* 2012;12(4):456–65.

60. Long T, Sque M, Addington-Hall J. What does a diagnosis of brain death mean to family members approached about organ donation? A review of the literature. *Prog Transplant.* 2008;18(2):118–25; quiz 26.

61. Singbartl K, Murugan R, Kaynar AM et al. Intensivist-led management of brain-dead donors is associated with an increase in organ recovery for transplantation. *Am J Transplant.* 2011;11(7):1517–21.

62. Palmer S, Bader MK. Brain tissue oxygenation in brain death. *Neurocrit Care.* 2005;2(1):17–22.

63. Diaz-Reganon G, Minambres E, Holanda M, Gonzalez-Herrera S, Lopez-Espadas F, Garrido-Diaz C. Usefulness of venous oxygen saturation in the jugular bulb for the diagnosis of brain death: Report of 118 patients. *Intensive Care Med.* 2002;28(12):1724–8.

64. Ingebrigtsen T, Romner B, Kongstad P, Langbakk B. Increased serum concentrations of protein S-100 after minor head injury: A biochemical serum marker with prognostic value? *J Neurol Neurosurg Psychiatry.* 1995;59(1):103–4.

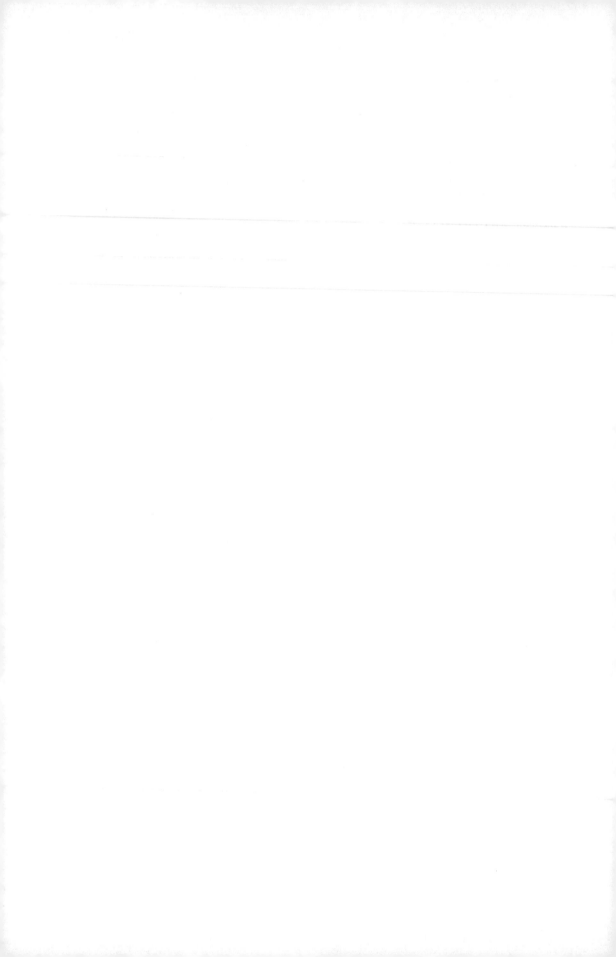

Index

T - #0500 - 071024 - C332 - 254/178/15 - PB - 9780367778590 - Gloss Lamination